Cash's Textbook of Neurology for Physiotherapists

CASH'S TEXTBOOK OF NEUROLOGY FOR PHYSIOTHERAPISTS

edited by

PATRICIA A. DOWNIE F.C.S.P.

J. B. LIPPINCOTT COMPANY

First published in 1974
by Faber and Faber Limited
Reprinted 1975, 1976
Second edition 1977
Reprinted 1979
Third edition 1982
Printed in Great Britain by
Fakenham Press Limited
Fakenham, Norfolk
All rights reserved

Distributed in the United States of America by
J. B. Lippincott Company, Philadelphia

ISBN: 0–397–58281–1

Library of Congress Catalog Card No. 81–82323

Book Code 65–73091

Contents

Contributors

Mrs H. W. Atkinson, M.C.S.P., H.T., DIP.T.P.
Principal Lecturer and Head of School
Coventry (Lanchester) Polytechnic School of Physiotherapy
Priory Street, Coventry CV1 5FB

Miss P. M. Davies, M.C.S.P., DIP.PHYS.ED.
Instructor, The Postgraduate Study Centre
Medical Department, Bad Ragaz, Switzerland

Mrs J. M. Dodgson, M.C.S.P., O.N.C.
Senior Physiotherapist, Department of Psychiatry
Queen Elizabeth II Hospital, Welwyn Garden City
Hertfordshire AL7 4HQ

Mr F. W. Frazer, B.A., M.C.S.P.
District Physiotherapist, South Birmingham Health District
Selly Oak Hospital, Birmingham B29 6JD

Dr R. B. Godwin-Austen, M.D., F.R.C.P.
Consultant Neurologist,
Nottingham University Hospitals *and* Derby Hospitals

Mrs B. Goff, M.C.S.P., O.N.C., DIP.T.P.
Senior Teacher, Oswestry and North Staffordshire School of
Physiotherapy
Robert Jones and Agnes Hunt Orthopaedic Hospital
Oswestry, Shropshire SY10 7AG

Miss M. A. Harrison, M.C.S.P.
District Physiotherapist, South Nottingham Health District
Queen's Medical Centre, University Hospital
Nottingham NG7 2UH

Mrs H. V. Haywood, M.C.S.P.
Superintendent Physiotherapist, The Ryegate Centre and
The Children's Hospital, Sheffield S10 5DD

Mr D. A. Hill, B.SC., M.C.S.P., DIP.T.P.
Reader in Health Sciences
Ulster Polytechnic, Newtownabbey, Co Antrim

Dr G. P. Hosking, M.B., M.R.C.P., D.C.H.
Consultant Paediatric Neurologist
The Ryegate Centre and The Children's Hospital
Sheffield S10 5DD

Miss J. M. Lee, B.A., M.C.S.P., DIP.T.P.
Principal, South Teesside School of Physiotherapy
The General Hospital, Middlesbrough TS5 5AZ

Miss S. Levitt, B.SC. (Physiotherapy) Rand
Supervisor of Therapy Studies, The Wolfson Centre
Institute of Child Health, London WC1N 2AP

Dr P. D. Lewis, B.SC., M.D., M.R.C.P., M.R.C.PATH.
Senior Lecturer in Neuropathology and Honorary Consultant
Neurologist
The Royal Postgraduate Medical School and
Hammersmith Hospital, London W12 0HS

Mrs O. R. Nettles, M.C.S.P., O.N.C.
Member of the National Committee of Paediatric Physiotherapy
The Association of Paediatric Chartered Physiotherapists
25 Goffs Park Road
Crawley, Sussex RH11 8AX

Miss M. I. Salter, M.B.E., M.C.S.P.
Superintendent Physiotherapist, Joint Services Medical
Rehabilitation Unit
Royal Air Force, Chessington KT9 2PY

Dr J. M. Sutherland, M.D., F.R.C.P.(Edin.), F.R.A.C.P.
Honorary Consultant Neurologist, Royal Brisbane Hospital;
Honorary Reader in Neurology, University of Queensland;
Visiting Neurologist, Toowoomba General Hospital

Miss J. M. Todd, M.C.S.P.
11 Alma Terrace
London SW18 3HT

Preface to the Third Edition

Advances in neurophysiology have so enhanced knowledge and understanding of the intricacies of the nervous system, that physiotherapists are now able to approach patients with neurological disorders in a much more effective manner.

Almost ten years ago Joan Cash decided that neurology must be allowed a textbook for itself. This third edition is a thorough revision, and aims to offer a comprehensive background to what is a most important part of a physiotherapist's work. As with the other volumes in this series, I have invited distinguished physicians to write the clinical chapters relating to specific diseases.

'No man is an island', so wrote John Donne and I have taken this advice literally and persuaded a distinguished neurologist now living in Australia to contribute the clinical chapter on Multiple Sclerosis. To Dr John Sutherland I offer particularly warm thanks.

Dr Paul Lewis has not only written the first chapter which outlines clinical diagnosis of neurological disease, but he has also provided the glossary at the end of the book. In addition he offered much help and advice and I am most grateful to him.

My thanks go to all the contributors for providing such excellent chapters, on schedule and in a splendid spirit of cooperation! I sometimes wish the reader could see the original roughs of some of the drawings from which Audrey Besterman produces the beautiful artwork which so enhances this text. To her and the various photographers who have helped individual contributors I can only offer the thanks of myself as editor and the contributors in general.

To you the reader, I hope you will not only extract much factual information but that you will also *enjoy* reading this volume.

P.A.D.
London, 1981

Chapter 1

Clinical Diagnosis of Neurological Conditions

by P. D. LEWIS, B.SC., M.D., M.R.C.P., M.R.C.PATH.

As in other branches of medicine, the art of the neurologist consists of making a diagnosis from the patient's own account of his illness and from a physical examination, aided by appropriate radiographic or laboratory tests. Once the diagnosis has been reached, suitable treatment can be given and the outlook predicted. What distinguishes neurology from its sister specialties is the degree of attention to detail in taking the medical history and in examining the patient. This quest for detail, often so mysterious to the non-neurologist, is linked to a wealth of knowledge of nervous anatomy, physiology and pathology, accumulated over more than a century, the application of which at the bedside often enables a precise diagnosis to be made. The meticulous enquiry into the patient's symptoms and search for physical signs was once the approach of all specialist physicians. However, as some diseased organs became easily and accurately studied by diagnostic tests (like chest radiographs), clinical methods in these fields of medicine became somewhat less important. Until quite recently, abnormalities of structure in the living brain could only be visualised by specialised radiological methods, sometimes carrying risks and sometimes needing anaesthesia. Now that computerised tomography (CAT-scanning) has become generally available, the brain can be x-rayed as readily as the chest, and it may be that in coming years the clinical neurological assessment will become simplified.

TAKING A NEUROLOGICAL CASE-HISTORY

For the neurologist, a complete and accurate history is essential. Very often a precise diagnosis can be made from the history, and examination is simply confirmatory; the converse, a physical examination which provides signs not predictable from the history, tends to come as a surprise. The description of the tempo of the illness – acute or chronic, coming on slowly or abruptly, steadily progressive or remitting, often suggests the type of pathological process. Vascular problems are usually of acute onset, tumour symptoms tend steadily to progress, demyelinating disease may remit. The characterisation of symptoms is then attempted, the neurologist assisting the patient with suitable questions. Headaches, 'dizziness' and 'fainting' are three of the most frequent problems dealt with in neurological clinics. It is the task of the neurologist to decide if the patient's headaches result from a brain tumour or simply (and as usually is the case) from muscular tension or from migraine. Dizziness may signify disease of the balance mechanisms in the ear and brainstem. Faints may or may not mean neurological disease: epilepsy may resemble fainting attacks, and careful enquiry with specific questions is often needed to obtain a clear picture of such episodes. Other symptoms of special significance to the neurologist include disturbance of memory or concentration; loss of vision; double vision; facial pain or weakness; difficulty with speech or swallowing; weakness, wasting, pain or numbness in a limb; abnormal movements; trouble with walking; and disturbance of bladder control. Each of these symptoms, described by the patient, has a range of possible causes which need to be considered; thus it will set in train a particular process of enquiry as the neurologist attempts – on the basis of the information given by the patient – to form a clear image of the nature and localisation of the underlying neurological disorder.

THE NEUROLOGICAL EXAMINATION

In some ways, the neurological examination begins from the moment the patient is first seen. Gait, attitude, alertness and speech may all give important diagnostic clues. However, the formal examination of the nervous system follows completion of history-taking. Testing of the head, trunk and limbs for motor and sensory function is preceded by an evaluation of mental state and intellectual level. The patient's overall appearance and behaviour, mood, orientation, thought processes, memory and intelligence may be affected in many brain diseases, and need to be assessed. A disturbance of speech may point to a disorder of the dominant cerebral hemisphere or of motor control.

The carotid arteries are felt and listened to in the neck to check on arterial blood flow to the brain, neck movement is tested and the skull is felt (and listened to for abnormal sounds). Functions of the cranial nerves are then examined in turn. Sense of smell (olfactory nerves); visual fields, visual activity, optic fundi – using the ophthalmoscope (optic nerves); examination of the pupils (oculomotor nerves) and of eye movements (oculomotor, trochlear and abducent nerves); facial sensation, corneal sensation and reflexes, jaw movement (trigeminal nerves); facial movement (facial nerves); hearing (auditory nerves); palatal sensation and movement (glossopharyngeal and vagus nerves); movements of sternomastoid and trapezius muscles (spinal accessory nerves); and tongue movement (hypoglossal nerves) are the major cranial nerve functions assessed in a full neurological examination. Abnormalities observed in any of these will suggest the anatomical basis of the patient's complaint.

The systematic examination of the trunk and limbs includes both motor and sensory testing; the patient's symptoms should suggest which of these is carried out first, since either can be tiring. In order to decide if muscle function is normal or abnormal the doctor must first carefully look at the limbs for signs of muscle wasting, abnormality of posture (suggesting muscular imbalance), involuntary movements (which may be a sign of extrapyramidal disease) and fasciculation (often a sign of damage to motor nerve cells). He then evaluates the tone of the limb musculature (the state of tension in the muscles, which may be increased or decreased under abnormal conditions), assesses power systematically, muscle group by muscle group, looks for signs of incoordination of movement, and tests the tendon reflexes (which can reveal derangement of function at or above or below the spinal segments each represents). Once again motor testing aims to localise the neurological abnormality.

Sensation from different zones of skin is conveyed to the nervous system via different spinal nerves and spinal cord segments, while distinct forms of skin sensation (e.g. pain and touch) have separate pathways in the nervous system. Clearly, careful sensory testing can also be of great localising value. In practice the neurologist will often test pain sensation with a pin, touch with a piece of cottonwool and joint position sense by carefully moving a finger or toe. He makes much use of the vibration of a tuning fork as an overall test of sensory function.

Further Tests

Even the most skilful and experienced clinical neurologist would not expect to make an accurate diagnosis in every patient on the basis of history and examination alone. Overall, perhaps 50 per cent of clinical diagnoses will be found to be correct. Accuracy is increased by means of special tests which aim to localise the abnormality in the nervous system or to define its pathology.

RADIOGRAPHS (X-RAYS)

These are invaluable for disease affecting the bones of the skull and the spine. They cannot however show the soft tissues contained inside. For these to be seen, it is necessary either to inject into the blood vessels of the brain or cord a substance which is opaque to x-rays (arteriography, angiography) or to outline the nervous tissue by defining the fluid spaces within and outside them, using air or an opaque medium (pneumo-encephalography or ventriculography for the brain; myelography for spinal cord). The selective uptake of radioactive isotopes by diseased nervous tissue can be used to produce images of the brain (isotope scans).

The CAT-scanner, mentioned earlier, has supplanted isotopic methods in those centres where it is available, and gives in many cases a definitive structural diagnosis. Its principle is the detection of minute changes of tissue density from point to point inside the head. In this way an x-ray picture of the brain itself, and not just the skull, can be assembled.

Electrodiagnostic Tests

These involve the amplification and recording of the electrical activity of nervous tissue and have certain diagnostic applications. Electro-encephalography is useful in the investigation of some epileptic patients, in some cases of coma and in certain forms of encephalitis.

Electromyography is described on page 89 and is an essential part of the evaluation of patients with neuromuscular disease. Measurement of sensory and motor nerve conduction is equally essential in the study of lesions of the peripheral nervous system.

Cerebrospinal Fluid Tests

These are important in neurological diagnosis. Lumbar puncture is the usual technique for obtaining a sample. It is a necessary procedure where meningitis or subarachnoid haemorrhage is suspected, and it may give useful information in certain inflammatory diseases of brain tissue.

The Tests of General Medicine

These include haematological tests, blood and urine biochemistry, and may give diagnostic information. Many generalised diseases have neurological complications, and the neurologist may be the first physician to see a patient whose disease has major effects on other parts of the body. The neurologist remains a physician, and for all his special skills he must not lose sight of the broad canvas of medicine. His history-taking, his examination and the laboratory investigations he chooses should be as generally comprehensive as appears to be necessary.

BIBLIOGRAPHY

Bannister, R. (ed) (1978). *Brain's Clinical Neurology*, 5th edition. Oxford University Press, Oxford.

Bickerstaff, E. R. (1980). *Neurological Examination in Clinical Practice*, 4th edition. Blackwell Scientific Publications Limited, Oxford.

Matthews, W. B. (1975). *Practical Neurology*, 3rd edition. Blackwell Scientific Publications Limited, Oxford.

Pansky, B. and Allen, D. J. (1980). *Review of Neuroscience*. Macmillan, New York.

Chapter 2

Applied Anatomy and Physiology

by H. W. ATKINSON, M.C.S.P., H.T., DIP.T.P.

The physiotherapist is frequently called upon to aid in the management of patients suffering from disorders of neurological origin. In order to give maximum assistance it is necessary for the therapist to understand certain basic physiological concepts and to have some knowledge of the general anatomy of the nervous system as a whole. Detailed anatomy and physiology is a preliminary subject in the training period and may be obtained from any of the standard textbooks. It is the intention in this section, therefore, to select only those concepts which are particularly applicable to therapy.

THE NERVOUS SYSTEM AS A TOOL

The nervous system is the tool used by the living creature in order to be able to react to its environment. The more complex the creature, the more complicated its nervous system and the more versatile are its reactions. The system is concerned with physical (motor, sensory and autonomic), intellectual and emotional activities and, in consequence, any disorder may involve any one or all three of these major functions.

Neurone

The nervous system is composed of an enormous number of neurones, connected together and following certain pathways, in order to make functional activity possible. The neurone is the basic unit of the nervous system and comprises the nerve cell and its processes. Each neurone has a cell body and two types of processes (Fig. 2/1), dendrites and axons.

Figure 2/2 shows how each ramus carries motor, sensory and autonomic fibres and the sympathetic ganglion communicates with those above and below it in level and also sends fibres to the visceral

Fig. 2/1 Structure of a
neurone

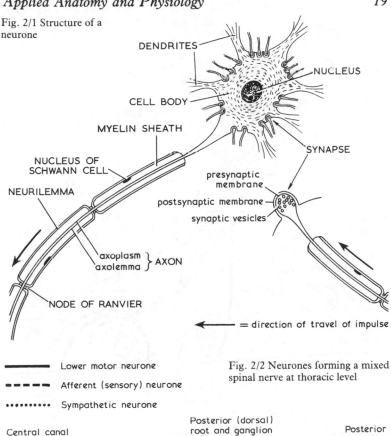

DENDRITES

NUCLEUS

CELL BODY

MYELIN SHEATH

NUCLEUS OF
SCHWANN CELL

NEURILEMMA

SYNAPSE

presynaptic
membrane

postsynaptic membrane

synaptic vesicles

axoplasm
axolemma } AXON

NODE OF RANVIER

⟵ = direction of travel of impulse

——————— Lower motor neurone

– – – – – Afferent (sensory) neurone

•••••••••• Sympathetic neurone

Fig. 2/2 Neurones forming a mixed
spinal nerve at thoracic level

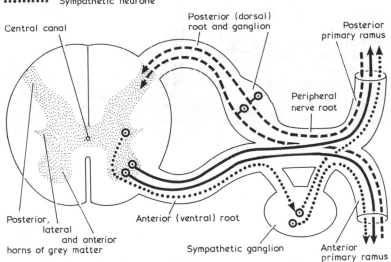

Central canal

Posterior (dorsal)
root and ganglion

Posterior
primary ramus

Peripheral
nerve root

Posterior,
lateral
and anterior
horns of grey matter

Anterior (ventral) root

Sympathetic ganglion

Anterior
primary ramus

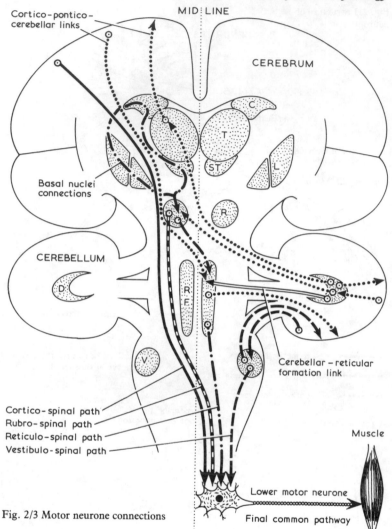

Fig. 2/3 Motor neurone connections

contents. Figure 2/3 shows that the corticospinal path represents the pyramidal system and other paths may be considered to be extrapyramidal.

The Synapse

This is the term used to define the area where the process of one neurone links with another. The synapse is a point of contiguity but not of continuity. Synapses may occur between the terminal parts of an axon and the dendrites of another cell or with the cell body. The number of synaptic areas may be very vast in any one neurone. The synapse enables impulses from one neurone to be transmitted to another neurone by virtue of chemical changes taking place which bring about an alteration in membrane potential on the receiving neurone. Synapses have certain properties which are of importance. Some of the more important ones are:

1. *Synaptic delay.* When an impulse reaches a synapse there is a brief time-lag before a response occurs in the recipient neurone. Consequently conduction along a chain of neurones is slower than along one single neurone. Thus monosynaptic pathways conduct more rapidly than polysynaptic routes.

2. *One-way conduction.* Synapses permit conduction of impulses in one direction only, i.e. from the presynaptic to the postsynaptic neurone.

3. *Vulnerability.* Synapses are very sensitive to anoxia and to the effects of drugs. Polysynaptic pathways are very susceptible to anaesthesia.

4. *Summation.* The effect of impulses arriving at a synapse can be added to by other impulses. For instance the effect of impulses could be subliminal (insufficient to bring about adequate chemical change for depolarisation of the postsynaptic neurone). If, however, another spate of impulses arrives before the effect of the previous one has subsided then the two effects may complement each other and the total change be sufficient to cause depolarisation. Such a phenomenon is called summation. There are two types of summation, the type just described being dependent upon a time factor and being called temporal summation. The other type is called spatial summation. It is the result of the adding together of impulses from different neurones which converge upon the postsynaptic neurone and bring about depolarisation of its membrane.

5. *Fatigue.* The synapse is thought to be the site of fatigue in nerve conductivity.

6. *Inhibition.* Certain neurones have an inhibitory effect upon the postsynaptic neurone, possibly because they use a different chemical mediator. Thus the effect of these neurones would be to discourage depolarisation of the postsynaptic cell membrane and would be antagonistic to influences exerted by excitatory neurones. These effects can summate in the same way as the excitatory effects. Many interneurones have an inhibitory effect.

7. *Post-tetanic potentiation.* This occurs across synapses which have

been subjected to prolonged and repeated activity. The threshold of stimulation of these junctions is thought to be lowered making transmission across it more easily brought about for a period of several hours. Facilitation of transmission is said to occur, and is an elementary form of learning and also forms an important part in the approach to physical treatment of patients with neurological disorders.

Supporting Tissue

Neurones are delicate, highly specialised structures and require support and protection. This is afforded to them in the nervous system by specialised connective tissue called neuroglia. If neurones are damaged and destroyed their place is filled by proliferation of neuroglial material.

The axons are surrounded by a fatty sheath called myelin which has an important effect on the conduction of impulses. Because of this sheath, bundles of axons give a whitish appearance and form the white matter of the central nervous system.

When the axon and its myelin sheath leave the central nervous system they become surrounded by a membrane called the neurilemma. This is of vital importance and it should be noted that the neurilemma is absent round the fibres of the brain and spinal cord whereas it is present as soon as they leave these areas.

Nerve fibres which are surrounded by neurilemma may regenerate if they are destroyed. Hence destruction of fibres in a peripheral nerve does not necessarily mean permanent loss of function whereas destruction of the fibres in the central nervous system will mean permanent loss of function of those fibres. It should also be noted that the nerve cell is resilient to injury and has considerable recuperative powers but, if it dies, it is incapable of being replaced. Thus destruction of cell bodies means permanent loss of function.

SOME PHYSIOLOGICAL CONCEPTS

Most patients suffering from neurological disorders show movement difficulties, and it is therefore important to consider the factors which are essential for the production of normal movement and activity.

Movement in its mature and skilled form is the result of complex teamwork between a multitude of muscles and joints so that balanced movement patterns are produced which can achieve an effect for the individual. Movement and postural attitudes are so closely related that it is impossible to distinguish one from the other.

The muscles concerned in the production of movement receive

their ultimate stimulation from the motoneurone pools or masses of cells housed in the anterior horns of the spinal cord or, in the case of the cranial nerves, in the motor nuclei of the brainstem. Axons from the motoneurone pools pass to the muscles and constitute the lower motor neurones or final common pathways.

Many neurones converge upon and synapse with the lower motor neurone, some coming from the extrapyramidal and pyramidal pathways, some being spinal interneurones and some coming direct from the peripheral afferent system. Whether or not impulses pass along the final common pathways depends upon two very important factors:

1. The integrity of the pathway
2. The influence exerted upon the cells of the motoneurone pool.

If the lower motoneurone pathway is not intact there is no route for the impulses to take. Fortunately each muscle is supplied by many neurones and only a severe lesion in the pathway would involve every lower motoneurone passing to any one muscle. However, this can occur and the result is a muscle which cannot be made to contract via activity in its own motor nerve supply and therefore one which is unable to participate in any team work towards functional activity.

Since many neurones are converging upon the cells in the motoneurone pools, including interneurones, it is possible that two types of influence may be exerted. These are *excitatory* – encouraging depolarisation – and *inhibitory* – discouraging depolarisation. The ratio between these two influences is the deciding factor as to whether the motoneurone pools are activated or not. The muscles they supply will, therefore, contract or remain inactive according to the balance of excitatory *versus* inhibitory influences being exerted upon their motoneurone pools.

When contraction occurs its intensity is dependent upon the number of muscle fibres brought into action. The number of fibres activated depends upon the number of cells in the motoneurone pool which have conveyed impulses. Thus the greater the excitatory influence on the motoneurone pool and the lower their threshold of stimulation, the greater the number of active motoneurones and the greater the resultant degree of muscle contraction.

The Factors Exerting an Influence on the Motoneurone Pools

These are many and varied. Pathways which are of importance are those of the pyramidal and extrapyramidal parts of the central nervous system which convey impulses resulting in volitional, postural and equilibrium reactions. Also of importance are the lower reflex pathways which give rise to withdrawal and stretch responses which are the result of more direct influences from the afferent side of the peripheral system. The interrelationship between one and the other is very important and can be illustrated by a simple account of the stretch reflex mechanism.

Skeletal muscles may be divided into two types of fibres. The large, ordinary fibres are known as extrafusal fibres and the smaller fibres which lie parallel to the extrafusal fibres and are encapsulated are

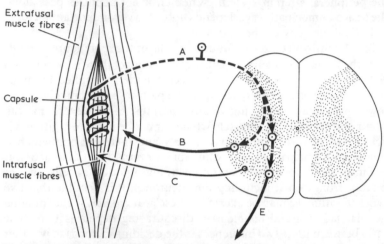

Fig. 2/4 The simple stretch reflex mechanism. A = Ia fibre; B = Alpha efferent; C = Fusimotor fibre (Gamma efferent); D = Interneurone; E = Motor neurone to antagonistic muscle

known as intrafusal fibres. The intrafusal fibres are part of the stretch reflex mechanism of muscle and the one illustrated in Figure 2/4 has a non-contractile part and a contractile part.

The non-contractile part of the intrafusal fibres is concerned with stretch reception and is linked to the central nervous system by an afferent neurone (called an Ia fibre) which makes direct synapse with a large anterior horn cell in the motoneurone pool of the same muscle to which the intrafusal fibres belong. Stretch to the muscle and therefore to the non-contractile part of the intrafusal fibre has an excitatory effect on the stretch receptor, and impulses travel along the Ia fibre to the motoneurone pool where the large anterior horn cell is stimulated and conveys impulses to the extrafusal fibres causing them to contract. The large anterior horn cell is said to send an Alpha efferent to the extrafusal muscle fibre. In this way the stretch on the intrafusal fibres is reduced. The afferent fibres also influence other associated motoneurones and by means of interneurones they may exert an inhibitory influence on the motoneurone pools of antagonistic muscles.

The contractile parts of the intrafusal fibres have their own nerve supply from the motoneurone pools by means of small anterior horn cells. The axons of these cells are called fusimotor fibres (Gamma efferents) to distinguish them from the fibres of the large anterior horn cells. Impulses passing along these fusimotor fibres to the intrafusal muscle fibres will cause them to contract and make them exert tension upon their own non-contractile areas. Thus they are able to make the intrafusal non-contractile area more sensitive to stretch by their activity or less sensitive to stretch by their inactivity.

In other words a bias can be put upon the sensitivity of the stretch reflex mechanism depending upon the degree of activity in the intrafusal contractile tissue and the fusimotor fibres. This bias depends upon the influences being exerted upon the small anterior horn cells which are particularly linked to the extrapyramidal pathways from the central nervous system, which in turn incorporates the balance and postural mechanism. Through this system the stretch reflex mechanism in muscle can be made more sensitive or less so according to the postural needs of the moment. Thus there is interaction between excitation and inhibition and between lower reflex activity and higher control.

The stretch reflex mechanism is in fact more complicated than this. There are at least two types of intrafusal fibres (nuclear bag and nuclear chain). There are also two types of stretch receptors, Ia and II, and there are at least two types of fusimotor fibres. This rather complicated mechanism makes the muscle sensitive to both velocity and degree of stretch, enables it to adjust its resting length and to be

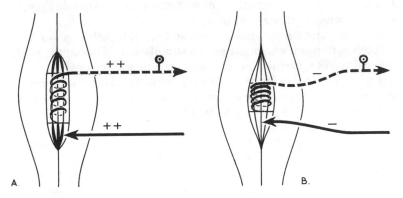

Fig. 2/5 Effect of activity of fusimotor (gamma) fibres

sensitive to stretch to a varying degree whatever its resting length happens to be. Figure 2/5 illustrates the simple stretch reflex mechanism and the effect of contraction of the intrafusal fibres.

Thus it may be seen that the influence of the fibres from the extrapyramidal system can adjust muscle activity to a fine degree and since certain righting, postural and equilibrium reactions are integrated into the extrapyramidal system it is not difficult to see that these reactions exert their influence upon the motoneurone pools via these fibres.

These postural mechanisms and reactions make possible a variety of automatic responses to various situations. The normal human being can, however, encourage or inhibit these activities at will and can carry out activities which are not entirely automatic but are dependent upon some automatic adjustments. When these background automatic adjustments are not available normal willed movement becomes incoordinate, posturally unsound and wellnigh impossible.

Some Useful Points to Note when Considering the Production of Volitional Movement

SENSORY INPUT

All volitional movement is triggered off as a response to some afferent information. Without input there can be no adequate motor output.

The types of afferent stimulation which give rise to movement are many and varied. The following few examples may be of some help in the appreciation of a need for sensory stimulus. We move if we feel discomfort, excessive pressure or insecurity; we move in response to basic needs such as hunger and thirst; we move if we see something we desire to investigate further; we move because of the stimulus generated by memory, thought or idea.

We must have stimulation to move and suitable pathways available to receive, transmit and interpret the stimulation. Without the available pathways movement would not occur to any purpose.

The importance of input is not fully appreciated until we consider its effect on where and how we move. Unless we have a knowledge of our position in space (conscious or subconscious) it is impossible for us to change our position.

If we do receive a stimulus to move we must know where we are in order to change our position, how we should feel during the movement and how the completed movement should feel. There has to be a constant 'feed-back' of information if our movements are to be successful.

AROUSAL OF IDEA OF MOVEMENT

The ingoing sensations must be able to arouse the idea of movement. This is probably done via the arousal part of the reticular formation which alerts the higher centres of the brain to the onslaught of ingoing information. It may also link with the non-anatomically defined centrocephalic area thought to be related to the initiation of the idea of movement. This area is connected with both the pyramidal and extrapyramidal cortical regions.

STIMULATION OF PYRAMIDAL AND EXTRAPYRAMIDAL
PATHWAYS

The pyramidal pathways need to be put into action but not before the extrapyramidal system has been informed of the intended movement. These two systems work closely together to give us the desired movement patterns with correct synergy and postural reactions.

Many theories have been put forward to explain the production of voluntary movement. The following factors are needed:

1. Initiation of the idea to move
2. Stimulation of the main motoneurone pools involved in the pattern of activity
3. Modification or controlled inhibition of the antagonists
4. Activation of synergistic and fixator muscles
5. The necessary postural adjustments and alterations in postural patterns to make the movement possible
6. Continuous 'feed-back' regarding progress.

The function of the pyramidal pathways. These are thought to be responsible for initiating the movement which has been conceived as an idea by the centrocephalic area. If these pathways worked alone without the aid of the extrapyramidal system the movement produced would tend to be a mass movement without synergy. Thus unwanted components might occur.

The function of the extrapyramidal pathways. The extrapyramidal cortical cells are thought to be also stimulated by activity in the centrocephalic area and as they are rapidly conducting they prepare the way for impulses passing down the pyramidal pathways. They send impulses to the extrapyramidal masses of grey matter (basal ganglia, red nucleus, substantia nigra etc) so that necessary patterns of excitation and inhibition of motoneurone pools are already initiated preparing them for action or preventing unwanted activity when the impulses via the pyramidal pathways reach them. In this way the appropriate excitation and inhibition of synergic activity may be brought about.

The extrapyramidal cortical cells also inform the cerebellum of intended activity via the cortico-pontico-cerebellar pathways. This enables the cerebellum to exert appropriate influences upon the red nucleus and brainstem nuclei helping the synergic selection activities and postural adjustments needed. A 'feed-back' exists between cerebellum and cortex via the thalamus.

To summarise this particular theory, it can be said that the pyramidal pathways will demand the main movements and extrapyramidal pathways will influence the motoneurone pools in such a way as to make the required movement possible without involving unwanted activity.

This gives rather a clear-cut difference between pyramidal and extrapyramidal systems which may be excessively dogmatic. The student must appreciate that movement is the result of an extremely complex combination of excitation and inhibition giving a desired effect.

SOME OBSERVATIONS ON REFLEXES

Reflexes and reactions play an important part in the activity of the nervous system. The reflex arc may be called the basic functional unit of the nervous system. It consists, essentially, of a receptor organ and its neurone which make synaptic connection with an efferent neurone which, in turn, connects with an effector organ. Such an arc would be monosynaptic and, in man, is only found in the phasic stretch reflexes of muscle, i.e. the so-called 'deep reflexes' elicited when a muscle is stretched by tapping its tendon such as the knee, ankle and elbow jerk.

Most reflex arcs are polysynaptic and because of this they are a little slower in conduction rate than those of the monosynaptic variety. Although the afferent supply enters the central nervous system at a given segmental level, according to the position of the receptor organ, the motor response may occur at many levels because of linkage by interneurones conveying impulses to many motoneurone pools at lower and higher levels. An example of such a reflex would be the protective withdrawal reflex which is a response to undesirable stimulation. The plantar reflex response to scratching the skin over the sole of the foot and the abdominal contractions following skin stimulation over the muscles would also be examples. These are commonly called superficial reflexes, due to the fact that the receptor organs lie at a superficial level.

There is only one reflex arc which involves one neurone only and it occurs outside the central nervous system. This is the axon reflex which is a protective mechanism against skin irritation.

Reflexes have been classified in many ways and it is not the intention to reclassify them in this particular work. Certain mechanisms will be named and some described in order to give the student a greater understanding of the problems faced by the neurological patient.

Normally the reflex mechanisms are kept under control and inhibited or semi-inhibited by higher reactions and volitional control. However, it must be remembered that the lower reflex mechanisms are like the bricks from which the foundations are made – not obviously useful by themselves, but, as built-in members of a whole, they are of vital importance. In certain neurological disorders the inhibitory and controlling mechanisms may be at fault and some of the reflex mechanisms may manifest themselves in an unrestrained way, dominating the activities of the individual.

The Segmental Reflexes

These are so called because they tend to have arcs in which afferents and efferents lie in the same segmental level in the central nervous system. The phasic stretch reflexes fall into this category.

The Intersegmental Reflexes

Here the arcs may travel by interneurones to different levels in the spinal cord and brainstem. The protective withdrawal reflexes are examples. The area and intensity of stimulus determines how far above and below segmental level it spreads. This is an important fact as it can have an important bearing on the management of patients in whom this type of reflex is relatively uninhibited.

The Suprasegmental Reflexes

These are mainly concerned with postural activities. Some are concerned with the maintenance of the upright position against gravity while others are concerned with the obtaining of the upright position and body alignment.

ANTIGRAVITY MECHANISMS

A. The myotatic extensor reflexes
These depend upon an intact peripheral system, intact spinal cord and intact brainstem up to and including the pons. The vestibular nuclei

are particularly important to the reflex arcs concerned, in that they have an excitatory influence upon the small anterior horn cells which supply fusimotor fibres to the intrafusal muscle fibres which, by their contraction, put a positive bias on the stretch reflexes of the extensor groups concerned.

Thus the responses are really those of stretch reflex of the tonic or static variety. Such reflexes include the extensor thrust (positive supporting reflex) which is the response of a limb to a compression stimulus preferably applied along their long axis, e.g. compression applied to the palmar surface of the hand and to the sole of the foot. Such stimuli encourage an extensor response or 'thrusting away' from the stimulus.

Under this heading would also come the crossed extensor response. This occurs when one limb is flexed giving an extensor response in the opposite limb to enable it to support the additional weight thrust upon it.

B. The tonic postural reflexes

These are many and include the following mechanisms which require the same amount of brainstem and spinal cord to function as those mentioned in the previous paragraphs.

1. The tonic labyrinthine reflex. The receptor organs in this case are the labyrinthine canals of the inner ear. The afferent pathway influences the vestibular nuclei and causes these neurones to send excitatory impulses to the fusimotor fibres of the extensor muscles so contracting their intrafusal fibres and making them more sensitive to stretch stimuli. This reflex, therefore, increases extensor activity. The position of the head has a profound effect on this reflex since the labyrinths are lodged in the skull. The receptor organs are most intensely stimulated when the face is directed upwards and forwards at about 45° to the horizontal regardless of the position of the rest of the body (Fig. 2/6(i)).

2. The tonic neck reflexes. These relate to the position of the cervical spine wherein the receptor organs are considered to lie. The afferents influence the vestibular nuclei as before but the pattern of increase in tone differs as follows:

(a) *The symmetrical tonic neck reflex*. This occurs if the cervical spine is flexed or extended. If it is flexed, extensor tone increases in the lower limbs and decreases in the upper limbs which flex. If it is extended, extensor tone increases in the upper limbs and decreases in the lower limbs which, therefore, now flex (Fig. 2/6(ii)).

(b) *The asymmetrical tonic neck reflex*. This is related to rotation of the cervical spine. If the head is turned to the right there is an increase

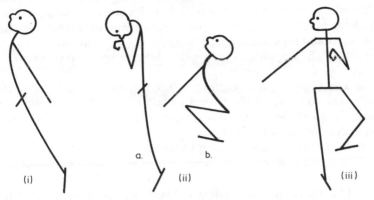

Fig. 2/6 (i, ii, iii) Patterns of increased activity imposed by some tonic reflex mechanisms

in extensor tone in the limbs of the right side (jaw limbs) and a decrease in extensor tone and therefore a degree of flexion in the limbs of the left side (skull limbs). If the head is turned to the other side the situation is reversed (Fig. 2/6(iii)).

REFLEXES CONCERNED WITH OBTAINING AN UPRIGHT POSITION
AND BODY ALIGNMENT

These are termed righting reflexes and require the peripheral system, the spinal cord and the brainstem up to and including the red nucleus, to be intact. The vestibular nuclei and reticular formation are very important grey areas. A combination of righting reflexes constitutes a righting reaction and enables an animal to obtain an upright position from any position of recumbency and very closely influences the rotational elements in movement. These are noticeably absent in certain neurological disorders.

The righting reflexes have been listed as follows:
1. the labyrinthine righting reflex
2. the neck righting reflex
3. body on head righting
4. body on body righting
5. optical righting (not complete at brainstem level).

The receptor organs required are the labyrinths, the muscles and joints, the skin and the retinae.

1. The labyrinthine righting reflex. This is the reflex which brings the head into the accepted upright position with eyes facing forward and eyes and ears level. Thus many pathways are involved.

2. The neck righting reflex. Rotation of the head or movement of the cervical spine stretches the neck muscles and triggers off a reflex mechanism to bring the body into alignment with the head so that shoulders and hips face forwards in complete harmony with the face. Obviously the response of the head to labyrinthine righting may, in turn, trigger off this mechanism.

3. The body on head righting reflex. Pressure on the side of the body will cause the head to right itself even if the previous two mechanisms are destroyed. It is a response to tactile stimulation and is dependent upon skin sensation.

4. The body on body righting reflexes. This is the response of the body to pressure stimulation. It will right itself whether the head can do so or not.

5. The optical righting reflexes. These require the presence of the visual cortex and are therefore more complex. Man particularly makes use of these reflexes but can manage without if need be. If there is a deficiency in the other reflexes, because of break in the arcs, man will substitute by using the optical righting mechanism almost entirely provided this is intact. This reflex fails him when it is dark or his eyes are closed.

It should be noted that these righting mechanisms work in conjunction with each other. The receptors and arcs concerned with the one response work to endorse or countermand another. The pathways linking the receptors for neck, optical and labyrinthine responses are carried in the medial longitudinal bundle of nerve fibres which link appropriate cranial nerve nuclei.

The righting reactions also work in conjunction with the tonic reflexes and segmental mechanisms. This interaction and integration of reflex mechanisms to gain functional adjustment is largely the function of the cerebellum working in conjunction with the cortical originating extrapyramidal system.

EQUILIBRIUM AND TILTING REACTIONS

These also need consideration. They are very complex mechanisms. The normal human reactions to disturbance of balance depend upon many factors among which are the following:

    (a) the state of maturity of the central nervous system

    (b) the mobility of the joints of the limbs and vertebral column

    (c) the relative muscle power in different parts of the body.

These reactions have been grouped in many ways and the following is only one approach.

1. Those which widen the base and lower the centre of gravity. These include the use of the arms in protective extension (sometimes called the parachute reaction). Both arms or one may be used passing in a forwards, sideways or backwards direction. These occur in response to a shift of the centre of gravity in the appropriate direction. They are rather primitive reactions since they prevent the use of the hands for skilled activity because of preoccupation with equilibrium.

2. Those which move the base to keep it under a moving centre of gravity. These include the stepping reactions in which stepping may occur forwards, backwards, sideways and across midline. Also in this category come the hopping reactions which particularly occur when only one limb is free to receive weight. The placing reactions related to skin contact with obstacles (e.g. if the dorsum of the foot strikes an object, the foot is lifted to prevent tripping) may also be included here for want of a better place.

3. Those which endeavour to keep the centre of gravity over the base. These include the movements of upper and lower limbs and trunk in order to adjust the relative overall position of the centre of gravity. Also included are the torsional movements of the vertebral column which are closely related to the righting reactions.

The last two groups can be considered to be more mature than the first group. Any reactions which leave the upper limbs free from obligation to equilibrium and therefore available for skilled function are relatively mature in nature.

In the normal course of events these reactions occur in conjunction with each other all the time and the vestibular apparatus, cerebellum and extrapyramidal system are all involved in their control. Each individual gives a reaction to any given disturbance of balance in his own individual manner, which is dependent upon the three factors mentioned above.

There are other reflex mechanisms and reactions which have not been mentioned. Some of these will be dealt with in other sections of this book and those particularly relevant to the developing child will be considered in Chapter 3.

Chapter 3

Developmental Background to Physiotherapy

by H. W. ATKINSON, M.C.S.P., H.T., DIP.T.P.

Chapter 2 has discussed the complexities of the nervous system and the way in which the ability to perform movement is brought about. However, we are not born with the ability to perform skilled movements. These have to develop gradually over a relatively protracted period of time.

At birth the central nervous system is not completely myelinated and it is therefore incapable of functioning in a mature manner until this process is complete. It may be said that maturation of the nervous system is dependent upon myelination. Connections between the mid-brain and cerebral cortex are not complete and, for this reason, the newly born child is inclined to behave in a manner which indicates that its reactions are being controlled by the subcortical regions. Movements tend to be relatively random and purposeless and specific reflex responses may be clearly demonstrated.

As the nervous system starts to develop shortly after conception it should be remembered that early reflex activities and movement responses develop long before birth. The child is, in fact, adapting his reactions to his environment right from the start. The influence of gravity upon the unborn child is not strong because of the fluid medium which supports and protects it in the uterus. This, added to the effect of the tonic labyrinthine reflex (which is quite strong at this stage), may explain why the child has so much difficulty in countering the effect of gravity during the early months of postnatal life.

As the nervous system matures some reflex pathways become more dominant for a period of time before becoming modified and integrated into more mature movement patterns. There are many early reflex mechanisms which are well developed in the full term infant and are very important to it for survival.

(a) **The rooting reflex.** This is a mechanism whereby the child can find a source of nourishment. It is a response to the touch stimulus applied to the outer aspect of the cheeks, lips and nose. The motor response is to 'root around' until the lips contact the nipple of the mother's breast. The reflex then gives way to the sucking reflex.

(b) **The sucking reflex.** This is a response to stimulation of the lips and in particular to their inner aspect. It gives rise to a sucking activity which in turn will trigger off the swallowing mechanism.

(c) **Swallowing.** This is a response to stimulation of the soft palate by the fluid which has been sucked into the mouth. The motor response is the contraction of the muscles which guide the fluid into the oesophagus and temporarily close the glottis.

(d) **The grasp reflex.** This is a mechanism whereby touch stimulus in the palm of the hand encourages flexion of the fingers giving the infant a grasp which clings to whatever touched the hand. In this way the child may cling to the mother's clothing by the same mechanism as a baby monkey clings to his mother's fur.

(e) **The traction reflex.** This is often associated with the grasp reflex and is a mechanism whereby traction applied to the limbs encourages a flexion response. It is often demonstrable by placing the fingers of the demonstrator's hands into the palm of the hands of the infant. The child will respond with a grasp reflex. If traction is now exerted by lifting the child with its grasping hands the degree of grasp will increase, and flexor tone in the upper limbs will increase to counter the traction. Many children can be made to support their own bodyweight for a minute or so by means of this grasp and traction mechanism.

(f) **The startle reflex.** This occurs in response to a loud noise or a jerk of body position. It is basically an extensor response. The upper limbs are carried upwards and outwards while the lower limbs extend and the head jerks into extension.

(g) **Reflex stepping or the walking reflex.** This occurs if the infant is supported in standing and his bodyweight is gently pushed forwards. The child will respond by stepping forwards in an exaggerated walking pattern. This reflex is present prior to birth and may well influence the position of the child in utero.

(h) **Placing reactions.** If the dorsum of the foot or hand is touched or placed so that it touches an obstruction the limb will be flexed and placed onto or over the obstruction.

Many of these primitive mechanisms are apparently lost during the first few months of life. Some become apparent again in a modified and integrated form while others may reappear under conditions of duress.

The postural reflexes, righting and equilibrium reactions are by no means completely developed at birth and many of the infant's activities are related to the development and integration of these, so that they are eventually able to give the correct malleable postural background to all our mature activities. The child has to develop the mechanisms and gain control over them before they can fulfil a useful function. Thus much of the maturation process is related to the ability to inhibit or modify the unwanted, while allowing desirable activities to occur.

CEPHALOCAUDAL DEVELOPMENT

It should be remembered that the maturation process occurs in a cephalocaudal direction. This means that the ability to control the posture and movements of the head, upper trunk and upper limbs occurs before control of the lower trunk and lower limbs. It is also true to say that control extends proximally at first and proceeds distally.

The fact that the child develops in a cephalocaudal direction means that control of the head, neck and upper limbs will always be in advance of the lower limbs and that the upper part of the body may be entering one phase of development while the more caudal area is still trying to develop a more primitive stage.

Early development is directed at reducing the dominance of the flexor muscle groups and gaining the ability to extend. At first only the cervical spine extends, but, as the child matures, the upper limbs, upper trunk and lower limbs all go into extension. When this occurs in prone lying the child is said to show a Landau reaction (Figs. 3/1, 3/2 and 3/3). This response is gained by pressure on the anterior aspect of the thorax, as might occur if the child is placed in prone lying or supported by placing a hand under the lower thoracic region. Such a response is unlikely to occur before four to five months of age and will not be available in full strength until about the tenth month after which time it subsides and becomes integrated into the general body patterns. The exact time and age at which any activity develops is not so important as the order in which it develops. The following paragraphs give an abbreviated outline of some of the landmarks in development.

FIRST SIX WEEKS

During this time the child is influenced quite strongly by the asymmetrical tonic neck reflex and by the neck righting reflex. Both of these have been described in Chapter 2. In addition to these the child is influenced by primitive grasp and traction, rooting, sucking, startle and stepping reactions. The child may be said to be in a stage of asymmetry. He is unable to keep his head in midline and thus the head

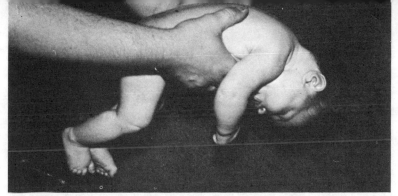

Fig. 3/1 Child aged 5 weeks. Ventral suspension; Landau response not yet available

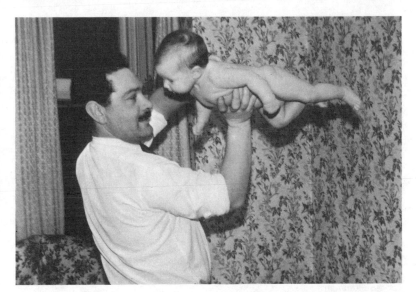

Fig. 3/2 Child aged 3½ months. Ventral suspension; Landau response developing well

Fig. 3/3 Child aged 7½ months. Ventral suspension; Landau response well developed

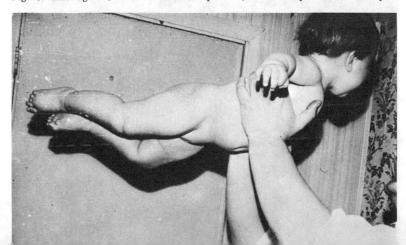

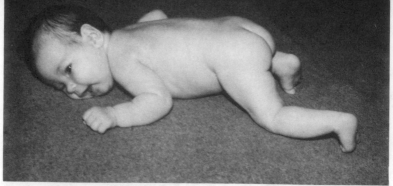

Fig. 3/4 Child at 5 weeks in prone lying. The effects of the asymmetrical tonic neck reflex can be seen in the limbs – it is particularly clear in the lower limbs

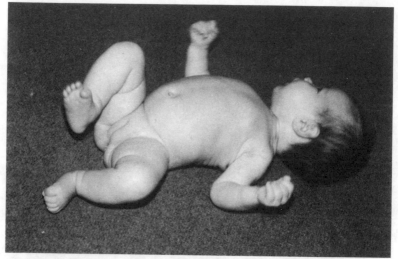

Fig. 3/5 Child at 5 weeks in supine lying. The physiological flexion of the limbs is very predominant

Fig. 3/6 Child at 5 weeks: sitting

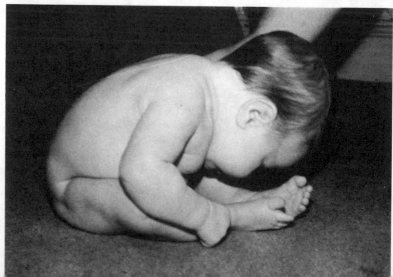

is turned to one side or the other. There tends to be a preferred side in many children. The limbs often adopt the asymmetrical tonic neck reflex posturing and this appears to show more often in the lower limbs than in the upper, possibly because the control of the lower limbs is less mature (Fig. 3/4). Movements occur in rather an asymmetrical and random manner using stereotyped mass flexion or extension patterns.

The neck righting reflex which is present means that the child will turn from supine to side lying if his head is turned towards the side (Fig. 3/5). The trunk follows as a whole and there is no spiralling at this stage.

In prone lying the hips and knees still retain a degree of flexion but the child will attempt to prevent himself from suffocating by turning his head away from the supporting surface (Fig. 3/4). In addition the labyrinthine righting reflex is beginning to develop and this means that the child will try to bring his head towards an upright position. Success is a long way off at this stage but the attempt is there. Ventral suspension does not give a Landau response (Fig. 3/1).

In supine lying the child may be pulled by the hands towards sitting. There will, however, be a complete head lag indicating no control over the head position at this stage (Fig. 3/6).

SIX WEEKS TO THREE MONTHS

During this period the strong influence being exerted by the asymmetrical tonic neck reflex gradually weakens while the symmetrical tonic neck reflex gains in strength. The neck righting mechanism is still quite strong and the labyrinthine righting mechanism is steadily gaining in strength. Because of these facts gradual changes in the child's abilities begin to occur.

Placed in prone lying the child will gradually begin to be able to lift his head further from the supporting surface and also to bring it towards midline. By three months the head and shoulders may be lifted and the elbows used to support the shoulders. The lower limbs may still show traces of the influence of the asymmetrical tonic neck reflex pattern, but this will not occur so frequently. Head lifting is

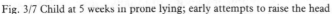
Fig. 3/7 Child at 5 weeks in prone lying; early attempts to raise the head

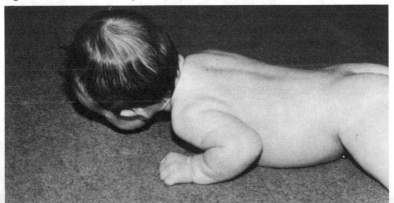

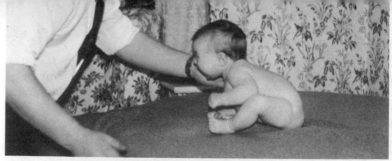

Fig. 3/8 Child at 3½ months: sitting. Note the head control

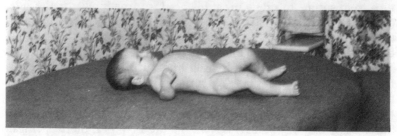

Fig. 3/9 Child at 3½ months: supine. Note the symmetry and reduction of physiological flexion in the limbs

brought about by the labyrinthine righting reflex and the extension produced may also influence the movements of the hands and feet (Fig. 3/7).

Placed in supported sitting the head will drop forwards frequently but towards the third month the child will be lifting the head and holding it steadily (Fig. 3/8). If, however, the trunk is inclined backwards from sitting towards supine lying, there will be a considerable head lag.

Because the child is gaining more head control in midline he is able to use his eyes for watching objects held for him to see. He is also able to place his hands in midline and can observe them, thus building up body image.

The gradually rising influence of the symmetrical tonic neck reflex encourages symmetry and the child is often said to be entering a stage of symmetry for this reason (Fig. 3/9). Because of this the ability to respond to primitive stepping or walking gradually subsides. If weight is put onto the feet the lower limbs go into bilateral extension and cannot work reciprocally.

FOUR TO SIX MONTHS

During this period the asymmetrical tonic neck reflex is still weakening in its influence while the symmetrical tonic neck reflex is gaining in strength. The labyrinthine righting reflex is strong but neck righting is gradually coming under some degree of control. The Landau reaction is beginning to be demonstrable (Fig. 3/2).

When placed in prone lying the child is able to rest on his forearms with his head lifted high (Fig. 3/10). He will occasionally lift the forearms clear and extend the head, shoulders and arms, supporting his weight completely on the lower thorax. This is an attempt at a Landau reaction. During this process the hips and knees also extend.

When in supine the head is held in midline and often lifts forward. The hands meet in midline and attempts are made to grasp objects when the hands are free.

Placed in sitting, the head is held well and only the lumbar spine shows flexion (Fig. 3/11). There is now no head lag if the child's trunk is inclined backwards or if the child is pulled towards sitting (Figs. 3/12 and 3/13).

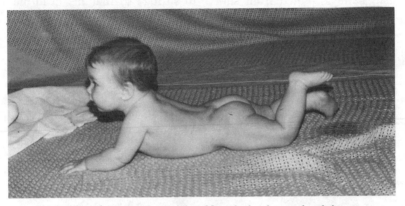

Fig. 3/10 Child at 5½ months: prone lying. Note the head control and the weight-bearing upper limbs

Fig. 3/11 Child at 5½ months: sitting. Note the head and upper trunk control and the participation of the upper limbs

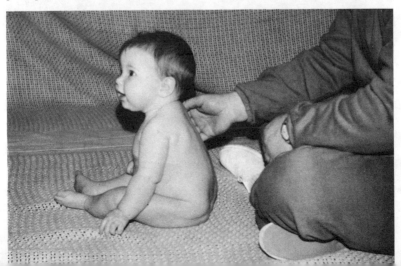

At this stage the child gradually develops the ability to grasp objects deliberately. This is only possible because the grasp reflex has now been integrated so that release of grasp can occur in order to open the hand prior to closing on the desired object.

SIX TO EIGHT MONTHS

During this period many interesting things are happening. The neck righting reflexes, which have become weakened in dominance, work in conjunction with the stronger labyrinthine righting mechanisms and also with the symmetrical tonic neck reflex to make rolling from prone to supine possible, and later from supine to prone (Fig. 3/14). At the same time the important body rotating activities also develop giving a special action to rolling over.

The child is now doing many different things (Fig. 3/15). He will help if he is pulled from supine to sitting, so that his head and

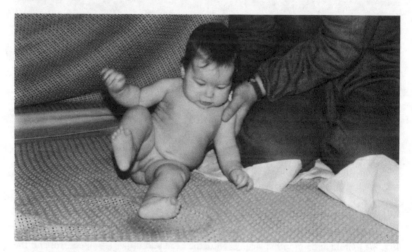

Fig. 3/12 Child at 5½ months: sitting. The balancing reactions are developing well

Fig. 3/13 Child at 5½ months: sitting. More balance reactions

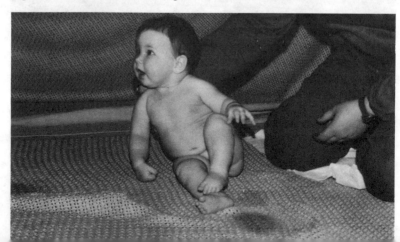

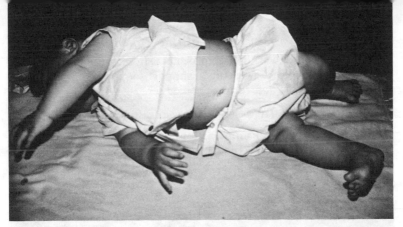

Fig. 3/14 Child at 8 months: spiral rolling

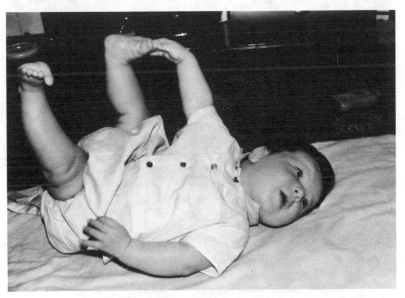

Fig. 3/15 Child at 8 months: supine. Playing with his toes – 'inverted sitting'

shoulders come forward. If he is placed in sitting he is able to balance by placing his hands in front of him with extended elbows.

If he is placed in prone he will bear weight on extended elbows and will weight-bear on one arm while reaching forward with the other. Thus he is developing equilibrium reactions. The Landau reaction occurs frequently (Fig. 3/3). He may attempt to creep using flexed elbows and allowing his legs to follow as passengers (Fig. 3/16). Nearer to the end of this time the legs may attempt to participate using rather primitive patterns. His elbows will be now extended, and the upper limbs will be working reciprocally. He may then be said to be crawling when his knees are able to support some weight and his legs are able to progress in a reciprocal manner.

EIGHT TO TEN MONTHS

The righting and equilibrium reactions are developing rapidly at this stage. They become available to the child in a variety of ways and equilibrium reactions may be seen in prone lying, supine lying and in

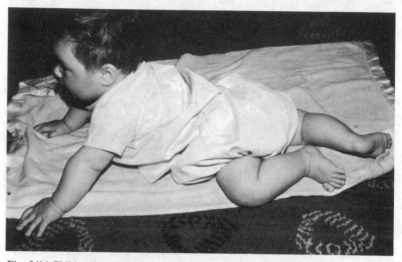

Fig. 3/16 Child at 8 months: prone. Head and upper trunk and limb control maturing well. Lower limbs still showing more primitive patterns

sitting. At first the child could only lean forward in sitting but by this time he is able to support himself with a sideways extension of the upper limb.

This improvement in balance enables the child to move from prone lying to sitting and vice versa. Body rotation becomes very important. As the child is able to roll over and sit up quite early in this period he is also able to sit up and rotate freely without hand support before the tenth month. This enables him to play in sitting and to investigate toys and objects around him. He will pick them up, investigate them by mouth and hand before casting them aside. Mouthing is important as an afferent stimulus as the tongue is a highly sensitive structure and plays an important part in the learning process. Casting away of objects helps in gaining spatial perception and is therefore another form of learning.

The weight is borne on upper and lower limbs (Fig. 3/17); crawling is gaining as a method of progression and many children change to the pattern of walking on hands and feet (bear walking). The child is also likely to attempt to stand using his hands to help pull himself up and may begin to lift one foot off the ground so long as he has hold of his support. He is now developing equilibrium reactions in standing.

Some children do not crawl but develop a method of progression which can only be described as shuffling along on the bottom! Provided no other abnormality is present this is acceptable and is then designated as benign shuffling.

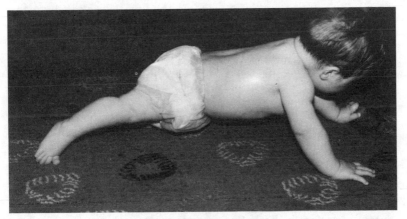

Fig. 3/17 Child at 9 months: prone. Weight on upper and lower limbs

TEN TO TWELVE MONTHS

The child is still likely to walk on hands and feet and when standing he may cruise around furniture. By this stage the child's upper limbs have gone from a period of behaving in a rather reciprocal manner to a period of freedom. The lower limbs are still learning reciprocal activities and for this reason balance in standing is not yet secure and walking may be delayed until reciprocal stepping activities are available again.

As the righting and equilibrium reactions become fully integrated the child's ability to walk unaided develops. At first a wide base is used and the hands may be held upwards or the scapulae retracted with elbows flexed. As balance becomes more secure and movement patterns more available the child ceases to use a wide base and adopts body rotation as a means of maintaining walking equilibrium.

At first the child will rise into standing by rolling to prone and then progressing upwards. Later he will half turn before rising and eventually he will rise symmetrically as in adulthood. The symmetrical method may not develop until he is about three years of age.

Steps and stairs present a problem. At about one year of age the child will virtually crawl up, while at two years he may ascend one step at a time, one foot coming up to join the other. He may well be four years of age before he is able to go up and down steps in a truly reciprocal manner. The ability to descend always lags behind the ability to ascend.

Maturation of movement continues for a protracted period of time. The most rapid progress occurs within the first three years but complexity of movement continues to improve throughout adolescence into early adulthood. It has been found that although stimulus and environmental influences may stimulate the perfection of activities they in no way affect the rate of myelination. In other words the child will not roll over unaided until the nervous system has sufficiently matured to enable the pathways to be used no matter how much external environmental pressure is exerted. Equally well demonstrated is the fact that if the child is held fixed and prevented from demonstrating movements to which its nervous system has matured they will be produced immediately the body is free to respond.

The above summary by no means covers all the aspects of motor development. It should be noted that mature movements are complex permutations of the basic flexion and extension synergies. Until the child can mix flexion and extension components of movement, only mass patterns can be produced. The ability to stabilise the trunk and proximal part of the limbs while allowing distal parts to move is important where skilled activity is concerned and cerebellar activity is very important to this. Equally well, the ability to retain a fixed distal extremity while the proximal segments and trunk move over it is also essential. Much of the child's developmental progress is related to the ability to produce these two varieties of movement, not only as distinct entities, but going on at the same time.

Let us take two examples to illustrate the points mentioned above:

1. *The mixture of flexion and extension components*. A simple example may be seen when the sitting position is considered. This requires *extension* of the vertebral column, but *flexion* of the hips and knees. If it is impossible to extend the column unless a total extension pattern is used then the child is unable to maintain a sitting position.

A more complex example may be seen if the lower limbs are considered in the walking synergies. Mass movement patterns of a more reflex variety follow certain stereotyped synergies. When the hip and knee flex the lower limb also abducts and may laterally rotate and the foot dorsiflexes. However, to walk forward we require to flex the hip and knee while adducting the limb. This is followed by extending the knee while dorsiflexing the foot. Here, alone, are some interesting synergies. The leg then prepares to take weight, when it extends at the knee and hip and abducts to prevent a Trendelenburg sign (drop of the pelvis on the non-weight-bearing side) (Fig. 3/18) while the foot is dorsiflexed – another mixture of synergies. In Figure 3/18a the abductors of the weight-bearing limb are working to prevent the pelvis from dropping on the non-weight-bearing side. In Figure 3/18b the abductors are not working and so the pelvis has dropped into adduction on

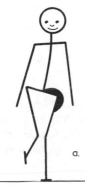 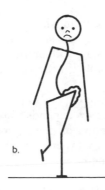

a.   b.

Fig. 3/18 (a) and (b) The role of the hip abductors in weight-bearing

that side, causing a compensatory lurch of the trunk. This is called a Trendelenburg sign.

The push-off requires more extension of the hip, flexion of the knee and plantar flexion of the foot. This is a very complex series of synergies. This ability is not immediately available. The child who has recently started walking flexes and abducts his hip. Only later does he keep it adducted as the leg comes forward.

2. *Proximal fixation and distal freedom and vice versa.* A simple example may be seen when we consider the child in prone lying. When he is able to take weight on one elbow while playing with a toy with the other hand he is demonstrating distal fixation of the supporting limb with the trunk free to move over it, while the free limb is moving distally against the proximal support of the steady trunk.

A more complex example of the same thing occurs with the much more mature pattern of writing. Here the supporting arm is offering distal stability to the trunk which is free to move over it. The hand which is putting pen to paper is working freely with a more proximal area of stability in the forearm. However, the forearm must also be partly free to move for each word and so movement at the shoulder has to occur. The shoulder is functioning as a stable and mobile structure at one and the same time against the stable background of the trunk which, in turn, is free to move over the other, or supporting limb. This is a very complex synergy. Little wonder that we cannot write at birth!

Many learning processes depend upon the ability to move. We require movement to be able to explore our environment and unless this is possible our mental processes cannot develop normally. Head control is essential to movement but is also essential for the ability to make maximum use of the sense of sight. If we cannot control our head position it is difficult to gain control over our eye activities. The eyes also need to have a stable base from which to work. Eye movements are similar to limbs. They can remain stable while the head moves, or they can move while the head stays still, or the two activities may go on at once. None of this is possible if head control is absent.

Assessment of spatial relationships depends upon movement. The relationship between hands and eyes depends upon the ability to move and explore, and the perception of depth, space, height, size and shape have all to be learned by experiences dependent upon movements of different areas of the body.

Balance activities basically start by the balance of the head upon the shoulders in prone lying. Progression is then made by balancing the shoulders over the elbows which offer a forward support in prone lying. In sitting it should be noted that the body is at first inclined forward so that head balance on the shoulders is still an extension activity and the arms are in a supporting forward position, but with extended elbows.

Later the ability to balance with the arms supporting sideways develops and much later the arms may support by being placed behind as when sitting in a backwards leaning position. This requires flexor activity in the head and neck to maintain the balance of the head on the shoulders.

Before the child is able to give a backwards support to the sitting position he is developing rotatory ability in the trunk which is the precursor to more skilful balance activities. Maturity of balance is seen when the upper limbs can carry out skilled activities, while the legs and trunk are dealing with maintenance of equilibrium without the aid of the upper limbs.

The development of motor skills is not complete until the hands can be used in prehensile activities and much work has been done by various authors on the development of prehension. As a summary it may be pointed out that the hand activities are inclined to develop from ulnar to radial side. The grasp and release activities of the early stages in development appear to commence with activity of the little finger and radiate out towards the thumb. Gradually the radial aspect of the hand becomes more dominant and eventually the pincer grasp between thumb and index finger develops while the ulnar side of the hand takes up a more stabilising function. Much more mature is the 'dynamic tripod' posture described by Wynn Parry in 1966 and explained by Rosenbloom and Horton in 1971. Here the thumb, index and middle fingers are used as a threesome to give fine coordinated movements of the hand. The classic example of the use of this tripod is in writing, although it may be seen in other functional activities.

The development of body image and awareness occurs in conjunction with the ability to move. At first, because of lack of myelination of the cortical pathways, the child is only able to know whether he is comfortable or not without necessarily knowing why. There is no discrimination of where the discomfort lies or what is causing it. Socially at this stage the child is only able to communicate by crying and consequently discomfort of any kind will be voiced by crying. Comfort or pleasurable sensation is indicated by a silent and contented-looking child.

Gradually the child starts to learn about himself. Body awareness develops cephalocaudally as one might expect and head control, hands in midline and the ability to bring the hands to the mouth give the child the ability to see and feel his hands and to become aware of them as part of himself. He may also be able to discriminate between the people who are handling him. Mother recognition comes fairly early and the child is usually able to register pleasure by this stage in the form of smiling at his mother.

The ability to discriminate between what is part of oneself and what is part of one's surroundings is an important part of perceptual development. Much is dependent upon the opportunity given to explore. When a child is being carried by an adult he often tries to explore the adult's face with his hands and can cause considerable discomfort doing so! This is his method of learning to perceive whether or not the face is his or someone else's. He cannot, at this stage, be expected to appreciate discomfort in others since he is not yet aware of it fully in himself. At the same time he will gain some social perception since there will inevitably be a reaction to his activities of some kind or another and early communication will occur.

As time passes the child becomes aware of other parts of his body and can often be seen lying with his feet lifted up towards his mouth where there can be contact between feet, mouth and hands. Incidentally, when he lies supine with his feet in contact with his hands he is also exercising his equilibrium reactions and can frequently be seen to roll from supine to side and back, still holding his feet. Control of trunk position is being developed while he is learning about body image.

By this time the child is more aware of his surroundings and able to communicate not only by smiling and crying but also by making gurgling noises, coughing, cooing, etc. He is also able to show likes and dislikes regarding food. The sense of taste and smell are early basic mechanisms and develop early in life. The child also learns to appreciate the tone used and the word 'No'.

The process of improving body image and social contacts continues for many months and the child is usually about fifteen months old before he is able to indicate discomfort regarding wet pants accurately to his mother. Since development occurs cephalocaudally this is hardly surprising. After this has occurred he is likely to learn gradually to control his bladder activities, but he may be three years of age before he is more or less reliable.

The physical, intellectual and social development of the child are so clearly linked with each other that it would take several volumes to give a complete and detailed account. (See Bibliography, p.147.)

The physiotherapist makes most use of the physical aspects of development but needs some understanding of the intellectual and social aspects to appreciate fully the whole problem.

As a brief summary it may be said that the process of integrating certain reflex mechanisms involved in movement occurs over a period of time and eventually makes controlled purposeful movement possible. The control develops in a cephalocaudal direction. It is closely linked with perception of body image, intellectual and social behaviour and, although it is not dependent upon environmental factors, these may influence the rate at which perfection develops. Motor development starts with control of the head position in prone with the upper limbs most able to take weight in a forward or elbow support position. Later development includes rolling and supported sitting with the weight supported forwards on the hands at first, and later at the sides and even later behind. Body rotation begins to be perfected as rolling occurs and limb rotation follows trunk rotation as a rule.

Movements at first follow primitive patterns of synergy but later the ability to combine flexion/extension patterns to give more complexity of movement develops. Ultimate maturity of movement is reached when the hands are totally free from an obligation to balance mechanisms, so that they can be freely developed as skilful tools and used in conjunction with visual and other sensory feed-back mechanisms.

It should be noted that the child's development mechanisms are so arranged that he is preparing for balance in a position before he is able fully to adopt the position and certainly before he is able to use it as a base for activities of his hands. Most usually the mother plays with the child so that he experiences advanced activities before he is able to perform them. In other words, he is being prepared for the activity in addition to making his own 'in-built' preparations.

Let us take an example. A child may be seven to eight months old before he is able to get himself into a sitting position. To sit in a balanced manner he needs to flex at the hips and extend at the trunk. He needs head control and the ability to support himself forwards on his hands. These are minimum requirements. He is prepared for this naturally by the early development of head control, the elbow and hand support prone positions, and by lying on his back playing with his feet. His mother also helps him by propping him into a sitting position so that he experiences it prior to achieving it. Help in this manner makes him experiment and he tries to balance when he is put into sitting and in fact learns to do so.

In the meantime his rolling and rotatory activities are developing. The child gradually develops the ability to get into sitting *after* he has learned to balance in that position.

The Clinical Value of a Knowledge of Developmental Sequence

When working with handicapped children and, in particular, with the very young, it is easy to see that this information is exceedingly valuable.

When treating babies with movement defects it is important to start as early as possible and to bear in mind the normal sequence of development so that one can, as far as possible, channel the child's reactions along suitable lines and encourage step by step progress without leaving gaps which may lead to abnormality. The earlier the abnormal child is given help the more successful is the treatment likely to be. It is much more difficult to correct abnormal habits than it is to prevent them from occurring. The child's nervous system is very malleable and able to adapt very readily. Consequently it can be most easily influenced before it is fully matured. It is a great mistake to wait until the child can consciously cooperate. By this time irretrievable abnormalities will have developed. The skilled physiotherapist is able to exploit her knowledge of the nervous system to stimulate suitable responses in the child long before it is aware of cooperating.

However, many physiotherapists deal only with adults or, at least, the greater bulk of their patient load is adult. Where then does this knowledge have value? The answer is simply that injury or disease to the central nervous system frequently brings about demyelination of certain areas and may damage or destroy the nervous pathways which have been used to control certain activities. The patient frequently shows a regression of motor skills to a more primitive level. Certain of the reflex mechanisms, which have hitherto been integrated into mature movement patterns, may be partly released from cortical control and may exert an excessive influence over the patient, dominating these movement patterns into abnormality or even preventing them from occurring at all. The patient will frequently show absence or disturbance of normal equilibrium reactions, poverty of movement synergy, perception difficulties and diminution of sensory discrimination. If the physiotherapist is going to help the patient to make full use of such nervous connections as are left, she is more likely to be successful if she has a knowledge of the way in which more skilled activities develop in the first place so that she can, to some extent, simulate the conditions to facilitate redevelopment. The following example illustrates this point.

A patient with neurological symptoms can often maintain a sitting position but, on attempting to stand, he pulls himself up by placing his hands on a rigid forward support or by pulling on a helper who is standing in front of him. Frequently the head is flexed forwards or, conversely, it may be thrown back so that the nose is pointing upwards. In the first instance the patient is using the symmetrical tonic neck reflex pattern to aid him into standing and in the second his legs are making use of the tonic labyrinthine effect. Neither of these is acceptable as the patterns are those of total reflex synergy and balance in standing will never be achieved using these patterns. Such a patient has his movement excessively influenced by the tonic reflex mechanisms and requires training to modify them and to start early balance activities. He requires help in receiving weight onto his arms in a forward position. Such activities as elbow support prone lying are suitable, progressing to hand support forward side sitting, leading to prone kneeling and hand support forward standing (standing but resting hands on a stool or low support in front of him). He needs to feel the sensation of weight being received forwards instead of pulling back. There are many other facets to this patient's problems which need attention but the above example makes the point.

Many head injury cases regress to an enormous degree and intellectual and social abilities regress also. Motor training along developmental lines is accompanied, in many cases, by a brightening of intellectual activities and the beginning of social communication. The patient may never achieve behaviour patterns which are mature but he is more likely to make balanced progress if a developmental approach is used.

REFERENCE

Rosenbloom, L. and Horton, M. E. (1971). 'The maturation of fine prehension in young children.' *Developmental Medicine and Child Neurology,* **13,** 3–8.

Chapter 4

Disturbances of Normal Physiology

by H. W. ATKINSON, M.C.S.P., H.T., DIP.T.P.

On reading the previous two chapters it will have become obvious that injury or disease of the nervous system may cause a wide variety of problems according to the area and extent of the lesion. This chapter will attempt to outline some of the more common problems which the physiotherapist may meet when dealing with this type of patient.

DISTURBANCE OF AFFERENT INFORMATION

Loss of, or imperfection in, afferent supply may give rise to several problems. It may be the result of definite interruption of afferent pathways, giving areas of anaesthesia or paraesthesia. If the interruption lies within a peripheral nerve then the area affected will be that specifically supplied by that particular nerve. If, however, it is more centrally placed the lesion may have more diffuse effects because many fibres from different areas tend to travel together in the spinal cord.

Sensory disturbance may be due to disease processes pressing on afferent pathways giving distorted input. It may be due to faulty linkage between thalamus and cortex, which would prevent discriminative assessment of sensory information.

Disturbance in the link between spinal cord and cerebellum would give rise to inadequate information to help the cerebellum in its postural activities.

One must also remember that visual, auditory and vestibular afferents may be affected in addition to those conveying joint sensation. These latter factors give rise to the most potent symptoms of disorientation and loss of body image.

The results of afferent disturbance vary from very slight effects to total loss of body image, disorientation and rejection of the affected area. Skin anaesthesia makes the patient vulnerable to injury since pain is absent and there is no withdrawal from harmful stimuli.

Patients with a reduction in afferent information may have difficulty with spatial perception. The relative positions, size, heights and depths of objects may be difficult for them to perceive. This, of course, is closely linked to visual impressions. Ability of hand/eye control depend to some extent upon binocular vision.

Appreciation of shapes, textures and weight is also important and depends upon eyes, hands and manipulative skills in addition to skin and kinaesthetic sensation. Loss of this variety of sensory perception magnifies he loss of body image and the patient may forget the affected area or even reject it.

Disturbance of sensory perception may, in some cases, be aggravated by lack of experience. If the patient is prevented from experiencing certain afferent stimuli because of the disability then some measure of deprivation must occur. For example, the human being normally carries the hand towards the face for a multiplicity of reasons. If the movements of the upper limb are so impoverished that this cannot occur then the link between hand and face becomes weaker and some degree of body image is lost due to lack of repetitive experience.

Conversely other disturbing things may happen. If a patient experiences an abnormal sensation often enough, he may well eventually accept this as normal and may resent any attempt to adjust or correct this. Let us take an example to illustrate: the patient's disability may make him inclined to lean his weight, when sitting, consistently on to one side. If this is allowed to continue he will accept the one-sided pressure as being natural and normal and interpret the position as being one of safety and one in which he feels secure. If attempts are then made to encourage him to take weight evenly on each side he will feel that he is leaning dangerously towards the side which has not been accustomed to receiving weight. He will not feel safe until he has regained his own 'normal' position. Thus he may reject attempts to correct his posture to a more normal one and much patience and understanding will be required to gain his cooperation.

Paraesthesia is a term used to signify disturbed and diminished sensory information. It refers to tingling and numbness of the affected area and may be the result of lesions of any part of the afferent system. However, it is most obvious in peripheral problems. Paraesthesia should not be confused with para-anaesthesia, which is a term used to denote *loss* of sensation in both lower limbs.

Dissociated anaesthesia refers to the loss of appreciation of pain and temperature while tactile information is still available. This is most often due to interruption of the lateral spinothalamic tracts within the cord and is seen in cases of syringomyelia.

Hypalgia refers to a reduction in sensitivity to pain. This occurs in certain disorders of the afferent system. Where all afferent information is reduced or lost there will obviously be hypalgia but it is most noticeable in association with dissociated anaesthesia. These two phenomena lead to damage as a result of major and minor trauma since they reduce the stimulation of protective mechanisms.

When afferent information reaches the brain it is received and interpreted. The brain processes the information so that appropriate reactions may occur. Any defect at this level makes the production of appropriate reactions difficult or impossible. The patient cannot recall, learn or relearn basic patterns of movement and may be very difficult to treat for this reason. It is important for the physiotherapist to appreciate this, since many patients are thought to be uncooperative or 'not trying', when in fact the problem is in the processing of afferent material.

ABNORMALITIES OF MOVEMENT

These may take several forms according to the area of damage.

Muscle Flaccidity or Paralysis

This is the result of disturbance in the lower motor neurone. The muscle or group of muscles affected may be totally paralysed if all their available neurones are put out of action. If, however, only some anterior horn neurones are involved the muscles will show partial paralysis and will appear to be very weak. Any muscles affected in this way would be unable to function as members of a team and consequently movement synergies requiring their participation would be abnormal and substitute patterns would be produced. If only a small muscle group is affected in this way the abnormalities are minimal, but if many groups are involved, substitution can be grotesque or even inadequate, in which case the subject is rendered relatively helpless.

Totally flaccid muscles have no lower motor neurone supply because of damage or injury to all the cells in their motoneurone pools or to all the fibres passing peripherally. Such muscles cannot be brought into action voluntarily, or as an automatic reaction or in a reflex action. They feel soft and flabby to the touch, are non-resilient, offer no protection to the structures adjacent to them and are unable to support the joints over which they pull. Because of lack of use, and therefore of blood supply, they atrophy quite rapidly losing the greater part of their muscle bulk.

Hypotonia

This term is used here to denote the reduction in preparedness for action found in the muscles when there are defects in certain areas of the extrapyramidal part of the central nervous system. In this case the excitatory influence exerted by the extrapyramidal system upon the motoneurone pools is diminished and, as a result, the muscles show a reduction in sensitivity to stretch. This may, at first sight, be confused with muscle paralysis because the muscles may appear to be totally or almost totally flail. It is, however, very different. The muscles have a normal lower motor neurone supply but the factors exerting an influence upon the motoneurone pools are seriously disturbed. There is a reduction of excitatory influence upon the small anterior horn cells which give rise to the fusimotor fibres. Because of this the fusimotor fibres are inactive and therefore activity of the intrafusal muscle fibres is diminished. Thus the muscles are less sensitive to stretch – particularly if it is applied slowly. Quick, exaggerated stretch will bring about a response via the spinal stretch reflex but the bias on the receptors is low. If the muscle is stretched by distortion of its tendon, as in the knee jerk, the response will occur but will not be quickly checked by a reciprocal response in the hamstrings because their stretch reflex mechanism will also be sluggish. The lower leg will swing backwards and forwards like a pendulum before it finally comes to rest again.

Hypotonia never affects muscle groups in isolation because it is not a peripheral problem. It is usually found as a general feature or, in some cases, it may be unilateral. The most common reason for hypotonia is disturbance in function of the cerebellum. It may be the result of damage or disease in the cerebellum itself or in the links between the cerebellum and the brainstem extrapyramidal mechanisms.

The cerebellum is thought to exert its influence upon the postural reflex mechanisms by its link with the extrapyramidal system. If it fails to encourage excitation in these tonic mechanisms the fusimotor system will fail to function adequately and the stretch reflex bias will be low. This gives a background of postural instability and makes proximal fixation for distal movements unavailable. Movements therefore tend to be slow in forthcoming and when they do commence they are of an unstable, ill-controlled nature, inclined to overshoot the mark and show intention tremor. This term is used because the tremor occurs when a movement is being carried out and is not present when at rest.

Balance reactions are also disturbed and when they occur they are inclined to overcompensate. The patient may, in fact, fall because of his exaggerated balance reactions. These are occurring against a background of unstable postural tone due to diminished fusimotor activity.

Ataxia

A patient who has hypotonia inevitably shows a form of ataxia. The symptoms described under the heading 'hypotonia' are also those of ataxia. Ataxia means that movements are incoordinate and ill-timed, giving a deficiency of smoothness of movement. Ataxia related to hypotonia occurs partly because of the defective postural tone as a background and partly because of the phenomenon of dyssynergia.

Dyssynergia is the term used to describe the loss of fluency in a movement. The balance of activity is upset because of faulty synergy. The teamwork between muscles is lost, giving a jerky appearance to the movements, which may well be split up into a series of jerky, separated entities. Both stopping and starting of movements are difficult and overshooting occurs.

These symptoms may also be noted when hearing a patient speak. Speech is a very mature ability, requiring intricate control of coordination of the appropriate muscles. Dyssynergia and accompanying problems lead to speech being broken up in the same way as was described for movement. Speech affected in this way is said to be 'scanning'.

Ataxia may also be linked with the sensory problems mentioned earlier in this chapter. It may be due to deficiency of afferent information to the cerebellum and to the cortex, making the individual unaware of his position in space. In this case the cerebellum cannot bring about the necessary postural adjustments, nor is the central nervous system receiving a feed-back regarding the success of the movements. A person with this problem will show very similar symptoms to the previous form of ataxia, but he may be able to mask his problem by using his eyes and ears to excess as substitutes for his loss of skin and joint position sensation. If he is temporarily deprived of the use of his eyes – as in the dark – or of his ears – as in a noisy environment – he may be much more ataxic than when he is able to make full use of them. This is often called rombergism.

The ataxias are often accompanied by *nystagmus*, which is a form of dyssynergia in the eyes.

Occasionally ataxia may be accompanied by vestibular disturbance which gives rise to vertigo. This is a condition in which the patient's appreciation of head position is disorientated. The subject feels giddy and nauseated. These symptoms can add greatly to the problems of the ataxic patient.

Dysmetria is a term often applied to the ataxic patient. It refers to the difficulty in assessing and achieving the correct distance or range of movement. It is seen in the overshooting symptoms mentioned earlier.

Hypertonia

This denotes the opposite state of affairs to hypotonia. In this case the excitatory extrapyramidal influences upon the motoneurone pools are present to excess and the stretch reflex excitatory bias is high. The muscles are therefore more sensitive to stretch and are said to be hypertonic.

Let us refer back to the stretch reflex mechanism. Muscle spindles contain stretch receptors which can influence the large anterior horn cells in the motoneurone pools by means of the Ia afferent fibres. Stimulation of these stretch receptors creates impulses which pass via the Ia fibres to the motoneurone pools where they stimulate the large anterior horn cells to convey impulses to the extrafusal muscle which contracts in response to these impulses.

In addition to the extrafusal muscle fibres there are intrafusal fibres which form a contractile element to the stretch receptor. Their function is to keep the stretch receptor in a receptive state whatever the length of the extrafusal muscle fibres. To do this they require to be held in a state of contraction sufficient to keep the stretch receptor area sensitive to stretch. They receive a nerve supply via the small anterior horn cells of the motoneurone pool. These nerves are called fusimotor fibres and are influenced by the extrapyramidal system.

If the inhibitory influence is dominant the stretch receptors are less sensitive because the intrafusal fibres are less active. This is what happens in hypotonia.

If the excitatory influence is dominant then the stretch receptors are much more sensitive because they are being held taut by the contracting intrafusal fibres. This is the situation in hypertonia.

Under normal circumstances an appropriate balance of excitation and inhibition is maintained to keep the stretch receptors suitably sensitive according to the circumstances of the moment.

There are some additional factors which should now be mentioned. In addition to the Ia fibres from the stretch receptors, there are secondary receptors in the spindle which give rise to fibres belonging to a group known as group II. These are also sensitive to stretch and if stimulated they have been found to inhibit slow-acting motor units and facilitate fast-acting motor units.

Another factor which has so far not been introduced is the Ib group fibres, which arises from the tendons or aponeuroses of muscle. These fibres arise from sensory receptors in the musculotendinous junction (Golgi organs) and are receptive to stretch. They are known to have an inhibitory effect upon motoneurone pools of their own muscle supply – an autogenic effect. These effects of inhibition are brought about via interneurones.

In order to appreciate fully the phenomenon of hypertonicity it is necessary to consider the stretch reflex in this way: the stretch reflex is said to have both phasic and tonic components. The phasic stretch reflex occurs when the muscle spindles are stimulated briefly and give rise to a synchronous motor response. The tonic reflex mechanism is the effect which is gained by a slow stretch of the muscle so that an asynchronous firing of motor units causes a sustained contraction of varying degree according to the sensitivity of the muscle to stretch.

There are two types of hypertonia, spasticity and rigidity.

SPASTICITY

As was stated before, the fusimotor system is rendered excessively active by the influence of the excitatory extrapyramidal system. The sensitivity of the stretch receptors is excessively high to both slow and quick stretch stimuli. In its milder form the sensitivity to quick stretch is most noticeable, when a 'clasp-knife' phenomenon may be demonstrated. In this situation the muscles respond to quick stretch in a phasic manner when there is synchronous firing of the primary receptors, which in turn gives a synchronous contraction of extrafusal muscle in response. The primary receptors fire synchronously because their threshold has been made low due to the excessive activity of the fusimotor system. The term 'clasp-knife' phenomenon is occasionally used because the opposition of the muscle to stretch seems to build up to a climax and then to subside suddenly. The sudden reduction in opposition may be attributed to the inhibitory influence exerted by the group Ib Golgi tendon organs, when tension is applied to the musculo-tendinous junction. Many explanations have been offered for this phenomenon and studies are not completed.

 The response to slow stretch is that of steady opposition to the stretch stimulus which, in some cases, may build up to a tremendous level whereas in other milder cases it may be very slight indeed. On the whole passive movements to joints, where the muscles are showing spasticity, are more likely to be successful if conducted slowly so as to avoid eliciting a phasic response.

This form of hypertonicity is associated with the release of reflex activity from cortical control. If the lesion has occurred at a high level in the central nervous system then the tonic postural reflexes may be released in addition to the spinal reflexes. The released reflexes will exert a relatively uninhibited effect upon the motoneurone pools and cause patterns of increase in tone relevant to the reflexes released. For example, the released asymmetrical tonic neck reflex will cause spasticity to show in the extensor groups of the limbs on the side towards which the face is turned and in the flexors of the opposite side. The tonic labyrinthine reflex will incline the patient to show spasticity in the extensor groups if his head is in the appropriate position. The symmetrical tonic neck reflex will cause appropriate spastic patterning according to the position of the cervical spine, i.e. if the cervical spine is flexed the upper limbs will flex and the lower limbs extend etc.

It is rare to find one reflex mechanism released in isolation and a confusion of patterns is more likely to occur. However, knowledge of these factors enables the physiotherapist to interpret what is happening at any one time more accurately.

Spastic patterning varies from moment to moment depending upon many factors. One factor is the general position of the patient. Another is the nature of the stimulus being applied to the patient and yet another is how much effort the patient is making to obtain a voluntary movement. Strong volition often simply facilitates the excitation of the spastic patterning. This is possibly because the threshold of the appropriate motoneurone pools is already low, due to reflex release, so that the slightest volitional effort triggers them into action.

If the damage to the central nervous system is lower in level so that only the spinal reflexes are released then the spastic patterning may well be more related to flexion withdrawal. According to the stimulus applied there may be flexion or extension patterning but flexion is more likely to be predominant. Withdrawal is a response to noxious stimuli, but in this type of case it can be the response to almost any stimulus: touching of bedclothes on the affected areas, vibration, noise, sudden movement. It is well to bear this in mind since such patients must be dealt with very carefully if flexion withdrawal is not to become a permanent position for the patient.

Spasticity is never isolated to one muscle group. It is always part of a total flexion or total extension synergy. Let us take a lower limb example. If the lower limb is in extensor spasticity it will tend to adopt hip extension, adduction and medial rotation, knee extension and foot plantar flexion. Thus if one detected spasticity in the adductor groups one should expect it in all the other groups in the pattern.

It should be noted that the limb is not put into a good weight-bearing position by this patterning. The heel is unable to touch the supporting surface and the adducted limb is unable to support the pelvis adequately. Thus the patient showing this patterning is not able to experience the appropriate stimuli which will give the slow-acting postural muscles the appropriate guidance to support the limb.

For sound supporting posture we require the normal afferent stimulus of compression upon the heel of the foot. In this way the appropriate malleable postural mechanisms giving balanced co-contraction of both flexors and extensors can be encouraged. If this occurs we do not show the hyperextended knee of the mildly spastic or the complete inability to get the heel on to the ground of the severely spastic case.

The spastic patient of this type may be deprived of experiencing the very afferent stimulation which could make his postural tone more normal. This occurs in many ways to the patient with this abnormal patterning and is an important factor in his treatment. The physiotherapist must help the patient to experience afferent stimulation which he is, by his condition, denied.

Reflex release mechanisms are more often than not incomplete. It is because this is so that many patients have interesting variations in patterning and also have some voluntary control. Obviously, the more control the patient has, the less severe is the residual problem. However, some patients require time to make use of such control as may be available and meanwhile bad habits, if unchecked, could mar the patient's eventual result.

RIGIDITY

In this type of hypertonicity the fusimotor system is also excessively active giving an increase in sensitivity to the stretch receptors in muscle. The disturbance is thought to lie at a different level from that causing spasticity since there is a considerable difference in the type of change in response to stretch.

It will be remembered that the subcortical nuclei comprising the basal ganglia are thought to help in the production of postural fixation by exerting their influence upon the stretch reflex mechanism via the reticular formation. They help to maintain adequate postural fixation while allowing the necessary malleability for voluntary movement. If, however, they become too effective as factors in postural fixation the stretch reflex mechanism may lose its malleability due to excessive fusimotor action. Damage in the area of link between the cortex and basal ganglia may well lead to excessive postural fixation to the detriment of volitional activity. The rigidity which ensues is different from spasticity in that it does not adopt the patterns of any particular reflex mechanism because the reflexes of tonic posture are not released. The pathways in the brainstem may still be intact and consequently some control of the stretch reflex mechanism may be available. The 'clasp-knife' effect seen in spasticity is not available in rigidity because phasic stretch does not appear to be suddenly inhibited. This may be because the control centres in the brainstem exert a suppressor action upon the inhibitory mechanisms.

In rigidity the muscles respond to slow stretch by steady resistance which does not particularly build up or relax off. There is a tremor which is said to give a 'cog-wheel' effect, or the limbs may feel like lead when moved, giving rise to the term 'lead pipe' rigidity. Explanations of this phenomenon are not complete and it must be remembered that, at present, there are many questions which remain unanswered.

Patients showing rigidity usually have lesions in the subcortical areas and show a typical posture which becomes progressively more flexed. They do not rotate in any of their movements and lack of axial rotation seriously interferes with their balance reactions.

The 'rigidity' patient shows movement problems in which auto-matic adjustment and activities do not occur freely and therefore voluntary movement is slow and impoverished because it is unaccom-panied by automatic balance reactions and because it occurs so slowly against the ever-resisting stretch mechanisms.

In spasticity movement impoverishment also occurs. Balance reac-tions cannot be produced against the spastic patterns and mature permutations of flexion versus extension patterns are not available, only the stereotyped reflex patterns being produced in voluntary movement.

Athetosis

When this occurs the patient shows disorder of movement because of fluctuation in the level of postural fixation. The patient adopts a succession of abnormal postures which may be quite grotesque. The condition is made more severe by excitement and emotional stress. It is thought to be due to lesions within the basal ganglia and in particu-lar in the putamen. In this instance the basal ganglia are failing in their ability to encourage adequate postural fixation and fluctuations there-fore occur.

Involuntary movements occasionally occur but the symptoms are always made worse by voluntary activity.

Choreiform Activity

This is a series of involuntary movements, which occur in the face and limbs. They are quicker than those of athetosis and are also made worse by voluntary movement. Many patients show a combination of choreiform and athetoid activities. The basal ganglia are considered to be at fault in choreiform problems.

Ballismus

This is a term used to describe wild flinging movements which may occur to such an extent that they throw the patient off balance. The condition usually occurs as a result of a lesion in the subthalamic region and only affects one side. In this case it is called hemiballismus.

Dystonia

This is a term used to describe an increase in muscle tone that is antagonistic to the intended movement. The symptoms tend to prevent movement and may pull the individual into grotesque postures. It may affect one part of the body or the body as a whole. Spasmodic torticollis is thought to be a type of local dystonia. The lesion is thought to lie in the putamen.

TENDENCY TO DEVELOP DEFORMITIES

Whenever there is a tendency to adopt habitual postures of one part of the body or many parts there is a danger of adaptive shortening of some soft tissues and lengthening of others. In this way joints may become stiff and give deformities which are very difficult to correct. The least vulnerable patients are the athetoids and choreiform types since these patients are rarely still, but the spastic, rigid and flaccid types of patient may develop severe deformities if left untreated.

VULNERABILITY TO INJURY

Sensory loss leads to obvious dangers. Pain produced by damage is a protection against continuation of the damage. If pain is not felt then damage can occur with no protective reaction. Many cases of skin lesion and ulceration are due to this problem.

Many of these patients have sphincter problems and are incontinent. This renders the skin soggy and even more vulnerable. Pressure sores are a common complication. If pain is felt and the patient is unable to move away from its cause damage will also occur.

Muscle flaccidity, dyssynergia, and spasticity may all lead to ill-controlled joint positioning so that joints are put to undue strain and ligaments permanently stretched. The hyperextended knees of extensor spasticity are an example of this. The joint distortion may in some cases be great enough to cause subluxation.

Malposturing may also lead to undue pressure on nerves and blood vessels. This may give rise to secondary neuropathy, defects of venous return and oedema.

CIRCULATORY PROBLEMS

These exist in various forms in most neurological disorders.

When muscle paralysis is present the muscle pump action is defective and venous return is reduced. This may not have a noticeable effect if only small groups are affected, but if large areas of muscle are paralysed the effect may be great enough to cause oedema and may have the effect of reducing the rate of growth in the child. A peripheral problem of this type also gives rise to autonomic defects involving the control of blood vessels and sweat glands. Skin changes corresponding to this occur. Atrophy of the skin may develop causing it to become dry, scaly, thin and more vulnerable.

Disorders of the spinal cord will interfere with the autonomic control of the blood vessels and may have a general effect on the patient's ability to give correct blood pressure adjustments. The higher the level of cord injury the more severe the effect. This is seen most dramatically in paraplegic and tetraplegic cases.

Hypotonia will also give rise to defects of muscle pump activity although the effect may not at first be noticeable because it is more general and there is no 'normal' for comparison.

RESPIRATORY PROBLEMS

The patient may show paralysis in the respiratory muscles and will then obviously have respiratory difficulties. Those who have paralysis or severe hypotonia in the throat musculature will also have difficulty, since the inspiratory movements tend to suck the walls of the pharynx inward unless muscle tone braces against this effect. Thus the patient may choke for this reason or because the throat muscles are incoordinate in swallowing so that inhalation of food occurs.

Respiratory movements may be so impaired as to make speech

difficult and coughing impossible. Communication is therefore a problem and lung secretions gather.

The patient showing rigidity may have impaired respiratory function due to the difficulty in obtaining thoracic mobility.

SPEECH DISORDERS

These may be the direct result of respiratory problems, due to paralysis of speech muscles, or due to more complex problems of dyssynergia, spasticity and speech perceptual problems. A patient is said to be *dysphasic* when he has incoordination of speech and is unable to arrange his words in correct order. He is said to be *aphasic* when he is unable to express himself in writing, speech or by signs and is unable to comprehend written or spoken language. There are many different forms of aphasia and each one is very distressing to the patient.

DISTURBANCE OF EXERCISE TOLERANCE

This is inevitable. Only the most minor neurological changes would leave this undisturbed. The dysfunction of normal movement necessitates uneconomical substitute movements which undermine exercise tolerance. If this is not apparent because the patient is relatively immobile due to his disorder, his exercise tolerance will be reduced because of lack of exercise. The chair-bound patient who is wheeled about by relatives, quickly loses such exercise tolerance as he had because his circulatory and respiratory mechanisms are not put to any stress. Added to this he may be inclined to overeat and will put on unnecessary fat which will further reduce his condition of tolerance.

Any patient whose respiratory capacity is reduced must have diminished exercise tolerance.

Since there are many reasons for this problem they should be noted by the physiotherapist who may be able to minimise them in some cases.

PAIN

This is a factor in neurological cases but is not so prevalent as might at first seem likely. Pain can only be felt if there are pathways to convey the sensation.

Pain is most likely to occur in irritative lesions when the threshold of pain reception is low. Thus pain is a feature of neuritis. Other reasons are those connected with raised intracranial pressure giving rise to headache and throbbing sensations.

Some patients with lesions in the thalamic region show intractable thalamic pain which is difficult to understand until it is appreciated as a centrally placed lesion and is not due to damage in the peripheral area from which the pain is interpreted as coming.

Discomfort and pain from habitual bad posturing also occur and patients who have sudden waves of increase in muscle tone will complain of pain.

Referred Pain

This is a term used to denote pain interpreted as arising from an area which is not, in fact, the site of the trouble. For example pressure on the roots of origin of cervical 5 and 6 spinal nerves can give pain which is referred to their dermatomes, myotomes and sclerotomes. The patient will complain of pain over the deltoid area, lateral aspect of forearm and over the radial side of the hand. He may complain of deep pain over the scapula, lateral aspect of humerus, radius and over the bones of the thumb. The site of this problem is, in this case, in the cervical region but the patient suspects disease or injury where he feels the pain. This type of referred pain is often called root pain.

Referred pain does not always relate to surface structures but may also relate to viscera. For example, in cardiac disease pain may be referred to the left shoulder.

It is well known that pain in the otherwise normal individual will give rise to protective muscle spasm and abnormalities of movement and posture. It must, therefore, be appreciated that pain will do the same to the neurological case provided the nervous pathways are available to react. Thus the abnormality induced by pain will be superimposed upon those already existing.

Causalgia

This is a term used to describe a severe sensation of burning pain which accompanies some peripheral problems. The patient shows hyperaesthesia or increased sensitivity, trophic changes and over-activity of the autonomic supply of the area.

The pain is aggravated by exposure and heat or cold and also by emotional crises. Because of the hyperaesthesia the patient protects the affected area to an extreme degree and does not move it at all. Even cutting the fingernails, if the hand is affected, may prove too painful and gloves, shoes and stockings and other items of clothing may be intolerable.

The skin shows atrophy and scales, and vascular changes occur ranging from vasoconstriction to vasodilation. The skin appearance will relate to the condition of the vessels. If vasoconstriction is present the skin is mottled and cyanotic and usually moist due to activity of the sweat glands. If the vessels are dilated the skin will be pink, warm, dry and later may become very glossy.

Muscle atrophy and joint stiffness are frequent in these cases and osteoporosis may be evident.

The exact cause of this condition is not fully understood. It is known to occur when the peripheral injury is incomplete and may be due to deflection of nerve impulses from efferent nerves to afferents so that more impulses are reaching the posterior nerve roots. This could happen in a nerve crush situation where the traumatised area may form a kind of pseudo-synapse between various nerve fibres. It is generally thought that the autonomic disturbances are secondary to the hyperaesthesia.

LOSS OF CONSCIOUSNESS

We are said to be unconscious when we are unaware of sensations such as seeing, hearing, feeling, tasting, smelling, etc. The reticular arousal system in the mid-brain and subthalamic region awakens the cerebral cortex to the reception of sensations. If this formation is damaged or if the cortex is diffusely damaged we may lose consciousness.

Sudden changes in movement may cause temporary loss of consciousness by causing torsional strain on the mid-brain. Space-occupying lesions like tumours and haemorrhages may press upon the mid-brain either directly or indirectly.

The reticular arousal system is very sensitive to deficiencies of oxygen and also of glucose and these may therefore bring about unconsciousness.

It is most important to realise that there are various levels of unconsciousness and that many patients who are apparently totally unconscious are, to some extent, aware of their external environment. They do not appear to be aware of it because they cannot react, but they may have a level of consciousness which makes them semi-receptive.

Careless management of such a patient could be detrimental to his recovery. He may hear discouraging information about himself or be treated in a way which he may resent. He should always be talked to when he is being handled and in an adult manner so that he may as far as possible understand what is happening around him. The physiotherapist should never talk about the patient in front of him.

EPILEPSY

This is a recurring disturbance of cerebral activity in which there is a sudden flood of discharge of impulses from neurones which have, for some reason, become uninhibited. If the area affected is near the reticular arousal area consciousness may be lost. Exact events depend upon the area affected.

Seizures may be major or minor in nature and may complicate many neurological problems, particularly those related to head injuries and tumours.

LOSS OF NORMAL FUNCTIONAL INDEPENDENCE

This is likely in most neurological problems except in the most minor. In slowly progressive disorders loss of function appears late since, subconsciously, the patient substitutes for each disability as it appears. In sudden disorders functional loss is dramatic, since the patient has suffered sudden physiological trauma which requires time for adjustment in addition to the psychological trauma associated with sudden disability.

Many patients show rejection of the area most severely affected or at least disassociation from it and they manage as best they can with what is left. Sometimes this is a necessity but there are occasions when such a drastic adjustment is detrimental to the ultimate result and should therefore be discouraged.

Simple functions may be lost because of lack of balance reaction or postural fixation.

The patient may not be able to move around in bed, transfer himself from bed to chair, dress, wash or feed himself.

If functional independence is permanently lost a great burden is placed upon the relatives and on the community as a whole. The patient may live an excessively confined life and have, therefore, limited horizons. This must be avoided and dealing with this aspect plays a large part in the patient's treatment programme.

Urine Retention and Incontinence

These distressing problems may complicate some of the more severely affected patients.

Sphincters may remain closed leading to retention of urine, which eventually leaks out due to overfilling of the bladder. Such a condition often gives the appropriate stimulus for flexion withdrawal and may increase flexor spasticity.

The recumbent position added to urine retention may lead to back pressure into the kidneys with further complications. It is always wise to allow such patients to adopt a vertical position periodically to relieve this effect.

Incontinence of urine may lead to skin breakdown since, inevitably, the skin will become soggy and more vulnerable.

Some patients may develop 'automatic' bladder-emptying mechanisms but others may have to have some permanent help in the management of the problem.

There may also be problems related to defaecation although these can often be managed by careful control of the intake of food and fluids in addition to developing a routine of timing of likely bowel activity.

Chapter 5

Assessing the Patient

by H. W. ATKINSON, M.C.S.P., H.T., DIP.T.P.

This is a most important aspect of the management of the neurological patient since the ultimate goal and treatment programme to obtain it depend upon the findings.

It is worth spending two or three treatment sessions in obtaining an assessment, particularly if the patient has widespread problems. Indeed most workers find that they are learning new facts about their patients all the time and adjust their approach accordingly.

It is necessary to have a period of initial assessment with all patients and to have intermediary assessments at intervals of a suitable length throughout the whole period of time during which the patient is receiving help.

A final assessment should be made at the time he ceases to receive any further help so that should he later be thought to have deteriorated since discharge, there is some record of his condition at that particular time.

Emphasis will be placed, in this chapter, on the assessments most suitably made by the physiotherapist. At the end of the chapter some of the more common medical and surgical investigations are indicated.

Prior to assessing the patient the physiotherapist should have studied the medical history and any pertinent aspects of the medical examination which will already have occurred.

The physiotherapist's assessment should include some or all of the following points depending upon the nature and extent of the condition of the patient.

A GENERAL IMPRESSION OF THE PATIENT'S CONDITION

It should be noted whether the patient is ambulant, chair-bound or confined to bed and whether he requires any assistance if he is ambulant or chair-bound. His general appearance should be observed for build, muscle atrophy, skin colouration, signs of obvious ill-health or malnutrition and the overall condition of his hair, skin and nails. If he has any pressure sores or is likely to develop them his skin should be carefully examined and areas of breakdown noted.

At this stage it is also important to note the general impression of the patient's mental attitude to his problem and also whether he appears to be a social individual or more introverted in nature.

INTERROGATION OF THE PATIENT

This is an important part of the examination as the experienced person can learn a great deal from the patient at this time. He should be questioned about his own particular difficulties which are the result of his illness. It is very important to find out from the patient what he finds to be the most serious drawback since his views may be quite different from that of those who are examining him.

If the patient has noticed some difficulty in fulfilling a function it is most important to examine this carefully and to try to find some way of alleviating the problem in the treatment programme. In this way the patient's cooperation is much more readily gained for this and many other aspects of his management.

The patient's hopes and fears must be noted and some idea of what he himself wants to be able to do must be obtained.

The physiotherapist should find out details of the patient's occupation and get some idea of what it involves in the way of physical and mental activity. In some cases it may be possible to enable the patient to resume his normal work but in many instances this is not possible. It is important to avoid holding out false hopes to a patient.

There will be some information concerning the patient's family and responsibilities in the medical notes but, if this has been omitted, it may be wise to find out as much as possible and to note the patient's attitude to those members of his family he mentions. Family relationships can have an important bearing on the desire to recover some functional ability.

The patient should be asked about pain and discomfort and he should also be asked about its quality and when and where it is felt.

The patient must be given time to tell his problems since, if he is rushed, he may omit some very important fact.

While carrying out this interrogation the physiotherapist can note many other aspects of the problem without the patient being conscious of her doing so. She can notice any problems of speech or hearing and whether the patient is able to interpret her words easily and reply quickly, or slowly and with difficulty. She can note his respiratory control, expression changes on his face, whether he can control the saliva in his mouth and whether he is able to swallow easily.

The physiotherapist should also notice whether the patient can make automatic position adjustments while conversing.

It is not always possible to hold a two-way conversation with some patients since speech or hearing may be difficult. It may be necessary to arrange a signal system and question the patient on a yes/no basis. In some cases the written word may be of help.

If the patient is unconscious or too young to participate relatives may be needed to help to answer some of the queries.

Assessment of Hearing

This is not really the province of the physiotherapist but it is important for her to know whether the patient can hear ordinary speech or whether this is difficult. She also needs to know whether he can hear himself moving against the bedclothes or chair or his feet on the floor, since the ability to do so makes a difference to his ability to move in a coordinate manner and with assurance.

Assessment of Eyes and Vision

Although this is the province of the highly qualified specialist, it is helpful for the physiotherapist to know whether the field of vision is limited or full, whether the pupils are able to react to light and whether there arc incoordinate movements of the eyes such as nystagmus.

It is also important to know whether the patient has normal vision or requires the help of glasses to enable him to see near or distant objects. If the eyes are to be used to help in the production of movement it is important to know how much they can be expected to help. The medical notes may give most of the information that is required and should be studied carefully.

Visual fields can be roughly tested by holding two different coloured pencils some distance apart and asking the patient how many he can see. If he only claims to see one then the one he can see can be identified by colour (provided he is not blind to colour). This gives some indication of the visual field. The pencils can be moved about to find the extent of defect of field and the search can be narrowed down to the field of one eye by masking the other.

There is also the possibility of double vision and this can be assessed by holding up one object and asking how many the patient can see. If the patient has difficulty of convergence of the eyes he is likely to show double vision which can be distressing and make him insecure. Covering one eye will prevent double vision from being too troublesome and can be used to help patients who have no hope of correcting the problem in any other way.

ASSESSMENT OF OTHER SENSORY INFORMATION

Skin Sensation

It should be noted whether the patient can distinguish between different types of sensation such as blunt and sharp, hard and soft, hot and cold etc.

It is possible to map out areas of defect on line diagrams of either the whole patient or the part requiring attention.

Two-point discrimination can be assessed for some patients but it must be remembered that this is variable in accordance with the area being examined. In the normal person two-point discrimination is better on the palmar aspect of the hand that it is on the dorsum. Thus one must expect discrepancies even in the normal individual. By two-point discrimination is meant the ability to distinguish two distinct areas being stimulated at any one time and noting how close the stimuli can be to each other before they are interpreted as one.

Vibration

This can be applied by a vibrator or by a tuning fork and is detected as a sensation by receptors in skin and bone. Because vibration has been found to have an important influence on muscle activity this is an interesting test to try. After the vibration stimulus has been given muscles working over the vibrated area may be seen to contract although they have not been stretched or stimulated in any other way. It is thought that the vibration is transmitted to the muscle spindles via the bone and gives a rapidly repetitive mild stretch stimulus. This may, incidentally, be one reason for the need for compression force of weight-bearing (giving a vibration) if one wishes to encourage co-contraction of muscles over a joint.

Joint Position

This should be checked carefully and it may be done in various ways:

1. The patient may have the movements of a joint named for him – e.g. 'this is called bending the elbow and this is stretching'. Then he may be put through a passive range of movement while his eyes are closed and asked to state whether bending or stretching is occurring. When moving the joint passively the physiotherapist must not indicate change of direction by moving her hands as the patient could otherwise detect discrepancies in direction because of this and give a false impression of his ability.

2. If the patient is sufficiently coordinate he could be asked to keep his eyes closed and to move a free limb into the same relative position as a limb being moved by the physiotherapist.

3. His limbs and trunk could be positioned by the physiotherapist and the patient could be asked to draw a pin man diagram of his position or to put a 'bendy toy' into a similar position. A 'bendy toy' is a toy doll made of sorbo rubber round a malleable wire frame which can be bent to any shape. These last methods do more than test joint sensation – they test body image interpretation and are suitable for only certain disabilities.

Stereognosis

This is the ability to recognise objects by feel and manipulation. It requires the ability to feel with the hands and to assess size and shape by the position of the joints. It also involves the ability to move the hands over and around the object.

It can be checked by putting objects into a patient's hand or hands while he is blindfolded and asking him to state what they are. Everyday articles should be chosen such as money, buttons, pens etc.

Another method would be to put a number of simple articles into an opaque bag and ask the patient to bring out only the pen or coin or button etc.

Closely allied to stereognosis is the ability to recognise texture of material and weight of identical-looking objects. Thus the patient may be asked to identify different materials such as wool, silk, paper, wood etc. The patient may do so by moving his hands over the material or having the material placed into or moved over his hands or other part of the body. Identical looking objects but with different weights may be arranged in order of heaviness. This requires touch, pressure and joint sensation as well as some interpretation of the muscle activity needed to support the weight.

Areas of lost sensation should be recorded and also any areas of paraesthesia should be noted. Numbness and tingling give false sensation and dull sensory perception and so need to be taken notice of as they are indicative of disturbance occurring in sensory pathways (Fig. 5/1).

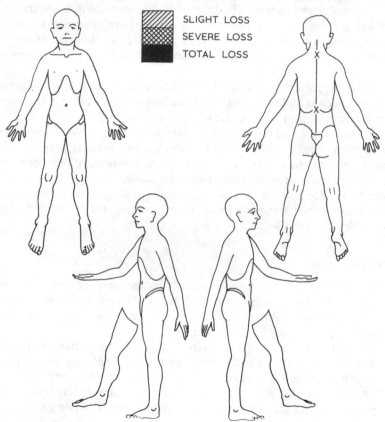

SLIGHT LOSS
SEVERE LOSS
TOTAL LOSS

Fig. 5/1 Chart for recording apparent information

JOINT MOBILITY AND SOFT TISSUE LENGTH

The available range of movement in the joints should be noted. In some cases the range should be accurately measured but in most cases of neurological disorder this is not really necessary.

Passive and active range should be assessed since many patients cannot move the joints because of muscle weakness, hypotonia or hypertonia. When assessing the passive movements available the physiotherapist should remember to check the biological length of two joint muscles as well as individual joint ranges.

If the patient is known to be spastic it should be remembered that certain positions of the head and neck could make movement of joints less available. For instance, supine lying could make hip and knee flexion very difficult for either the patient or the operator.

The physiotherapist should try to ascertain the reason for limitation of movement, note any fixed deformity and also any habitual posturing.

VARIATIONS IN MUSCLE ACTIVITY

Here the physiotherapist is looking for flaccidity, hypotonicity, hypertonicity and the fluctuations associated with athetosis and ballismus etc.

Some information will already have been gained if the other assessments mentioned above have been carried out. However, discrepancies in muscle activity can also be assessed in the following ways:

Passive Movements

Relaxed passive movements give the following information:

1. That the muscles are flail and are allowing movement to occur with no opposition and may even be allowing an excessive range of movement to occur. If many muscles are involved the limb may feel heavy as there is no support from normal muscle activity.

2. That the muscles are showing excessive opposition to stretch. If they are showing spasticity they may show the clasp-knife phenomenon and will certainly oppose movements away from the spastic patterns. If they are showing rigidity all movements will feel stiff and the cog-wheel phenomenon may be detected.

Passive movements should be performed both slowly and quickly to detect any difference in the response of muscles to slow and quick stretch.

If hypotonia is present the passive movements may feel similar to the effect given by flaccid muscle. However, quick passive movements to joints controlled by hypotonic muscles may initiate a stretch response which is not available in flaccid muscle.

Palpation

Handling of muscles in varying states of tone can give helpful information. The flaccid muscle usually feels non-resilient, soft and atrophied. The hypotonic muscle feels soft but not really non-resilient. It does not usually show much atrophy. The spastic muscle feels tight and hard particularly if it is put slightly on the stretch. Its tendon may be felt to stand out from underlying structures. Muscles showing rigidity feel solid and the limbs are rather leaden to move about.

Reflex Testing

This is a common method of assessing muscle tone and the condition of the various neurological pathways.

Superficial reflexes may be tested by scratching the skin over an area and watching for muscle contraction. If the skin of the abdomen is stroked the abdominal muscles contract. If no response occurs there is either an interruption of the lower reflex pathway or a state of central shock in which the motoneurone pools are not receptive to stimuli. The response may be exaggerated if flexor spasticity is present, sluggish if there is hypotonia, and difficult to see if there is rigidity because the muscles will not be adequately relaxed to start with.

Scratching the sole of the foot has a similar effect. There is a withdrawal from the stimulus involving dorsiflexion of the foot. In the normal situation the great toe of the mature individual will plantar flex while the rest of the foot dorsiflexes. However, if hypertonicity of a spastic nature is present there will be dorsiflexion of the whole foot accompanied by flexion of knee and hip. This is often called a Babinski sign. In hypotonicity the response will be sluggish and in the case of flaccid dorsiflexors there will be no response of these muscles but there may be flexion of knee and hip if these muscles are working and the limb is free to move. Again, as for the abdominal reflexes, if there is a state of spinal shock the reflex will be absent.

Tendon reflexes may be tested by tapping the tendon of a muscle. This does not stretch the tendon but, by putting a momentary kink into its shape and by vibrating it, the muscle fibres attached to the tendon are suddenly stretched. The normal response to this is for the muscle fibres to contract together giving a jerk of tone in the muscle. Hence we talk of the knee, ankle and elbow jerks. In these cases the patellar tendon, tendo Achilles and triceps tendons are struck once with a tendon hammer and the appropriate response is awaited. The lower limb, foot and forearm must be free to move if the full effect is to be observed. This method can be applied to any muscle tendon but these are the ones most commonly tested.

If there is no response there may be interruption of the motor pathway between the spinal cord and the muscle indicating a flaccid paralysis of the muscle. It is possible also that sensory interruption has occurred which may or may not mean flaccid paralysis depending upon whether the motor pathway is also involved.

No response will occur if there is a state of spinal shock which may occur temporarily in injuries to the brain or spinal cord.

If the response is exaggerated it means that an excessive contraction of muscle occurs, then some hypertonicity of a spastic nature should be suspected.

A pendular or oscillating response indicates hypotonicity and lack of postural fixation to steady the limb after the initial jerk. The limb swings back and forth several times before settling down.

If hypertonicity of a spastic nature is suspected the physiotherapist should look for dominant reflex patterning and could well make use of her knowledge of the tonic postural reflexes to assess the severity of the condition. By placing the patient in the various postures which will most readily elicit a static reflex response, she can assess the dominance of the reflexes by the spastic patterning which occurs or by the increase in tone she feels in the muscles. For example, if the patient is placed in supine lying and the tonic labyrinthine reflex is therefore allowed free rein, the patient showing spasticity will show an increase in extensor tone and flexion will be difficult. If the head is then flexed forwards there may be more extensor tone in the lower limbs but an increase in flexor tone in the upper limbs indicating a symmetrical tonic neck reflex patterning.

Head turning may give extension of the limbs on the side to which the face is turned and flexion of the others indicating the influence of the asymmetrical tonic neck reflex. It should be noted that full patterning into spastic patterns may not necessarily occur. There may be a simple, slight increase in tone into the patterns, or movement out of the patterning may just be made slightly more difficult in the milder cases.

Fluctuations of tone as seen in the athetoid, chorea and ballismus case can usually be readily seen as involuntary movements.

ASSESSING FOR QUALITY OF MOVEMENT

These assessments are most relevant to patients showing hypertonicity, ataxia and hypotonia, athetosis, chorea and ballismus.

Assessment is made of the patient's ability to give various permutations of movement, to balance adequately with suitable equilibrium reactions and to carry out smoothly coordinate movements with suitable postural background (Chart 1 pp.91–94).

Movement Permutations

By this is meant the ability to mix flexion and extension movement components so as to get a balance of activity. It will be remembered that the spastic pattern of extension of a lower limb is extension, adduction and medial rotation of the hip, extension of the knee and plantar flexion of the foot. The reversal of this is flexion, abduction and lateral rotation of the hip, flexion of the knee and dorsiflexion of the foot. Mature movements involve a mixture of these two limb synergies so that every time the hip extends it does not also have to adduct but can remain abducted etc.

A quick method of assessing the patient's overall ability is to encourage movements through some fundamental and derived positions which are all, in fact, mixtures of flexion and extension synergies.

The quality of the movements and positions is the point to be observed. The positions most related to neurodevelopmental sequence are probably most useful. Let us take as an example the use of the lying position.

(a) Prone lying. Is the patient able to take up elbow support prone lying? If not can he be put into the position and is he able to hold it when he is placed there?

(b) Is he able to remain in prone lying with his legs abducted and laterally rotated?

(c) Can he roll from prone lying to supine, leading with different parts of his body, e.g. head and neck, arms, or lower limbs – and does his body spiral as he turns or is it a solid mass going over as a whole?

(d) Is he able to lie in supine with his legs abducted and laterally rotated and also his arms in a similar position?

(e) Is he able to roll from supine to prone, leading with different parts of his body?

(f) Does he have balance reactions in side lying if gently pushed backwards and forwards?

These points can be charted.

It must be remembered that disturbance in movement permutation need not necessarily be the result of neurological problem but may be related to an orthopaedic or traumatic problem or even simply to pain.

Assessing Balance

Good balance requires a well-integrated nervous system with adequate afferent information, mobile joints and sound muscles. Faults in any of these factors will influence the patient's ability to balance.

The ability to balance needs to be assessed in various postures and during movements from one posture to another. The earliest balance activity involves balancing the head over the upper trunk in prone lying and supported sitting, whereas a very advanced balance activity could be walking, carrying a tray full of glasses while avoiding and talking to people who are passing by! Obviously circus artistes perform many more advanced balance activities but few of us aspire to their heights.

Thus it would take a complete volume to assess every posture and movement for balance. However, having selected a position for assessment suitable for the patient the following procedure may be adopted:

(a) How much help does he need to maintain the position?

(b) Test his conscious balance responses by applying pressure and telling him to 'hold' or saying 'don't let me move you'. Give pressure in various directions and note his stability.

(c) Try the same approach with his eyes closed. If he has been relying on eyesight he will be less stable or may fall when his eyes are closed.

(d) Let him have his eyes open and test his automatic reactions to balance disturbance. Ask him to let you move him and tilt him backwards, forwards, sideways and rotate him – all gently – so as to disturb the position of his centre of gravity. Notice whether he moves his head, trunk, upper limbs or lower limbs or all of them to maintain his equilibrium. Try disturbing his balance this way by moving him at the shoulders, or using his arms as handles or by using his legs. The reaction you will get will depend upon what is available to the patient and what part of him you have left free to react.

(e) Try the same reactions with his eyes closed. Be careful to prevent injury should his ability be poor in this situation. Record the reactions you obtain and relate them to those which should be obtainable. For example you do not expect stepping or hopping reactions if you have tested the patient in sitting.

(f) Now test his reactions when carrying out a movement of some part of the body. For example in sitting, movements of the arms require balance adjustment. Try this with the eyes open and then closed.

(g) Objective activity test. This requires the use of the position for a function such as dressing or any simple activity which takes the patient's mind off balancing and puts it on to the fulfilment of purposeful activity.

The various reactions obtained will depend upon the condition being examined. If there are many flaccid muscles exaggerated reactions will be seen in the normal parts of the body as compensation. If there is hypotonicity balance will be precarious, reactions slow to occur but exaggerated when they do occur and of rather a primitive nature (putting hand down onto a support and using a wide base).

If there is spasticity, disturbance in balance will give exaggerated reactions to any normal part and spastic patterning of the rest of the body.

If there is rigidity, balance reactions will probably be almost entirely absent except for forward stepping and protective extension. The reactions will occur very slowly.

It must be remembered that balance reactions may be altered by joint stiffness and account must be taken of this in any patients who are likely to have limitation of movement.

Assessing Coordination and Precision

Well coordinated purposeful movement requires 1) a variety of movement permutations, 2) good balance reactions, and 3) the ability to stabilise one part of the body while moving another part so that movement occurs smoothly. In assessing (1) and (2) a large part of (3) has already been examined. However, smoothness of movement needs to be checked, the ability to move the trunk on the limbs and the limbs on the trunk needs checking, and the ability to stop and start movement is very important.

This can be done by examining the patient's ability to move from prone lying to supine and from supine to prone in a slow smooth manner stopping and starting on the way. If suitable, he may be required to take up side sitting from prone lying and then proceed to all fours, kneeling, half kneeling and standing with stops and starts throughout. While doing this, precision and smoothness are being checked and any tremor, overshooting or lack of precision is noted. These are gross coordinate activities and provided the patient is capable of coping with the various positions and movements they make a good starting point.

It should be remembered that slow movements are very often more difficult for the incoordinate patient and so both fast and slow movements should be assessed.

More detailed checks can be made regarding the abilities of the patient by placing him in a very stable position and asking for free movements of the limbs of a precise nature. The finger to nose test is the classic method of testing coordination. In this the incoordinate patient either misses the nose altogether or has much tremor before landing and he strikes it rather heavily. This indicates lack of postural fixation of the proximal joints. The patient with sensory loss shows a worsening of symptoms if the eyes are closed.

If the patient succeeds in moving the limbs well when the trunk is in a stable position, it should then be placed in a less stable position so that mechanical proximal fixation is no longer helping the patient.

The movements should be checked for smoothness, ability to stop and start, ability to occur as a whole and not be broken up into joint by joint activities. Later they should be checked as purposeful actions in which the patient's mind is not on the movement but upon the purpose of moving.

Obviously such functions as walking must be involved if the patient is sufficiently able to do so.

Coordination between hand and eye can be checked by asking the patient to reach out and take objects of various sizes and shapes and to give them back to the physiotherapist. Objects such as balls can be rolled to the patient for him to take as they arrive, later they can be thrown to him and smaller balls can be used. Shapes and sizes and coordination can be tested by asking the patient to put objects of certain shapes through appropriate slots. This requires extremely good hand coordination, coordination between hand and eye and also sensory perception.

ASSESSING MUSCLE POWER

This assessment is most applicable to the lower motor neurone problem as seen in peripheral nerve lesions, peripheral neuritis or in anterior poliomyelitis.

The classic method of assessing muscle power is to relate the ability of the muscle to move the appropriate part of the body against the force of gravity. The Medical Research Council assessment gradings from 0–5 are assigned as follows:

0=No contraction felt or seen.
1=Flicker of activity either felt or seen.
2=The production of a movement with the effect of gravity eliminated.
3=The production of a movement against the force of gravity.

4=The production of a movement against the force of gravity and an additional force.

5=Normal power.

It is usual to start assessing for grade 3 and be prepared to move up or down the scale. Obviously the specific action of the muscle to be tested must be known since positioning the patient must be related to the effect of gravity on the movement to be produced.

It is important to note that a muscle can only give its best performance if its synergists are also participating. For example deltoid is an abductor of the arm and requires a stable shoulder girdle if it is to be successful in this action. It particularly requires the activity of serratus anterior and trapezius as fixators of the scapula to prevent the inferior angle of the scapula from swinging medially as the arm tries to move sideways. Unless these muscles work with deltoid it is unlikely to succeed in producing abduction.

If the physiotherapist is testing a weak deltoid it is important that she checks the abilities of the synergists and fixators to see that the weak muscle gets adequate chance to show its abilities.

If the scapula is not fixed by the patient's own muscles then steps must be taken to fix it manually or mechanically before assessing the power of deltoid. This is, of course, true of all muscles – deltoid has only been taken as one example.

There is not usually much difficulty in coming to conclusions about grades 2, 3 and 4 in this method of assessment. Grade 1 can be difficult and so can grade 5. Before deciding that no flicker is available and therefore scoring 'o' it is wise to try maximum facilitation and see if some activity can be encouraged. In that case grade 1 can be awarded provided it is made clear that it was only achieved with maximum facilitation. Grade 'o' should never be awarded until maximum facilitation has been tried and failed.

For grade 5 the muscle must be compared to the normal side if there is one. It must be remembered that different activities use different levers and that movements against gravity can be done as weight-bearing and non-weight-bearing activities. Thus, for instance, the hip abductors cannot be graded as 5 unless they can function correctly to prevent a dropping of the pelvis towards the non-weight-bearing side (Trendelenburg's sign) while receiving weight in walking, running and jumping (if these last two are applicable to the age of the patient being examined).

These readings can be charted.

Other methods of assessing power include the use of a grip dynometer in which the patient is asked to grip a rubber bulb which is filled with air. The pressure exerted gives a pressure reading which is shown on a scaled dial. This, of course, assesses the power of the finger flexors and the efficiency of their synergists.

Static muscle power can be assessed by using spring balances arranged in series to pulley circuits so that the pull exerted can be recorded.

Dead weights may also be used and increased until the maximum load moved by the patient is found and recorded.

ASSESSMENT OF SPEECH, TONGUE MOVEMENTS AND SWALLOWING

This is largely the province of the speech therapist but the physiotherapist may need to check some points for herself. The early interrogation will have given some indication of the patient's problems and speech patterns will have been noted.

The physiotherapist also needs to know whether the patient understands the spoken word even if he cannot reply. This can be assessed by asking the patient to make a signal if he understands what is being said. The signal requested must be one of which the patient is capable. It must be appreciated that many patients know what they want to say but can only say one phrase or word which may come out every time they try to speak. Thus they may say 'no' if this is their only word when they mean 'yes' or 'it doesn't hurt' or 'hello'! If this is the case yes/no signals need to be devised and questions worded so that yes or no is the only answer required.

Tongue movements are essential for speech, mastication and deglutition. The physiotherapist can assess the availability of tongue movements by using any of these functions but if they are absent she may need to use a spatula or ice cube to encourage tongue movements while urging the patient to cooperate. It must be remembered that the tongue musculature is attached to the hyoid bone and if the synergists which control the position of the hyoid bone are not working control of tongue movements will be difficult. The infra- and suprahyoid muscles are important and may be paralysed. Equally, a patient with poor head control may well have infra- and suprahyoid synergy difficulties.

The ability to swallow involves complicated synergy of tongue, infra- and suprahyoid muscles and pharyngeal activity coupled with the maintenance of the closed mandible and closed lips. The muscles need power and coordination to be able to achieve the function.

Swallowing is most easily carried out in an upright position and is much more difficult if the patient is either recumbent or if the neck is extended.

It is important to remember that repetitive swallowing is self-limiting so the patient should not be asked to repeat the activity very often in quick succession.

RESPIRATORY FUNCTION

This may seem remote from neurology but it must be remembered that respiratory capacity depends not only upon lung field and thoracic mobility but also upon the muscle power and coordination of the respiratory muscles which include those of expiration as well as inspiration. Measurements of vital capacity using a spirometer can be graphed and give some idea of the power of the muscles and mobility of the thorax. Consecutive measurements at intervals give an idea of progress or rate of deterioration. A measurement of forced expiratory volume is one method of assessing the power of the expiratory muscles. This group includes the abdominal muscles.

ASSESSMENT OF FUNCTIONAL ABILITY (see Chart 2, p.95)

This section has been deliberately held separate from the section on quality of movement since it is important that the two are in no way confused with each other.

When assessing function the physiotherapist is assessing the patient's ability to be independent and this need not, necessarily, be also an assessment of movement quality. In fact many patients with appalling quality of movement may be able to be relatively independent, provided normality of movement is not required.

Such functions as the ability to move about in bed, the ability to transfer from bed to chair, the ability to transfer from chair to toilet seat and to the bath are all included. Dressing, washing and other toilet activities should be assessed. The patient's ability to walk, climb stairs, manage in the home environment, cope with rough surfaces, cross roads, get on buses and even drive a car can be assessed.

If the patient is a wheelchair case then his ability to use his chair must be assessed. His ability to transfer from his wheelchair into a car and out again should be checked.

Functional assessments are best done in conjunction with an occupational therapist since this is also part of her work. In many cases a home visit may be required to relate function to home environment and in some cases a visit to places of employment may be needed. Achievement charts may also be used (p.170).

ELECTRICAL TESTS

Strength Duration Curves

These are done as part of the assessment of a patient suffering from a peripheral nerve lesion. Representative muscles of the affected group are stimulated by stimuli of different durations ranging from 300ms pulses down to 0.01ms. As is mentioned in Chapter 6, p.114, denervated muscle is only capable of responding to the longer duration stimuli because the shorter stimuli are too fast for muscle tissue unless very high intensities are used. The shorter stimuli are usually only transmitted via a nerve supply and thus only the innervated muscle can respond to such stimuli.

The term strength duration relates to the duration of the stimulus and the strength of the stimulus applied. More intensity is required for the shorter duration stimuli to produce a contraction even when there is a nerve supply. Thus a characteristic curve can be graphed relating stimulus duration and intensity applied to the contraction obtained (Fig. 5/2).

It is usual to attempt to obtain a minimal perceptible contraction using a long duration stimulus and then progressively shorten the stimulus duration. If the contraction disappears, the intensity is increased until a contraction of the same degree is obtained, a reading is then taken and recorded. This goes on until the shortest stimulus is reached. However, if the muscle is denervated the long duration stimuli only will be successful and no amount of increase in intensity for the shorter stimuli will produce a contraction. Thus the graph will not be complete for the denervated muscle.

A muscle containing some innervated and some denervated fibres will show a special type of curve with a 'kink' in it. It is a mixture of the short graph for the denervated fibres and the long graph for the innervated group (Fig. 5/2c).

Accurate strength duration curves are only obtainable after 21 days following injury. This is because denervation takes this time to be completed.

Rheobase is a term used to describe the lowest intensity which can produce a muscle contraction when a long duration stimulus is applied.
Chronaxie is a term used to denote the duration of stimulus which

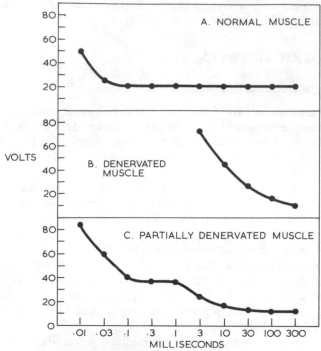

Fig. 5/2 Strength duration curves

requires an intensity equal to twice the rheobase level, before a contraction is obtained.

As a muscle becomes innervated the chronaxie should gradually be a shorter duration of stimulus and move to the left of the graph.

Nerve Conductivity

This is sometimes done to assess whether a nerve which has suffered compression is degenerating or not. The nerve is stimulated directly by a short duration stimulus along its course. When it is stimulated it conveys impulses to the muscles it supplies (provided it has fibres to carry them) and the muscles contract. If this is carried out at intervals from the time of injury the nerve will at first be hypersensitive and require a very low intensity. Later it may require more and, if it is degenerating, it will not conduct after about the fourteenth day. If, however, it does continue to conduct after 21 days the nerve has not degenerated and the injury is only a neurapraxia. In this case voluntary movement may be difficult or absent temporarily but recovery is likely eventually.

The above two tests can be carried out by the physiotherapist.

Electromyography

This is usually the province of the physical medicine consultant. It involves placing needle electrodes into the patient's muscles or using surface electrodes on the skin. These are attached to a highly sensitive piece of apparatus which amplifies and records electrical activities in muscle; these activities are recorded on a loudspeaker and as line graphs on an oscilloscope.

A muscle is electrically silent when there is no activity in the fibres. This occurs when it is fully relaxed. It creates sound and gives a graph when it is active. The sound and graph give a distinctive pattern.

If a muscle is fasciculating (which it does in certain muscular disorders and at certain stages of denervation), there is a different sound and visual pattern.

Such tests require great accuracy if they are to be valid since it is essential that the needle electrode is exactly in the muscle to be tested. Surface electrodes are not very accurate and there are many factors which can give artefacts in results. A shortwave machine working in the vicinity, for example, can cause interference if it is of unsuitable wavelength.

OTHER INVESTIGATIONS

Lumbar Puncture

This is a surgical procedure in which a sample of cerebrospinal fluid is extracted from the lumbar region below the termination of the spinal cord. If the needle is connected to a manometer it is possible for the cerebrospinal fluid pressure to be recorded. The sample of fluid can be examined for the presence of blood which could indicate a subarachnoid haemorrhage, for a high protein content, for high cell count, for a Wassermann reaction and sometimes for sugar and chlorides.

Other similar procedures are ventricular punctures and cisternal punctures.

Angiogram

In this procedure a radio-opaque dye is injected into the circulatory system so that the arteries show up on x-ray. The blood vessels can then be examined for defects such as aneurysms, the presence of constriction or blockage by thrombus formation. Displacement by tumours may also be seen.

Encephalogram

In this case electrical changes in the brain are detected by a sensitive piece of apparatus and graphed upon an oscilloscope screen. Surface electrodes on the scalp are used. Various wave patterns can be detected according to the activity going on at the time and related to abnormalities such as epilepsy.

Tests for Meningeal Irritation

NECK FLEXION TEST

If the patient is recumbent and the head is lifted so that the neck flexes, extensor spasm is produced which prevents flexion. Neck rigidity is said to prevent movement. This together with headache, photophobia and vomiting is indicative of meningeal irritation.

KERNIG'S SIGN

The hip is flexed slightly and any attempt then to straighten the knee causes pain and is restricted.

Both of these tests involve flexion of the spine and the rise in pressure in the vertebral canal is likely to be the chief factor in causing pain and muscle spasm.

SUMMARY

When the assessment has been made the patient's treatment programme can then be mapped out. It is helpful to have in mind:
1. An immediate aim
2. An ultimate aim.

In all cases the immediate aim will change as time progresses. As each aim is achieved a new one has to be made. It may also be necessary periodically to review the ultimate aim as the patient may progress further than originally expected. It is better to set one's sights low and progress, than to aim too high at first only to be disappointed.

If a patient is heavily handicapped it is wise to have a relative present at his final assessment before discharge so that the relative knows how much or how little help the patient needs. It is so easy for good work to be undone by over helpful relatives who undermine the patient's independence. At the same time it is important that the patient is able to obtain such help as he does need.

Chart 1. For use in assessing for quality of movement (see p.79)

PHYSIOTHERAPY DEPARTMENT

Quality of Movement

The chart is intended to record the *quality* of the movements performed. All variations from normal patterns should be observed and noted.

This chart is *not* intended to record functional ability since functions can often be achieved with grossly abnormal patterns.

NAME   REFERRED BY

ADDRESS   DATE

OCCUPATION   HOSPITAL NO.

Date of assessments

KEY

0 = Impossible
1 = Can be placed in position or moved passively
2 = Can assist when helped into position or through movement
3 = Cannot offer balance reactions
4 = Can produce the position or movement and react but abnormally
5 = Normal in all respects
A, B, C, D, E = Tick where appropriate

Test Applied	Score	A Tremor	B Weak-ness	C Stiff Joints	D Reflex Pattern	E Rigid-ity	Comments
Prone Lying Head turned, hands by side. Legs abducted and laterally rotated							
Obtaining elbow support. Prone lying							
Rolling Prone – Supine to right a) Head leading b) Upper limbs leading c) Lower limbs leading							

Test Applied	Score	A Tremor	B Weak- ness	C Stiff Joints	D Reflex Pattern	E Rigid- ity	Comments
Rolling Supine to Prone to right a) Head leading b) Upper limbs leading c) Lower limbs leading							
Rolling Prone – supine to left a) Head leading b) Upper limbs leading c) Lower limbs leading							
Rolling Supine to Prone to left a) Head leading b) Upper limbs leading c) Lower limbs leading							
Side lying Balance reactions a) Conscious volitional b) Automatic							
Supine lying move to right side sitting Supine lying move to left side sitting	Not always suitable for elderly						
Supine lying move to sitting over bed edge to right							
Supine lying move to sitting over bed edge to left							
High Sitting Balance a) Conscious volitional b) Automatic							
Right side sitting to prone kneeling Left side sitting to prone kneeling	Not always suitable for elderly						

Test Applied	Score	A Tremor	B Weak- ness	C Stiff Joints	D Reflex Pattern	E Rigid- ity	Comments
Balance in prone kneeling a) Conscious volitional b) Automatic							
Sitting move to hand support and forwards stoop standing							
Left side sitting to kneeling upright Right side sitting to kneeling upright	Not always suitable for elderly						
Balance in kneeling a) Conscious volitional b) Automatic							
Kneeling – change to right half kneeling							
Kneeling – change to left half kneeling							
Balance Right half kneel a) Conscious volitional b) Automatic							
Balance – Left half kneel a) Conscious volitional b) Automatic							
Right half kneeling move to hand support forwards stoop standing							
Left half kneeling move to hand support forwards stoop standing							
Upright Standing a) Stride b) Walk c) Oblique walk							

Test Applied	Score	A Tremor	B Weak-ness	C Stiff Joints	D Reflex Pattern	E Rigid-ity	Comments
Balance reactions in standing a) Conscious volitional b) Automatic							
Walking a) Forwards b) Sideways c) Backwards							
Right step Standing							
Left standing							
Stairs a) Up b) Down							

Chart 2. For use in assessment of functional ability (see p.86)

PHYSIOTHERAPY DEPARTMENT

Gross Functional Ability

NAME	REFERRED BY
ADDRESS	DATE
OCCUPATION	HOSPITAL NUMBER

KEY

0=Not possible
1=Possible with assistance but difficult
2=Possible with some assistance
3=Possible without assistance but difficult (stand-by needed)
4=Possible without assistance
5=Normal

Bed examination	Date						
Turn over: prone to supine supine to prone							
Move to side of bed							
Move up bed							
Move down bed							
Sit over bed edge							
Balance in sitting							
Transfer: bed to chair chair to bed							

Wheelchair examination	Date						
Apply brake Release brake							
Propel chair on level: forwards backwards turn							

Wheelchair examination	Date						
Negotiate doorway							
Slopes: up down							
Kerb: up down							
Transfer: chair to chair chair to toilet seat chair to floor floor to chair chair to bath or shower bath to chair							

Examination of gait	Date						
Balance in standing Stand up Sit down Get on to floor Get up from floor							
Walking – Crutches On level Slope up Slope down Rough ground							
Walking – Sticks On level Slope up Slope down Rough ground							
Walk – No sticks or crutches On level Slope up Slope down Rough ground							
Stairs 6 inches up 6 inches down 10 inches up 10 inches down							

Chapter 6

Principles of Treatment – 1

by H. W. ATKINSON, M.C.S.P., H.T., DIP.T.P.

Many factors influence the management of patients suffering from neurological disorders. There are many views on appropriate action and treatment, some of which are complementary while others may conflict to some extent.

The greatest conflict occurs when the need for urgent independent function is taken as top priority when perhaps a little delay in independence could lead to more adequate adjustment of the patient. There are arguments for both sides. It must be remembered that, while early functional independence may de-congest hospital wards and outpatient departments, this approach inevitably encourages the development of undesirable abnormalities of movement. These are substitutes for those normal activities which have now been temporarily or may be permanently made unavailable.

If a patient's potential is really quite good, given adequate time to redevelop along more normal lines, it may be quite seriously detrimental to him to allow substitute abnormalities to become a habit. Compromise is not always the answer since the result is often that of 'falling between two stools'.

Thus, the teamwork between consultants, nurses and therapists in addition to other workers is vital. There is nothing more detrimental to the patient than conflicting views between the team members dealing with his own particular case.

The physiotherapist's part in the management will be considered under similar headings to those used in Chapter 4 so that some correlation between the two chapters may be maintained. Aspects other than physiotherapeutic may be mentioned in passing but will not be discussed in detail.

DISTURBANCE OF AFFERENT INFORMATION

This can complicate the progress of the patient considerably and must always be taken into consideration.

Loss of Afferent Information

This may be local and specific if the problem is a peripheral one or it may be diffuse if the problem is more centrally placed. In either case there is much in common from the physiotherapist's point of view.

INJURY TO THE AFFECTED AREA

This is an important aspect in the management of such cases since cutaneous loss, in particular, is likely to make the patient vulnerable to cuts, burns from fire and steam, frictional abrasions from contact with harsh surfaces and pressure sores from prolonged contact with a supporting surface.

All patients with this problem should be made aware of this danger and it is the job of all concerned with the patient to ensure that he fully appreciates the dangers.

Obviously avoidance of injuries is to be encouraged and the patient should be told to use substitute measures to enable him to detect hazards. His hands are particularly vulnerable if they are involved since it is hard to avoid injury when the hands are so often used as tools. He must always use his eyes to detect hazards and beware of likely problems ahead of their occurrence so that complications do not arise.

Frictional abrasions and pressure sores can be avoided by adequate padding of areas likely to be subjected to friction and by care over the tying of such things as shoelaces if there is sensory disturbance in the skin of the lower leg and foot. The application of sheepskin cushions and mattresses for the more heavily disabled is valuable so that the patient is 'cushioned on air' trapped in the wool. Ripple beds and frequent turning are necessary for the severely handicapped patient.

To some extent the patient should be responsible for his own safety. He must be warned to inspect his skin for signs of injury and to take steps to relieve pressure whenever possible. For instance the patient who is confined to a wheelchair should endeavour to lift himself up in the chair by using his arms to relieve the weight and pressure on the buttocks frequently. He will most particularly need to be reminded to do this if he has lost sensation in the buttock region since he will not then receive the uncomfortable stimuli which would normally encourage him to change position.

LOSS OF BODY IMAGE AND REJECTION OF THE AFFECTED AREA

This can be quite a difficult problem and to achieve any measure of success it is important to remember that we develop a knowledge of body image by being able to move, touch and feel objects in close proximity to us and by being able to touch different parts of ourselves. It will be remembered that, as far as the hands are concerned, contact with the face, nose, mouth and hair is important. Thus we may be able to prevent loss of body image and rejection of parts of the body by using passive movements which are directed to simulating some of the more natural activities, e.g. taking the hands to the face and running the fingers through the hair, allowing the affected area to come into contact with more normal parts of the body and vice versa.

The patient may be positioned so that he can see the affected part and have his attention drawn to it frequently.

In some problems this aim of treatment is more important than in others. Permanent rejection is unlikely to occur in the localised peripheral problem but it is very common in the more centrally placed lesions.

If rejection and loss of body image have already occurred by the time the patient is receiving physiotherapy then the task is much more difficult to deal with. Sometimes exaggerated application of stimuli helps and heavy compression force repeated with the affected limb in a weight-bearing position may help. Constant handling of the area and helping the patient to simulate normal activities with the affected limb may be of value. Much patience and tolerance is needed in these cases.

The use of mirrors is sometimes of value and of particular importance is the need to encourage the patient who is showing signs of improving.

If the patient is accepting an abnormal position as being normal this must be pointed out to him and explained in such a way that he understands. He must then be allowed to experience the more normal position with the help of the physiotherapist who must, of course, ensure that he is safe and secure in his new normal position.

Mirrors again may be useful as an adjunct since the patient may need to use his eyes as substitutes for defective afferent information regarding general position. Even if the eyes are not needed for this purpose he may need convincing that the new posturing is more normal since it will 'feel' abnormal to him. Once the patient has appreciated the difference he must always be encouraged to adopt the more normal posturing in preference to the abnormal.

In cases of defects of sensory perception of this kind and in cases where loss of ability to move inevitably encourages the immediate adoption of abnormality, the patient must be treated as early as possible to avoid bad habits taking hold. For example, a patient who has had a cerebrovascular accident of such severity that he awakes as a hemiplegic, starts to develop abnormalities *as from that moment*. He substitutes and quickly accepts disability on that side of the body which for a time is virtually useless to him. Very soon it seems 'normal' to carry that half of the body as a passenger and to depend solely upon the non-affected side. This will be perpetuated unless some measures to prevent this occurrence are taken very quickly.

DISORIENTATION DUE TO FAULTY INFORMATION

This can occur if afferent information is not completely cut off so that faulty impressions are being received. For instance, some patients may have diminished touch and pressure sensation. If this occurs in the soles of the feet it gives rise to a 'cotton wool' sensation when the foot contacts a hard surface and very little sensation at all if a soft surface is contacted. This can make life very difficult for the patient. He may develop the type of gait which involves lifting the knee high and forcing the foot down hard on to the floor in order to obtain an exaggerated effect. This method of walking also makes a noise which tells the patient when he has landed. He may also have to look where he is walking all the time.

In this type of problem, substitution would have to be encouraged particularly if the disorder is permanent. Such a patient may have to be advised against wearing cushioned soles and heels since he cannot hear these land on the floor. He may have to wear studded shoes which make more noise than normal when he walks. He would have to be encouraged to use his eyes as substitute sensory organs.

As far as possible his high-stepping, exaggerated weight-bearing should be avoided since this could cause joint injury.

There are special methods of helping the movement problems of such cases. These will be considered under the heading relevant to movement abnormality.

Vertigo is another problem associated with faulty afferent information. As was stated in the previous chapter the patient may feel giddy and nauseated due to disorientation of the position of the head in space. The fault lies usually in the vestibular pathways or in the vestibular organs themselves. Any movement of the head or even of the eyes may make the patient feel symptoms. Impressions from the eyes and vestibular apparatus are so closely associated with each other that disturbance in one can give problems to the other.

The patient may have to be trained to rely upon the information he is receiving from his joints and skin and from his eyes since these are more reliable than the vestibular impressions. This takes time and while help from certain drugs is available to the patient, helping to reduce the feeling of nausea, he will still need help in movement activities.

Such patients frequently show a very fixed posture of the head and shoulder girdle because movement of the head is known to trigger off the symptoms.

The more unfortunate patient may well have vertigo in addition to faulty position sense. This makes life very difficult since substitution information is less available. Many patients with multiple sclerosis show these mixed problems and they may also have defective vision to complicate their problem even further.

The method of approach to the movement problem associated with vertigo will be considered under the appropriate heading (p.122).

DISORDERS OF MOVEMENT

The average person has very little appreciation of the complexity of performing an apparently simple function. All the necessary reactions are built in so smoothly that the timing and synchronisation of muscle and joint activity escapes notice. Throughout activity movement occurs against a background of malleable postural tone adjusted to maintain the equilibrium of the individual in all eventualities. In this way movement flows in a smooth, coordinate and purposeful manner.

Even less appreciated is the importance of afferent information. If there is no appreciation of the position in space the necessary steps to alter it cannot be taken. Moreover, if inadequate information is forthcoming during the performance of the movement it can be nothing but crude and wide of the mark since no corrective measures can be taken.

For normal function to occur the nervous system must be in sound order from the receiving, correlative and transmission aspects. There must be adequate mobility available in the joints of both the trunk and the limbs and the muscles must be healthy and able to respond to the activities of the nervous system. It is only under these circumstances that appropriate muscle synergy will be forthcoming giving the common movement patterns associated with normality.

The more common movement patterns incorporate a balanced mixture of the movements seen in the more primitive mass flexion and mass extension patterns. Primitive mass flexion and extension patterns may be seen in the young child but even these are more refined than those seen in the patient whose central nervous system is grossly disordered.

The tiny child does have some control over his reflex mechanisms which gives him the ability to modify these effects to some extent. Although the normal child does show a poor vocabulary of movement when compared with the normal adult, he does have the basic foundations upon which to build the permutations of movement with which we are familiar in the mature individual. Skilled activity is dependent upon mature movement permutations and therefore mature muscle synergy.

Since all human beings are built along essentially the same lines and all require to be able to achieve similar basic functions, certain movement permutations are common to all. During the development of these permutations the child repeats a movement until it can be achieved with ease, thus illustrating the phenomenon of physiological facilitation. Repetitive use of a neuromuscular pathway lowers the threshold of synapses involved and makes it easier for the pathway to be brought into use. Thus the pathway is said to be facilitated.

Since movement involves excitation of some muscle groups and inhibition of others, it is important to remember that we are facilitating both excitation and inhibition when we facilitate a neuromuscular pathway so that a movement occurs. The word 'facilitation' means 'to make easy' and it is in this context that the word will be used throughout this chapter.

The physiotherapist who undertakes the problem of movement re-education in a disabled person is accepting an enormous responsibility. Not only must she be able to detect and assess the degree of, and type of, abnormality presented, but she must have the necessary knowledge and skill to guide the patient towards normality while recognising the limitations set by the nature of the disorder.

THE PROBLEM OF FLACCIDITY

This may be seen when there is disorder in the peripheral system. On referring back to Chapter 4 it will be noted that such a state of affairs is usually the result of damage to the motoneurone pools of the anterior horns or to fibres passing peripherally from these motoneurones towards the muscles they supply. If all the motoneurones supplying any one muscle or group of muscles are completely destroyed then the muscles concerned will be completely paralysed, become flaccid and show atrophy in which muscle bulk is markedly reduced offering no protection to underlying structures.

If the damage is complete and irreversible, no amount of physiotherapy will restore muscle action. However, if only part of the motoneurone pool is affected, leaving intact those cells which have a higher threshold of stimulation, certain physiological factors may be applied to increase the excitatory effect on the motoneurone pools. In this way the remaining cells and their fibres may be made to convey impulses to the muscle, by the process known as recruitment. Similarly, if the cells or fibres of the motoneurone pools have suffered temporary damage they may eventually regain their ability to conduct impulses to the muscles. This may, at first, be difficult because they may have a raised threshold of activity.

These recovered neurones may also be encouraged to become active more readily by the physiotherapist exploiting her knowledge of physiology so that the use of these pathways is facilitated.

In this instance the physiotherapist has to make use of all the methods she can devise to have an excitatory effect upon the offending motoneurone pool or pools so that each effect can be added together or summated to reach the threshold of excitation.

Methods of Excitation Which are Suitable

THE USE OF NORMAL MOVEMENT PATTERNS

This involves the use of muscles which commonly work with the muscle which is flail. This is of value because the neuromuscular pathways commonly used are facilitated during the developmental process by repetition. Volitional impulses are conveyed to the motoneurone pools of the whole pattern. Neurones influencing one motoneurone pool in the pattern are thought to branch and also influence the other associated motoneurone pools. By this spreading of effect the motoneurone pool of the weakened muscle will receive maximum volitional stimulation.

USING THE EFFECT OF STRETCH STIMULATION

The stretch stimulus applied to the muscles involved in the whole pattern will, by branching of the afferent nerves, stimulate the motoneurone pools of each other as well as those of their own muscle. The excitatory state of the motoneurone pools including that of the weaker member of the team will be increased for a brief period of time. If to this effect, is added volitional effort (by summation) the excitatory influence may be enough to cause the lower motoneurones to conduct impulses to the muscles showing weakness.

RESISTANCE

This is, in effect, a kind of continuous stretch applied to a working muscle and thus is a facilitatory method. The degree of resistance applied should be as great as the muscle can overcome and *no greater*.

In some instances suitable resistance may be appreciably high whereas in other circumstances it may be as little as frictional opposition offered by the joint being moved. The term maximal resistance is often used and this must always be related to the available power in the muscle under treatment.

THE USE OF TRACTION FORCE

Traction is applicable if the movement pattern to be produced is that of flexion. It simulates the natural influences upon such movements which are basically a withdrawal from the pull of gravity. This effect summated to stretch, resistance and volition will further alter the excitatory influence upon the motoneurone pools.

THE USE OF APPROXIMATION (compression through the joints)

This is a postural stimulus associated with extension and is thus suitable in any situation in which a weight-bearing stimulus could be applied. The extension patterns are most suitably facilitated by the application of approximation. This stimulus, like traction, could be applied to summate with resistance, stretch and volition.

THE USE OF TOUCH

This should be applied over the working muscles and/or to the surface against which the movement is to occur. This supplies skin stimulation which acts as a guidance to the movement and facilitates activity in the motoneurone pools.

THE USE OF VISUAL AND AUDITORY STIMULATION

A well-voiced command facilitates volitional effort. The patient's eyesight is of particular value if sensory information is otherwise a problem.

The timing of the use of stretch, traction or compression and the use of auditory stimulation is of vital importance. These should all be applied together, simultaneously, if they are to offer maximum facilitation to the patient's volitional effort. Use is made of both spatial and temporal summation. Misuse of the timing of the application of various stimuli can lead to a reduction in effect.

THE USE OF COLD

Short duration applications of cold in the form of crushed ice over suitable dermatomes can be used to cause excitatory influences to occur at the appropriate motoneurone pools. A time-lag is usually necessary between the application of the stimulus and expecting a result so, consequently, this is a stimulus which can be applied prior to the other methods and it will then be able to add its effect by summation with the other stimuli.

THE USE OF BRUSHING

This can be applied to encourage excitation if it is carried out briskly over the appropriate dermatome. Usually there is a delay in response of up to 20 minutes, so this can be applied prior to the other stimuli.

THE USE OF RIGHTING AND EQUILIBRIUM REACTIONS

These can be applied if the patient is placed in such a position that balance is rather difficult. The postural and equilibrium mechanisms will influence the motoneurone pools of the muscles concerned in implementing the reaction and if these include the weakened group of muscles the influence applied may well have the necessary excitatory effect.

To use these reactions effectively the physiotherapist must have a knowledge of the most common reactions and which patterns of muscle activity they are likely to stimulate. It is possible to add to this effect by applying approximation through the appropriate limb or limbs and trunk and by commanding the patient to 'hold' while counter pressure is applied in different directions.

THE USE OF OTHER PARTS OF THE BODY AS A PRELIMINARY PROCEDURE

When other parts of the body are used, strongly associated reactions can be seen in those parts not being directly stimulated. This may occur because the nervous pathways controlling the movement influence the motoneurone pools of counterbalancing muscles or other associated groups. This is another form of spreading. Thus, if the affected muscle is in the right leg, it would be quite feasible to work the left leg or either of the upper limbs or even the head and neck or trunk first in order to have an irradiation effect upon the motoneurone pools of the affected limb.

THE USE OF REVERSAL PATTERNS

also include diagonal + rotational components along with flex + ext. + F.R.O.M

Sherrington found that the flexor withdrawal reflex was stronger if the extensor thrust reflex preceded it. The phenomenon became known as that of 'successive induction'. This phenomenon also seems to relate to volitional movement. If a movement is preceded by the exact opposite one the final pattern is produced more strongly. Thus it is physiologically sound to precede a flexion pattern by an extensor one in order to obtain a stronger flexion pattern. This method would be reversed if it was desired to use this phenomenon to facilitate extension.

Emphasising the Weaker Team Members

When using the above methods to facilitate activity in the weaker members of a muscle team it may be found that the weaker member does show activity. This should then be exploited. One method of doing this is to maintain activity in the muscles concerned in the rest of the pattern by making them hold the pattern strongly. The weaker member of the pattern should then be stimulated, by stretch and command, to participate concentrically, repeatedly through a suitable range. In other words, the total pattern is held in a suitable range and movement is only allowed to pivot about the joints controlled by the weaker member of the team. This approach is often called 'timing for emphasis'.

Let us take an example: the weakened muscle group is that supplied by the musculo-cutaneous nerve of the upper limb. Thus biceps brachii, brachialis and coracobrachialis muscles are involved. The most appropriate movement pattern for involving these muscles is called the flexion, adduction and lateral rotation pattern of the upper limb which would be combined with elbow flexion. In this pattern the wrist and finger flexors would be used and flexion would be accompanied by radial deviation. The forearm would supinate, the elbow flex and the shoulder flex, adduct and laterally rotate so that the hand would be carried towards the face and may progress obliquely across. The scapula would protract and laterally rotate carrying the upper limb into elevation across the front of the face.

Let us suppose that the efforts of biceps and brachialis as elbow flexors are to be emphasised. The patient is commanded into the pattern with the physiotherapist using the appropriate grasps, traction and stretch stimuli. The biceps and brachialis may be participating weakly and may need help to produce the elbow flexion. At the point in range where they offer the most activity the patient would be commanded to hold the pattern and pressure would be applied to make the shoulder, wrist and finger muscles hold a strong static contraction while stretch stimuli and command to bend the elbow would be repeated again and again to get maximum effort out of biceps and brachialis as elbow flexors. As appropriate, the range of the holding of the pattern may be changed until the two muscles are participating well throughout.

It may, of course, take many treatment sessions to achieve full range participation.

Such an approach may be applied to any muscle group involved in any pattern and may even be used to facilitate a weak pattern of one limb as a whole by making the other limb, limbs or trunk hold appropriate patterns while the weaker limb is encouraged to move through some range. This method of approach is exploiting the spreading effect of branching neurones which influence their own specific motoneurone pools and those of associated groups. Thus, volition directed to the weaker groups may be more effective since the excitatory threshold of these motoneurones has been, to some extent, prepared and lowered.

The above methods form an ideal way of: a) initiating activity in the weakened groups of muscles and b) of building on the activity obtained. This second point is very important.

When trying to initiate activity the physiotherapist must be prepared to go to a great deal of trouble to obtain the maximum facilitation and may have to try several methods before a result is achieved.

When activity is seen to occur the physiotherapist must exploit it to the full and try not to lose any ground she has gained. Thus repetition is vital. The more often the volitional impulses are able to cross the synapses and be transmitted the more readily can they effect a crossing. Thus, once activity is seen it must be repeated again and again until it becomes relatively easy to produce. Progress is then made by reducing facilitation and expecting an equally good action to be produced.

Once the weakened member has been made active, encouragement should be given to getting it involved in as many functions as are appropriate so that it is no longer allowed to become a passenger but has to participate.

These methods are particularly appropriate in the lower motoneurone problem because they make use of strong volitional effort in addition to other stimuli. Since there is nothing wrong with the 'computer' system but only with the external connections strong volition is unlikely to lead to undesirable associated movements. In fact, as has been said before, the associated movements may be highly desirable in this case and can be exploited to good effect.

When the weakened muscles are participating well in pattern with minimal facilitation, muscle strengthening techniques of a standard variety may be used quite effectively. Progressive gravity-free to weight-resistance exercises may be given either in patterns or in a more isolated manner to build up muscle power and endurance. Deep pool therapy may be of particular value. Movement patterns may be quite effectively produced in deep water and the efforts of the patient may be directed to moving the limbs about the stationary body or the body about the limbs.

Pool therapy is of particular value if the patient has large muscle groups involved, when the limbs and trunk may be particularly heavy and unwieldy in a dry land environment. If, however, the muscle weakness is associated with severe reduction in afferent information, as may be the case in polyneuritis, then deep pool therapy may not be so appropriate. Many patients of this type find the weightlessness and lack of sensory information which is associated with immersion in a deep pool, very frightening. They already have sensory loss and do not know their position in space when gravity is being fully effective. If they are then put into a pool where the effect of gravity is minimised then disorientation may be intensified to an alarming level. Each patient must be considered as an individual and assessed and treated to his best advantage.

In this section emphasis has been placed upon the exploitation of physiological factors while using movement patterns. The patterns which are most effective are those described by Dr Kabat, Margaret Knott and Dorothy Voss. They are of a diagonal nature and include rotational components which are of great importance (see Bibliography p.147).

The patterns used are described through full range and are most commonly used through full range during certain aspects of treatment. This gives maximum facilitation. Functional daily activities which include these movement patterns through a lesser range are also encouraged in the patient's treatment programme. Eventually, it is hoped that the patient will gain maximum participation of the affected muscles without having to have maximum facilitation on their motoneurone pools.

It is important to note that the use of movement patterns themselves only offers some help to the affected motoneurone pools. Much more is to be gained by exerting the additional physiological influences which can summate with the patient's volitional efforts to produce the movement pattern. In other words the patterns are there to be used, they are not sufficient in themselves.

The techniques described can be applied to straight movements, and even to individual muscle action if the physiotherapist so desires but they are not as effective used in this way because the patient is really using a pattern of muscle synergy which is new and alien to him, and pathways which have therefore not been physiologically facilitated during their early developmental processes.

Following this account it may be helpful to consider one lower motoneurone problem in a little more detail. Let us consider that the patient has had an axillary nerve lesion and that the deltoid muscle is at present not participating at all in any movements although the nerve injury has not been severe enough to disrupt completely the continuity of the nerve fibres. The problem is one of neurapraxia and the nerve fibres are showing a very high threshold of activity.

To deal with this satisfactorily the physiotherapist must have a knowledge of the functional significance of the muscle and how it participates in many simple daily living activities.

Deltoid must be recognised as having the following functions:

1. It is an abductor muscle of the upper limb.

2. Its anterior fibres flex and medially rotate the humerus.

3. Its posterior fibres extend and laterally rotate the humerus.

4. It commonly works with trapezius and serratus anterior to elevate the upper limb.

5. It becomes involved in any functional activities in which the arm is taken away from the side of the body.

6. It counters traction force applied by gravity to the upper limb by supporting the humerus up into the glenoid cavity. It is helped in this function by biceps brachii, triceps (long head), coracobrachialis and the smaller rotator cuff muscles in addition to the clavicular portion of pectoralis major.

7. It helps to stabilise the shoulder in weight-bearing activities and is particularly active if weight is being taken on one arm in the prone kneeling position when it acts as a supporter of the shoulder girdle in the same way as the hip abductors support the pelvic girdle when the opposite limb is taken off the ground. It may be seen working strongly in side sitting particularly if the body is being pushed away from the supporting arm. It moves the arm away from the body or the body away from the arm if the hand is fixed.

8. It becomes involved in balance reactions when the body is pushed sideways. One upper limb may move outwards to be placed upon a support at the side of the individual while the other may lift sideways in an effort to readjust the overall position of the centre of gravity. In both instances deltoid is involved.

9. It becomes involved in stabilisation of the non-weight-bearing arm when hand skills are being carried out. It may be felt and seen to be functioning in many fine skills of the hand as a stabiliser and/or adjuster of the gleno-humeral positioning.

10. It is involved in turning over movements, when moving up and down the bed and from side to side, walking with free swinging arms, carrying the shopping, doing the hair and putting on the hat.

In fact there are so many functions which involve this muscle that a book could be filled with an account of them.

The physiotherapist must have a knowledge of these functions and also a knowledge of the most appropriate movement patterns which may help to facilitate early activity. Probably the most appropriate patterns are the flexion, abduction and lateral rotation pattern and also the extension, abduction and medial rotation pattern.

Method of Approach

1. Make the patient aware of the reason for his movement difficulties. This can be done by comparing the activities of the affected limb with those of the normal side.

The patient may also be shown, by using mirrors, the lack of muscle bulk of deltoid and the trick movements which he is inclined to produce due to lack of participation of the muscle.

2. Make the patient as aware of the muscle as possible. This may be done by using simple methods such as handling the muscle and moving it over the underlying bone using a mixture of kneading and picking up massage manipulations while talking to the patient about the muscle. This, incidentally, distorts the muscle fibres and may be a start to offering sensory input which may help to bring about excitation of the motoneurone pools. Light clapping over the muscle may also help in awareness and will stimulate the sensory area in the immediate vicinity which may be of value. It is also possible to apply electrical stimulation which will have a similar effect. This will be considered in a later section of this chapter (p.114).

3. Start trying to initiate activity. This may be done in many ways and the physiotherapist should try many before giving up. Some suggestions are as follows:

(a) Use the normal limb and have the patient in a lying position. Give strongly resisted flexion, adduction, lateral rotation, reversing with extension, abduction and medial rotation patterns. While doing this watch for associated activity in the affected limb. It is likely to produce a reciprocal extension abduction pattern of the affected limb reversing with flexion adduction. There will not be much movement but a pattern of tone may be noticeable. If this appears to bring about extension abduction and medial rotation of the affected limb then give repeated contractions into the pattern on the normal limb which is getting the desired associated action. This may build up the associated activity. Then, without wasting any time, give flexion, adduction and lateral rotation as a resisted movement to the affected limb and follow this immediately with a reversal into extension, abduction and medial rotation. If a result is obtained give repeated contractions into this pattern.

(b) Another possibility would be as follows: Have the patient in high sitting leaning onto the hand of the affected side or in side sitting with the supporting hand being on the affected side. Stroke over the dermatome of C5 and 6 on the affected side with a piece of ice and then work the normal limb strongly by giving resisted flexion and abduction with repeated contractions into the pattern. The cold will take about thirty seconds to be of value so work the normal limb for about thirty seconds and watch the abnormal deltoid all the time. Action of its motoneurone pools is being facilitated because of the compression force through the shoulder which stimulates stabilising activity, and because of stimulus of the cold and the effect of spreading from the voluntary activity of the normal limb (Fig. 6/1).

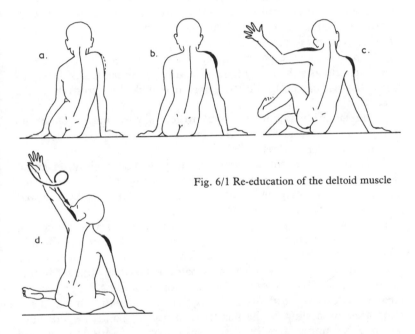

Fig. 6/1 Re-education of the deltoid muscle

If the muscle responds then make the patient hold the normal limb against opposition in flexion and abduction and apply compression force through the shoulder on the affected side. Sway the patient in many directions and ask him to 'hold' his position. This may further activate the muscle.

There are many other methods which may be used to initiate contraction in this muscle. These approaches are only offered to give a general concept.

4. Follow the contraction which has been initiated into a functional

activity. For example in approach (b) the deltoid was used as a stabiliser of the shoulder while weight was put through the upper limb. If the muscle has become active in this way it may be worth using lateral displacement of body weight to get a balance reaction and stabilisation activity.

Have the patient in high or side sitting. Gently pull the bodyweight laterally using the affected limb and place it in a supporting position. Repeat this sideways sway several times and allow the limb to receive a little compression force from the bodyweight each time the limb is in a weight-bearing position.

Gradually take the help of the physiotherapist away and displace the body laterally without helping the arm, watching for deltoid activity. As the body sways laterally gravity will help the arm to move sideways but deltoid is needed to prevent over-shooting when the weight of the body arrives onto the upper limb.

The patient can then be encouraged to push himself back to neutral using the arm as a thrusting tool. If he uses too much trunk substitution resistance can be applied to the trunk to make help from the arm a necessity.

At this stage it may not be possible to get full participation of deltoid in these activities, but it should be encouraged to participate as much and as often as possible.

5. Later progress could involve a short period of maximum facilitation as a 'warm-up' method followed by some further functional activities to encourage easy natural usage. This could then be followed by more specific strengthening techniques.

From the moment the patient starts treatment simple functional habits should be corrected and, as appropriate, functional use should be encouraged. For example, the patient with severe weakness in the deltoid muscle may also have had a painful shoulder injury. He will almost certainly have adopted the bad habit of holding his upper arm strongly adducted into his side even if, additionally, it has been supported by a sling. If he has tried to use his hand, he will have steadied his upper arm by, even more firmly, adducting his arm against his body. This habit is very undesirable since it will not only lead to a stiff shoulder joint but will also actively **inhibit** the deltoid muscle and so undermine any progress the therapist may hope to achieve. Thus the habit of 'clamping' the arm to the side must be stopped forthwith and, instead, relaxation, either into the sling or just into a normal postural pattern, should be insisted upon and, indeed, should take priority over every other treatment measure. Unless this re-education of body image and postural pattern occurs quickly the use of any recovery may be seriously delayed.

Similar problems occur when any other muscle group becomes severely weakened and the physiotherapist must become familiar with the most likely pattern abnormalities which are inclined to be associated with weakness of any of the major muscle groups. A sound knowledge of functional anatomy is essential and the therapist must expect to go on developing this knowledge for the whole of her working life.

In the case of the weakened deltoid, early functional activities can be encouraged as soon as a flicker of contraction is available and the patient has learnt to relax the adductors. Relaxed arm swinging, when walking, is one of the easiest early activities and this should become established as a habit as soon as possible. Simple stabilisation of the shoulder *without adduction* during the performance of hand skills should be encouraged next. An example of a suitable situation for the involvement of the muscle in such activity occurs when the subject leans forward to tie up a shoelace while the foot is on the floor or supported on a stool in front of him. In this example the effect of the force of gravity is minimal and deltoid needs only to contract very gently to carry out its stabilisation function successfully.

Balance activities involving the upper limbs may later be added and active participation in rolling activities and weight-bearing on elbows and hands can be expected as the muscle becomes more active. The therapist must make a real effort to help the patient involve the muscle in suitable ways. The patient cannot be expected to do this automatically. He will have had to substitute for deltoid deficiency for so long that he will not necessarily realise that he is continuing to do so and neither will he know when, or how, to involve the muscle without a great deal of help. In the author's view this part of the re-education programme is more important than any of the progressive strengthening exercises recommended, since regular involvement in everyday activities will automatically improve the overall performance of the muscle group as a whole. Strengthening exercises, alone, do not guarantee involvement of the muscle in daily activities.

Specific strengthening could include repeated contractions with emphasis on deltoid in appropriate patterns through different ranges. It could include the use of pulleys and weights as resistances to the pattern of movement and progressive resistance could be applied.

Strengthening could also involve pool therapy in which the limb is abducted, flexed and extended, using the influence of buoyancy as a support or resistance. On the other hand the limb could be held stable by the physiotherapist and the patient asked to move the bodyweight away from the limb, the body being supported all the time by the water.

Suspension therapy can be used as a substitute for water and can be made very progressive by some enthusiasts.

6. As the muscle gains enough power to lift against gravity it should require less initial 'warm-up' facilitation and should also be expected to participate in antigravity functions. Such things as prone kneeling, changing to side sitting on alternate sides use deltoid in fairly easy weight-bearing activities. Crawling forwards is more difficult because the weight-bearing arm has to support the shoulder girdle of both sides and the non-weight-bearing arm has to lift forward against gravity.

Balance reactions may be given in which the deltoid is expected to help in lifting the affected limb sideways and forwards in an effort to adjust the overall position of the centre of gravity. Overhead arm and hand activities should be encouraged and light shopping may be carried by the affected limb.

Strengthening techniques should be carried out against the force of gravity and resisted movement patterns may have to be done in the sitting position or some other suitable position so as to involve gravity also. Progressive resistance exercises should include antigravity activity.

7. Eventually the patient should not require any preliminary facilitation methods and should be encouraged to participate in sporting and daily activities which will involve the affected limb totally.

The patient may do some activities as a member of a group in the gymnasium, and have some individual attention but, most important of all, he should be advised on suitable home activities. Eventually he has to manage his own limb entirely. Home activities are always available and should be exploited.

The above outline is not intended to be specific. It is used to give a concept and there are many variations to any one theme. The physiotherapist is not a technician. She must have a concept of aim, try to fulfil it and be observant of results so that she can adjust her method. No patient is exactly the same as any other and no patient can, therefore, be treated in exactly the same way as anyone else with the same problem.

Maximum sensory input in these cases will give maximum motor output. This fact must be exploited in the early stages of treatment and modified as the patient progresses.

Electrotherapy in the Lower Motoneurone Problem

If a peripheral nerve has been injured in such a way that the pathways will be disrupted for a prolonged period of time prior to being able to conduct again, it may be advisable to make the muscle contract artificially. This is in order to maintain its mobility against underlying structures and to minimise the rate of atrophy and loss of bulk by promoting the circulation through the muscle itself. In this way the muscle is maintained in a sound condition until such time as the nerve fibres are able to be functional again.

In order to influence as many muscle fibres as possible it is usual to place an electrode at each end of the muscle belly. Modified direct current is used and trapezoidal pulses of long duration (30–300ms) are given. These pulses are used because they are less likely to stimulate muscles which have a nerve supply, since they rise and fall slowly and the nerves going to the normal muscles will accommodate to them. Muscle does not have such good powers of accommodation and since the electrodes are placed over the muscle which has, at present, no nerve supply this is the muscle most likely to respond. Shorter duration pulses are not suitable as muscle tissue is unable to respond and only those muscles which could receive the stimulus via their nerve supply would be able to contract.

Apart from keeping the muscle in good condition electrical stimulation may also help to keep the patient aware of the muscle and its actions.

It is also possible to use electrotherapy as a re-educative measure. When the nerve has repaired but voluntary effort is still having difficulty in producing a contraction, it may prove helpful to use the faradic type of stimulus to help in the initiation of activity. In this situation a train of short duration pulses are delivered to the muscle via its nerve supply. The electrodes are therefore placed one over the motor point of the muscle and the other over the nerve trunk or nerve roots. Voluntary effort on the part of the patient is requested at the same time as electrical stimulation is given and the patient is asked to maintain the contraction when the electrical stimulation is reduced or ceases. This is a method of reeducation and it can be helpful in certain circumstances.

Biofeedback

Biofeedback equipment has now been developed which uses the basic principles of electromyography and can involve the use of surface electrodes applied to the patient by the therapist. This has the value of feeding back, to both the therapist and the patient, information regarding the successful contraction of muscle during a movement activity. The apparatus is neat and compact and can be strapped to the completely mobile patient without any difficulty. The electrodes are placed over the relevant muscle and the electrical discharges issued by the contracting muscle are picked up and converted into audible signals. In this way the therapist and patient are informed that the muscle is active and success or otherwise can be monitored. The threshold of muscle activity required before a signal is heard can be varied by programming the apparatus to be more or less sensitive to the electrical changes within the muscle. In this way even the patient with extreme muscle weakness can be informed if his effort has been successful. As the muscle participation improves, the equipment can be made less sensitive so that more activity is required to raise a signal. This equipment is not yet available in all hospital departments but, used skilfully, could be of great value to both therapist and patient.

Chapter 7

Principles of Treatment – 2

by H. W. ATKINSON, M.C.S.P., H.T., DIP.T.P.

THE PROBLEMS OF HYPOTONIA AND ATAXIA

Hypotonia and ataxia are so closely allied that they may be considered together. The bias on the stretch receptors is low and there is deficiency of activity of the excitatory extrapyramidal system. This is therefore a central and not a peripheral problem. There is lack of synergy and postural co-contraction of muscles round joints so that precision of movement and stability of posture is lost. Equilibrium and righting reactions are slow in being produced and inclined to over-react when they do occur. Movements are inclined to be slow to start and to be jerky and ill coordinated.

The physiotherapist has to attempt to redevelop the patient's movements along more normal lines and to keep him aware of normal movement patterns and normal posture and balance.

It is most advisable to make use of knowledge of developmental sequence in these cases and to encourage the development of postural stability and coordinated movements along these lines. The patient should progress from a position in which the centre of gravity is low and the base wide to the use of positions where less stability is offered.

It is very easy to use basic functional positions and movements following the developmental sequence since this inevitably complies with the low centre of gravity and wide base principles of progression.

If approximation is applied in the direction of weight-bearing, the stimulus already being applied by gravity will be reinforced. This tends to encourage extrapyramidal activity and gives rise to co-contraction of the muscles supporting the joints over which the weight is being placed.

The stimulus of gentle swaying may be applied at the same time to encourage activity in the appropriate patterns. This helps to elicit postural and righting reactions. The patient may be asked to participate volitionally by adding instructions which would be combined with manual pressure in all directions. The instructions would be to 'hold' or 'don't let me move you' as rhythmical stabilisations are carried out. These will further encourage co-contraction and combine automatic reactions with volitional effort.

Let us take as an example a patient whose condition is so difficult that he is unable to balance the head in a stable posture over the shoulder girdle because of hypotonia. To start with he would be most suitably positioned into prone lying with the elbows and forearms supported over a small bolster of pillows so that he is in a supported, elbow support prone lying position. If this position is too uncomfortable for the patient because of age or joint stiffness then a supported elbow support sitting could be used as a substitute (Fig. 7/1). In this

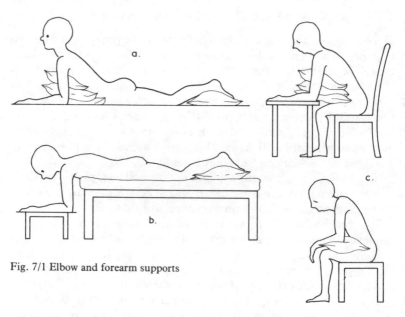

Fig. 7/1 Elbow and forearm supports

position all that has to be supported by the patient is the head. The physiotherapist can then help the patient to raise the head and, still assisting, can apply gentle approximation through the head and cervical spine while encouraging the patient to hold the position. She can take her support away and re-apply it in a rhythmical manner to allow gravity to have a frequent momentary influence upon the supporting muscles giving them a repeated small stretch. In this way a co-contraction can be built up encouraging the patient to be responsible for his own head position.

It should be remembered that while applying sound mechanical principles here, sound neurodevelopmental physiology is also being applied since control of the head position first shows itself as head lifting from prone lying.

Progress can be made by encouraging the patient to lift the head actively either by using resisted and commanded movement patterns of extension with rotation reversing with flexion with rotation or by making the patient follow moving objects with the eyes in appropriate directions. Holds should be given in various positions so that the patient learns to maintain suitable co-contraction wherever the head happens to be.

As improvement is noticed the patient can be encouraged to be responsible for the stability of the upper trunk and shoulders. The pillow support is taken away so that the patient is in an unsupported elbow support prone lying. The physiotherapist may need to apply quite vigorous and repeated compressions through the shoulder and elbow at first to gain some activity and then may stimulate the action by swaying the patient's weight from side to side and forwards and backwards to encourage excitation of the co-contracting muscles. It may help to use rhythmic stabilisations again here by pressing on the shoulders and commanding 'hold' and 'don't let me move you'.

When balance on the elbows is fairly secure the patient may be encouraged to rise from complete prone lying into elbow support prone lying and return down again. This requires a remarkable amount of postural and balance control and can be quite difficult for the patient.

The patient can then be encouraged to bear weight on one elbow while using the other limb or pushing on the other hand so that the trunk is rotated towards a more supine position.

Balance activities in this situation can be exploited. The patient periodically is lifted off the almost free hand and pushed down on to it again and made to hold with rhythmic stabilisation. In this way the upper trunk rotation components are now being involved and becoming more able to stabilise.

When the patient has reached this stage it is time to start encouraging head control with emphasis on the flexor muscle groups. The patient may be in a supported sitting position with the head in such a situation that gravity would gently pull it backwards into extension. It can then be worked upon as before encouraging a 'hold' and co-contraction round the neck and shoulder girdle region.

Trunk stability is most important in these cases and the rolling activities from side lying are particularly valuable. Spiral trunk rotation should be encouraged and resisted movements of rolling leading with the head and upper trunk and also leading with the legs and lower trunk should be encouraged, provided the patient does not show signs of going into abnormal patterns. Static holds and rhythmic stabilisations can also be of value to give trunk stability.

The natural progression from here is to make the patient stable in side sitting or in an arm forward support sitting prior to expecting him to be able to take up the position for himself.

The continuing progress would take the patient through prone kneeling, kneeling, half kneeling and standing. In such case the patient should be encouraged to learn to balance in the position before moving into it unaided and before using the position for functional activities.

Patients can be prepared for kneeling by being placed in prone lying with the knees flexed. Co-contraction round the flexed knees can be encouraged by giving compression sharply repeated through the heels and lateral aspects of the foot. In some cases voluntary rhythmical stabilisations may also be used. Half kneeling positions can also be adopted in side lying to accustom the patient to the limb position before being put into a difficult balance situation.

While the above progress is being made it should be remembered that we must also be able to carry out skills with free hands and even free feet and so far the limbs have primarily been used as weight-bearing structures. Thus the patient needs help to move the limbs on the trunk as opposed to moving the trunk over the limbs.

There are many ways of helping the hypotonic patient with this problem. The above approach will help to some extent since it gives the appropriate postural background.

Resisted limb patterns performed against moderate resistance at first quickly and then progressing to slower movements are of value. The emphasis should be placed on smoothness and precision of patterning. Reversals without rest are valuable and starting and stopping with holds in mid-pattern are also useful. At first the trunk should be in a position of supported stability but later progress can be made by making the patient support her own trunk.

The range of the reversals may be gradually reduced and the activity changed to static reversals and eventually to rhythmical stabilisations in different ranges.

It is also possible to train proximal stability for distal movements by using 'timing for emphasis' techniques. The patient is made to 'hold' the proximal part of the patterns while moving the distal parts. Resistance in these cases should be light as it is being used primarily as guidance. Gradually the guidance should be removed and the patient left free to move by himself.

It may be of value to use Frenkel's precision exercises in these cases and, in fact, the principles of these can be added to the above account. Movements in pattern may be done to counting in a rhythmical manner and even mat activities such as moving from side sitting to prone kneeling can be done to counting, using markers on the floor as guides.

When the ataxic symptoms are related to sensory loss as well as to hypotonia, the above suggestions are still applicable but more care must be taken to help the patient with afferent stimuli.

Frenkel's approach may be emphasised more, still using patterns. Mirrors may be a necessity and the patient must be allowed to use the eyes and ears as substitutes for other afferent information. Hard surfaces help this patient more than softly cushioned ones and often the stimuli applied have to be exaggerated to have their effect. Movements carried out to counting or other rhythmical sounds are likely to be more successful than silent performances. All patients showing ataxia have to use cortical control for many of their problems and this can hamper their activities, since movement has to become a conscious activity instead of an automatic one. However, with continuous repetition automaticity can be achieved and automatic balance reactions should be encouraged to occur in a controlled manner.

As the patient gains postural stability he should react in a more controlled manner to gentle, unexpected disturbance of balance. Attempts should be made in all positions to get gentle reactions to body sway, controlled stepping reactions and the use of the hands as a support in standing and sitting only as a last resort. So long as the hands do not have to be used for balance they are free for skills.

It is most important to note that many patients showing hypotonicity may also have an underlying tendency to adopt spastic patterns of movement, mass flexion or mass extension. It is therefore most important to keep a wary eye on the use of volition to see that its excessive use is not encouraging the use of undesirable patterns. If it does, then emphasis on volition should be reduced and more automatic methods adopted to gain the same result.

These patients should not be encouraged to use their upper limbs in 'pulling' functions since this may encourage them to use the arms in a mass flexor manner to pull themselves into standing. They will never gain balance in this way and for this reason such activities should be discouraged. Thus such a patient, if confined to bed, should not be supplied with a monkey bar to help him to move around in bed. It will encourage reflex patterning which is undesirable.

Functional Activities

As with the lower motoneurone problem, functions within the
capabilities of the patient should be encouraged. Suitable functions
should be found relevant to the patient's ability. If good movement
re-education is to occur, it is most important that excessive demands
are not made upon the patient since abnormalities will inevitably
appear which might otherwise be avoidable.

Walking will possibly be a goal and this should be encouraged *after*
the patient has the ability to balance in standing. At first some support
by the hands may be necessary using walking aids of some kind and
only when the patient is secure should he be encouraged to walk
without using the upper limbs as balance mechanisms.

It must be borne in mind that perfect functioning is unlikely in
these cases and the physiotherapist must be aware of the likely limitations. Occupational therapists and physiotherapists can often work
well together with these cases provided each respects the other
person's aim for the patient. The goal must be discussed and re-set as
progress is observed.

The patient's hopes must not be raised excessively and every step
forward must be noted by both the therapist and the patient. Every
member of the team should be prepared to meet each problem as it
arises and no one should expect too much.

There are other problems with these patients but they will be
considered under the appropriate headings since they are common to
most neurological patients.

Vertigo

Patients with this particular sensory problem have to learn to rely
upon joint and skin sensation and those sensations from sight rather
than those from the vestibular apparatus. As has been mentioned
earlier the giddy sensation and sickness are also accompanied by an
active inhibition of movement since movement of the head gives rise
to increase of the dizziness and nausea. The head and shoulders show
rather a fixed posture and the patient is afraid of movement.

Such is the link between eyes and vestibular apparatus that eye
movements may even trigger off the symptoms. Thus the patient need
not be moving at all but could be watching a moving object and would
have symptoms similar to those which would occur if he had been
moving.

Re-education of this patient involves giving him confidence in moving and helping him to take notice only of the reliable sensory or afferent information.

He should be treated at first in a fully supported semi-recumbent position so that head movements are unlikely to occur. Relaxation of the head, neck and shoulders should be encouraged and the patient asked to use his eyes only at first. His attention should be drawn to the sensation of complete support that his position offers so that he is aware of the unlikelihood of moving at that moment. He should look at a stationary object which is a comfortable distance away from him and be asked to focus upon it. When he has it in full focus the object should move slowly while he follows it with his eyes. If he feels dizzy then he should close his eyes and feel the stationary condition of his body. At first the object should only move as far as his eyes can travel but as he progresses head movements may also be involved, and later still, head movements with closed eyes should be encouraged in order to help him to rely only on joint and position sense.

As he progresses the patient may adopt less stable starting positions and exercise the eyes, head and trunk progressively until he can move fairly freely without suffering from excessive symptoms. Gradually he should progress to using hand/eye activities without losing his balance. Such activities as throwing and catching a ball in all directions are suitable. Standing and walking are advanced and the patient must be made accustomed to having objects moving in relationship to him. It is particularly important that stairs are included in his treatment programme, since the sides of a staircase can appear to be moving in the corner of the eye and can give vertigo symptoms in even quite normal people.

As the patient progresses he should be involved in group activities so that people and things are moving about him at the same time as he is moving himself. This does to some extent prepare him for coping with crossing roads and traffic. His treatment is not complete without postural correction and mobility exercises of head, neck and shoulder girdle and at some stage he must be taken in among traffic on foot and given the confidence to cross the road.

THE PROBLEM OF HYPERTONICITY

Spasticity

As described in Chapter 4 the patient will demonstrate at least partial release of certain reflex mechanisms from cortical control and hence difficulty in producing movement patterns other than those produced by the released reflexes. The stretch reflex mechanisms will be extra sensitive particularly in patterns dominated by the released reflexes.

The normal malleable postural background will not be present having given way to stereotyped patterns of a reflex nature. The patient will show poor vocabulary of movement patterns and of quality of control.

There is frequently a lack of synergy, evidence of instability of joint control coupled with lack of righting and equilibrium reactions.

The patient develops a pattern of spasticity related to the dominating reflexes. The reflexes most likely to exert their influence include the tonic labyrinthine, the symmetrical tonic neck reflex and the asymmetrical tonic neck reflex.

These reflex pathways are present in all of us and by the process of maturation of the nervous system their effect becomes integrated into the general control of all our movements. It is only when they are released from integration that they cause disturbance of movement pattern.

A study of these reflexes will show that the position of the head and neck is very important and that if care is taken to control their position and to encourage the patient to control it, excessive domination by the static postural reflexes can, to some extent, be avoided. Careful positioning of the patient can make management easier for the physiotherapist and the nurse and, at the same time, make movement more possible for the patient.

A study of the more dynamic righting reactions is also of extreme value. These reactions enable the individual to obtain the upright position and the spiral movements of the head and neck, trunk and limbs are related to them. It is thought that they may have an inhibitory effect upon the static postural mechanisms. The reduction in spasticity which is seen to accompany trunk and limb rotation may occur for this reason although there is, as yet, no proof that this is so. However, rotation of the trunk and limbs, when trying to reduce spasticity, is a very valuable asset and emphasises the importance of treating the whole patient instead of dealing only with the offending part.

When treating a patient who shows spasticity it is necessary to carry out three important aims:

1. Inhibit excessive tone as far as possible
2. Give the patient a sensation of normal position and normal movement
3. Facilitate normal movement patterns.

INHIBITION OF EXCESSIVE TONE

Earlier in this chapter it was pointed out that inhibition could be facilitated as well as excitation. In cases of spasticity it is important to facilitate the patient's ability to inhibit the undesirable activity of the released reflex mechanisms. As has already been mentioned the position adopted by the patient is important since the head and neck position can elicit strong postural reflex mechanisms. Avoiding these head and neck positions can facilitate the inhibition of the more likely reflexes and if the positions have to be adopted, then help in preventing the rest of the body from going into the reflex pattern thus elicited may be required by the patient. The patient cannot, of course, spend the rest of his life avoiding the positions which encourage dominance by reflex activity but, at first, this may be necessary until the patient has developed some control in the suppression of the effect of the reflex activities. As he develops this control then he can be gradually introduced to the use of positions which make suppression of reflex activity more difficult.

As an early introduction to treatment the side lying position, well supported by pillows, is very convenient since it avoids stimulation of the tonic labyrinthine reflex, and also as the head and trunk are in alignment, the stimulation of the asymmetrical tonic neck reflexes. It makes a good resting position for the patient with spasticity and also is convenient for the application of rhythmical trunk rotations of both a passive and assisted active form. These do help to encourage a reduction in tone.

The scapula is also readily available to be involved in the movements. The upper and lower limb of the uppermost side are also easily accessible for any passive, assisted active or automatic movements which may seem suitable.

Side lying is not always desirable because of respiratory problems in the older patient or because of the need to obtain a greater range of movement. Other attitudes are often very satisfactory such as crook lying or even with the knees as high on the chest as possible. These last two are helpful if there is flexor spasticity. As the trunk is rotated the legs are allowed to lower towards the extended, abducted and laterally rotated position. For older patients trunk rotation may have to be encouraged in sitting.

Limb rotations are also very effective in helping to give a more normal control of muscle tone to the patient.

These facts are of help not only to the physiotherapist but also to the nurse who may be concerned in moving the patient in bed or attempting to position the patient so as to avoid the development of deformities.

The important factors in attempting to gain control over muscle tone are:

1. Patterns of movement and posture associated with the released reflex mechanisms must be avoided and discouraged by positioning, guidance and using the inhibitory methods mentioned in this chapter.

2. Conditions which will facilitate control of tone should be given using the stimuli which will encourage normal patterns.

As an example of the above two points let us consider pressure applied to the undersurface of the foot. If it is applied to the ball of the foot it may well stimulate an extensor reflex in which a pathological pattern of extension, adduction and medial rotation of the hip is produced together with plantar flexion of the foot. This would be undesirable in a case of spasticity. If pressure is applied under the heel of the foot then a more useful co-contraction of muscle is likely to occur giving a suitable supporting pattern. The physiotherapist must become familiar with the stereotyped reflex patterning so that she can avoid permitting them to occur.

It is most important that the physiotherapist becomes familiar with the patterning of normal movements and postures so that she can help her patient to move using them in preference to spastic patterns. Help is needed to facilitate the movements by correcting weight distribution, head and shoulder positioning and encouraging suitable rotational balance activities. For example, when walking, the right leg cannot be moved forwards unless the left leg is receiving weight correctly and the body is balanced over it. Trunk rotations normally accompany the mature walking patterns as reciprocal balance mechanisms and should be encouraged. Standing from sitting cannot occur unless the head and shoulders are brought well forward so that weight is distributed to the feet. As the patient rises she may extend her neck and trunk too soon and throw her weight back so that she is not successful in reaching a standing position. The timing of neck and trunk extension may need to be assisted. All the necessary automatic adjustments are impoverished in these patients and help may be needed. Sometimes verbal help is needed but more often actual assistance by simply adjusting the movements and waiting for the patient to react may be more helpful. This enables the patient to feel and perhaps see the successful activity. At all times the effect on the whole patient must be observed since it is quite possible to be gaining more normal tone in one part of the patient at the expense of another.

Movement of a normal nature does appear in itself to reduce excessive tone and consequently this should be encouraged in the patient. However, care must be taken if conscious volitional movement is demanded. Due to reflex release, some motoneurone pools are already in an excitatory state and any volitional effort is likely to act as a triggering mechanism to those motoneurone pools giving associated muscle contraction in the spastic pattern. Such patients should not be encouraged to make strong volitional effort since this is inclined to facilitate the production of spastic patterning. Conscious voluntary activity should be kept to a minimum until it is not accompanied by undesirable associated activity. Instead, appropriate stimuli should be given to encourage more normal responses which will automatically help to reduce the patterns of spasticity.

Other methods of reducing spasticity include the application of heat or cold for relatively prolonged periods of time. These can have dramatic effects on some patients provided a large enough area of the patient is included. Total immersion in ice cold water has been recommended for some cases of multiple sclerosis who show spasticity and the author has seen very impressive temporary results from this approach. The patient who responds to this shows a marked improvement in movement ability for several hours before the process has to be repeated again.

Deep rhythmical massage with pressure over the muscle insertions has proved effective in some cases and many authorities advocate slow, steady and prolonged stretching. This last method does have its dangers since, if the stretching is forced against severe spasticity, the hyperexcitable stretch reflex reacts even more strongly and damage to the periosteum of bone may occur where excessive tension has been applied by the tendons of the stretched muscles.

Rhythmical, slowly performed passive movements through normal patterns may also be helpful and in the more moderate cases the patient may subconsciously join in and by his own activity a reduction in spasticity may occur. Quick movements, abruptly performed, and noisy surroundings are most detrimental as are excitement, anxiety or any form of discomfort.

SENSATION OF NORMAL POSITION AND MOVEMENT

This is of vital importance. A patient who is dominated by reflex patterns never experiences the sensation of normal movement and position unless helped to do so. He is denied normal stimulation and either cannot know or soon forgets the normal. Very quickly the abnormal feels normal and vice versa.

A patient showing extensor spasticity of the lower limb will most often hold the limb in hip extension, adduction and medial rotation, knee extension and foot plantar flexion, i.e. mass extensor synergy of the lower limb. Such a patient when standing or sitting may never be able to experience weight-bearing through the heel. When weight is taken through the heel the stimulus encourages a true supporting reaction which gives co-contraction of hip, knee and ankle muscles, flexors as well as extensors, in a malleable co-contraction suitable for normal weight-bearing. Thus there is no hope for the patient who is in extensor synergy unless some method of applying the more appropriate stimulus is found.

If an abnormal position makes a starting point for a movement then an abnormal movement must occur. Because of their spasticity many patients are forced by circumstances to repeat abnormal movement patterns. By repetition the nervous pathways used to cause these movements are facilitated and the abnormal movements therefore occur more and more readily. When this has occurred correction is difficult, if not impossible. Because of this it is important to give early treatment to the whole patient so that, as far as possible, the sensation of normal movement is retained.

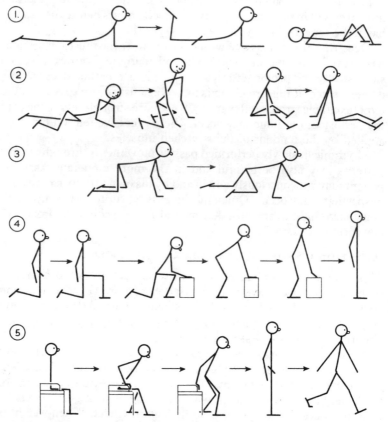

Fig. 7/2 Patterns of movement to be encouraged

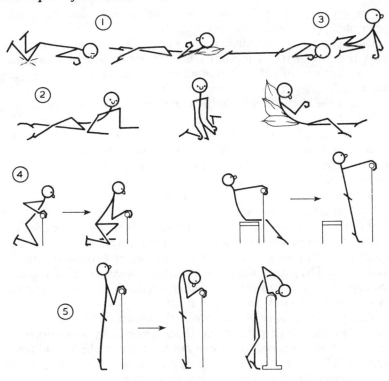

Fig. 7/3 Patterns of movement to be discouraged

Praise for a movement should only be given if it really is good because, having received praise, the patient will try to repeat the same performance. If it was a good movement the second attempt is also likely to be good, but if it was unsatisfactory at first the repeated movement will also be poor and this faulty pathway has been facilitated.

FACILITATION OF NORMAL MOVEMENT PATTERNS

More normal movement patterns can be produced when domination by reflex mechanisms is minimised. Thus, when the patient appears to be relatively free, movement should be encouraged. Movement itself will reduce spasticity if it follows normal patterns. Often automatic adjustment of position is easier to produce than conscious volitional activities. Figures 7/2 and 7/3 illustrate some movements and positions which are helpful if encouraged and some which should be discouraged. Rotational movements of the trunk and limbs are important and spiral rolling patterns involving head, shoulder girdle, pelvis and limbs should be encouraged.

In most cases it is helpful to follow a neurodevelopmental approach with these patients. They often have a vocabulary of movement pattern less versatile than that of a newly born child. Thus they are more likely to learn movement control if they are encouraged to follow the sequence of events seen in the movement patterning of a child.

Basic functional movements are the ones to encourage at first. The child does not develop skilled hand movements until the hands are freed from being props for balance. The same holds good for adults showing spasticity. One does well if the upper limbs can be trained to support the patient. The ambition to train skilled hand movements should be deferred until this is achieved.

It is important to appreciate that points (1), (2) and (3) (p.124) are best dealt with at one and the same time. In other words one does not arrange for the patient to fulfil the aim of reducing spasticity and then proceed to applying appropriate sensation and then re-educate movement. The patient should be placed in an area suitable for seizing the opportunity of moving as and when a reduction in tone is felt and as a suitable stimulus has had an effect.

The physiotherapist must constantly observe the effect of her efforts on the whole patient and if an opportunity arises to use a movement which is occurring in a normal manner she should use it without delay. For this reason a sample list of activities is impossible to offer since fixed methods are not applicable.

Functional Activities

It is in the field of spasticity that most controversy occurs regarding functions of daily living. If the aim is to normalise movement only those functions which do not produce pattern abnormalities should be encouraged and progress should be made relative to this. The physio-therapist should, in this case, be the person to decide which functions are suitable.

If however, the aim is to gain functional independence at all costs, then movement abnormalities may have to be ignored or even encour-aged in order to gain some sort of ambulation. Strictly speaking, the skill of a good physiotherapist should not be used for long if this is the aim, since well-trained aides could fulfil it quite adequately with guidance. It is most important that consultants and therapists exchange views and come to an agreement on which line of approach is to be followed and also when further attempts to help the patient are to be abandoned. Conflicting views can have seriously detrimental effects.

Use of Drugs

There are drugs available which will have an inhibitory effect on the stretch reflex. These mainly work by blocking the synaptic functions of internuncial pathways. If they are effective the patient is likely to be hypotonic with underlying movement patterns of the flexor/extensor synergies. Such patients are best treated as hypotonic patients but great care should be given if resisted exercises are used. Free active patterning with some automatic compression stimuli and gentle balance activities are more suitable.

Rigidity

In this situation the patient tends to show excessive postural fixation, axial rotation is non-existent and normal balance reactions do not appear to be available. The patient tends to adopt a fixed head and shoulder positioning and movements which would normally be those of trunk rotation either do not occur at all or occur by the patient moving round as a whole.

The face adopts a mask-like rigidity and the patient appears to be unresponsive to stimuli. A tremor is often present when resting, which disappears when purposeful movement occurs. All these symptoms are seen when the centres concerned with automatic reactions are the site of lesion, so that these reactions do not occur.

Increase in tone causes opposition to all movements, which are therefore slow in being produced and are not readily accompanied by automatic postural adjustments.

As in the case of spasticity the abnormality effectively prevents the patient from experiencing normal sensory information and he quite rapidly 'forgets' the normal and accepts the abnormality as normal.

The physiotherapist can help the patient in several ways, but she must always have the following aims at the back of her mind:

1. To encourage a reduction in the overall sensitivity of the stretch reflex mechanism

2. To help the patient to experience more normal reactions

3. To encourage movements to follow normal patterns in as wide a range and as freely as possible.

REDUCTION IN OVERALL SENSITIVITY OF THE STRETCH REFLEX
MECHANISM

There are several methods available to achieve this aim and the sooner
the patient is treated the more effective is treatment likely to be.
Methods include: teaching general relaxation in a comfortable, well-
supported, recumbent position; the application of rhythmical
massage of a sedative nature; and the use of rhythmical passive and/or
assisted active movements.

The most effective method is likely to be to give rhythmical passive
to active movements with the patient recumbent or semi-recumbent.

The movements which are of most value to the patient are those
which are not available to him. Trunk rotations are particularly
useful, and may be carried out through a small range at first, gradually
increasing the range and speeding up the rate of rhythm of the
movement as the rigidity subsides. Such movements can be done
passively by the physiotherapist, but she should not discourage the
patient from helping if he can. It is not total relaxation that is wanted
but only a sufficient reduction in tone to make movement more
possible.

Probably the side lying position is a most convenient one for this
purpose since trunk rotations can be most easily produced in this
position and can also be easily converted into rolling activities when
the patient has enough freedom to do so. In addition the patient's
scapula is freely available and can be moved prior to encouraging
greater range of activity in the whole body.

Since many patients showing rigidity are elderly, the fully recumbent position is not always suitable and rotations may have to be
performed in other positions. It is quite possible to help a patient to
rotate at the trunk in sitting by moving the upper trunk upon the
lower and one can even involve the trunk diagonal patterns of flexion
with rotation to one side, followed by extension with rotation to the
other.

Limb movements can be encouraged in a similar way involving the
diagonal patterns, if possible, and starting with a small range and
progressing to a larger range as the movement becomes more available. If the patient assists so much the better.

EXPERIENCING MORE NORMAL REACTIONS

Helping the patient experience the more normal reactions is very
much linked with the methods suggested in the previous section. As
the patient loosens up when the overall tone of the muscles is reduced,
opportunities to react to situations should be given and help to reach

and experience the reaction should be offered as needed. For instance if trunk rotation is being encouraged in side lying the patient will gradually loosen up and start to participate. The upper limb should then be encouraged to come forward to receive weight as the trunk comes forward ready for going into prone lying. If the limb does not react automatically the therapist can repeatedly encourage rotation and bring the patient's arm and hand forward into the supporting position. Gradually the patient will appreciate the sensation and will join in until all the physiotherapist need do is gently push the shoulder forward to initiate the reaction. A similar method of encouraging the appropriate lower limb reactions may also be used.

If the trunk rotations are being done in sitting, other balance reactions may be aided. Such reactions as hand support forwards or hand support sideways may be encouraged. Even the lifting reactions of the limbs on the side away from which the patient is shifted can be helped by the skilled physiotherapist in this way, so that the patient experiences the sensation of balance reactions.

By lifting reactions are meant the reactions of the body to displacement of weight sideways or backwards. If the bodyweight is displaced sideways the upper limb on that side moves sideways to receive some of the weight. The other upper limb lifts sideways to try to pull the body back to its original base. The lower limbs, if free, may also participate by rotating (Fig. 7/4).

Any sign of regression back into rigidity to an excessive degree should be countered by further rotations. Trunk rotations with rhythmic arm swinging can be very helpful and give the arm swing sensation required when walking. Many physiotherapists encourage this by having the patient sitting or standing holding one end of a pole

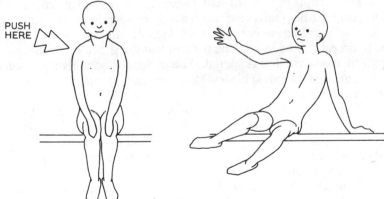

PUSH
HERE

Fig. 7/4 Reaction to lateral displacement of the trunk

in each hand. The physiotherapist is holding the other ends of the poles and using her arm swing she can encourage the arm swing of the patient.

ENCOURAGING MOVEMENTS TO FOLLOW NORMAL PATTERNS
IN AS WIDE A RANGE AND AS FREELY AS POSSIBLE

This automatically links with the previous two sections and has to some extent already been encouraged. Movement patterns may be encouraged with minimal resistance for guidance. The range should be small at first and slowly encouraged to larger range and faster movement. The patient has to be 'pumped up' to more rapid and fuller range of activity. This also applies to functions such as standing up and sitting down, rolling over and getting started with walking activities.

For the younger patient the author has found the following type of activities most successful:

1. Rhythmical rolling in a spiral manner, first helping the patient and later starting the movement for the patient and allowing him to react by following.

2. Encouraging the adoption of side sitting and moving on to all fours and then sitting on the opposite side. This is started on all fours and the patient sways rhythmically towards the side upon which he will eventually sit before rising back to all fours. At first he does not sit at all but gradually approaches the sitting position as a fuller range is available. This activity encourages trunk and limb rotation and if rhythmical it will help to keep the overall tone reduced.

3. Rhythmical crawling may also be encouraged by swaying the bodyweight forwards and backwards and eventually encouraging a step forward reaction of the limbs.

4. Hand support forward half kneeling, changing legs rhythmically, may also help and eventually leads to the adoption of standing.

5. The standing activities should include rhythmical walking, which is best started by rotating the trunk at the shoulders so that an easy arm swing rhythm is started. The patient's bodyweight is then pushed gently forwards at hip level to encourage a stepping reaction in the lower limbs.

6. The customary stooping position should be avoided and the patient encouraged to maintain as upright a position as possible. Many physiotherapists use poles as mentioned previously to initiate walking and do so by encouraging the patient to step forward with the right leg as the left arm comes forwards.

7. Gradually the walking should include turning and stepping backwards and also across the other leg. These activities may be done

as conscious volitional activities but, if possible, should eventually become an automatic response to disturbance of balance.

One cannot do quite such agile activities with the older patient and some of the following suggestions may prove helpful:

1. Sitting: assisted active trunk rotations to encourage a hand support sideways sitting position.

2. Hands supporting to one side: encourage standing up by leaning back to leaning forwards and standing up. Rhythmical swaying may be more suitable at first and then gradually changed to standing up.

3. Standing up to sitting down as before, progressing to standing up again with the hands supporting to alternate sides. This also involves trunk rotations which are so easily lost in these patients.

4. Arm swinging and walking can be encouraged as in the younger person.

In both types of patients limb patterns through full range should be encouraged in addition to functional mat type activities.

Patients' relatives can be taught to help reduce the rigidity at home by encouraging rotational movement and perhaps helping to give the necessary 'pumping up' procedures prior to achieving a particular function. It is most important to keep these patients as functionally independent as possible and relatives must be encouraged to give minimum assistance of an 'educated' nature.

The patient can help himself to a tremendous degree once he receives adequate guidance and provided he receives appropriate encouragement from his relatives. It can be helpful to allow him to have a period of intensive physiotherapy at intervals and to encourage him to be responsible for his own welfare ('movement-wise') in the periods when he has no formal treatment. An early morning 'warm up' exercise session involving trunk rotations and rhythmical swinging movements of arms and legs can be very valuable when he is otherwise receiving no treatment.

Odd jobs about the house which require movement are more suitable than those which can be done sitting down. They may take a longer time for the patient to perform but they are a treatment in themselves.

Static activities are undesirable and rhythmical stabilisations do not usually help these patients and so should be avoided if possible.

Drugs are available to reduce rigidity and some surgical procedures have given a measure of relief. The patient may then show variable movement problems and has to be dealt with according to individual peculiarities.

It cannot be emphasised too much that the earlier the patient receives treatment the more effective it will be. When a patient is first suspected of showing rigidity symptoms he is unlikely to show gross abnormality and will not have so much underlying joint stiffness or have 'forgotten' normality to such a degree. He is therefore more able to be receptive to help. This is directed at helping him to help himself. He may then well be able to minimise his symptoms more effectively for longer.

If the patient is very rigid when he first receives help he may also have painful joint stiffness and have mechanical difficulty in addition to physiological problems. Normal movement will be very unusual to him and the likelihood of his being able to help himself adequately is considerably more remote.

THE PROBLEMS OF ATHETOSIS, CHOREA AND BALLISMUS

These three movement abnormalities are grouped together since all show the presence of involuntary activity and fluctuations of tone. The physiotherapist has to meet problems with these patients when they appear. At one time she may be required to encourage stability in the same way as she would a hypotonic patient and at another time she may have to help in the inhibition of abnormal activities while encouraging normal purposeful movement patterns.

Excitement should be avoided at all costs since this increases the symptoms.

Athetoid patients frequently have problems with body image and steps must be taken to improve this by experiences of normal activities and stimuli.

Many athetoids are helped in stability by compression forces being applied through weight-bearing joints. Some children benefit by wearing little leaded caps which add to the weight of the head and give compression force to the vertebral column. This helps to stimulate stabilisation. Much of the action advised in preceding sections is useful for these patients and the physiotherapist must use her ingenuity in selecting those activities which help and discarding those which do not. She must receive a constant 'feedback' from the patient and adjust her stimuli accordingly.

Drugs and surgery have been used to control the symptoms of these disorders and have met with varying success. In such circumstances the patient is still left with movement abnormalities which have to be assessed and treated accordingly.

Biofeedback equipment as mentioned at the end of Chapter 6 may also be of value to the therapist treating problems discussed in this chapter. The signal of muscle activity can be used to indicate successful patterning to the patient or, more negatively, it can be used to indicate unwanted activity.

PROBLEMS OF DEFORMITY

Adaptive shortening of soft tissues is likely to occur when habitual posturing is adopted by patients who have any disease or injury problem. In neurological problems it is particularly likely to occur when no movement is available to the patient and when there is imbalance of muscle pull.

There are many methods of preventing the onset of deformities of this nature. These include:

Passive Movements

These were already suggested in an earlier section as being helpful in the maintenance of a knowledge of body image. When used to prevent deformity the physiotherapist must bear two facts in mind:

1. She must maintain the biological length of the muscles which work over the joints she is moving. This means that her passive movements must involve elongating the muscle over all its movement components. For example, to maintain the length of gastrocnemius she must dorsiflex the foot and extend the knee and her return movements should be plantar flexion of the foot and flexion of the knee. In that way she has fully lengthened gastrocnemius which pulls over the back of the knee and ankle and she has also put it into its most shortened position.

2. She must maintain the biological pliability of the ligaments of the joints she is moving. This means that she must be cautious when moving a joint over which a 'two joint' muscle works since it could restrict the range of movement available before the ligaments are fully elongated. For example, ankle dorsiflexion is limited by gastrocnemius if the knee is held extended as the ankle is dorsiflexed. Therefore the ligaments of the joint are not fully elongated by the time movement has stopped. Thus in this case the tension should be taken off gastrocnemius by flexing the knee before dorsiflexing the foot. A greater range will then be found to be available.

Careful Positioning of the Severely Disabled Patient

This should be done in such a way that constant adoption of one position is avoided. Limbs and trunk should be supported in a variety of positions throughout the day. Extreme positioning of any joint should be avoided.

Splintage

This is most helpful in patients with peripheral problems as it prevents the flaccid muscle groups from being constantly stretched by normal opposing muscle action. Splints should never be left on permanently but should be used as resting splints when the patient is likely to adopt a prolonged poor position of the joints concerned. Lively splints are very useful since they allow movement to occur and simply return the limbs to a normal position at the end of the movement. They are more functional than the simple rest splints.

Many people use splintage with central nervous system problems but it should only be used in certain well-considered circumstances. Splints applied to such cases effectively prevent normal movement patterns and pressure from the splint may actually increase the spastic patterning. For example a plaster cast applied to the lower leg and foot to keep the foot in dorsiflexion may effectively stimulate (by pressure on the ball of the foot) an extensor response which will take the form of mass extensor synergy. This could be undesirable and worse than no splintage at all. Only in some circumstances is splintage helpful in these disorders.

Use of Bed Cradles

These are very helpful. They lift the weight of bedclothes off the limbs, which may be paralysed, and therefore the bedclothes do not force the feet into plantar flexion.

The cradle is also useful when hypertonicity is a problem since the constant irritation of bedclothes can stimulate withdrawal reflexes which encourage flexion deformities.

If deformity is already present by the time the patient comes for help, the problem is much greater. The patient may require more help to counter the problem such as traction, manipulation, and surgery. In the latter case tendons may be divided and lengthened or muscles are disattached and left to re-attach in a more suitable position.

The physiotherapist may be able to help in some cases by the application of serial plasters designed to correct deformities gradually.

Some patients, particularly those with lower motoneurone problems, develop adaptive shortening of the muscles antagonistic to those which are paralysed. The physiotherapist can help considerably here to encourage a new resting length for these muscles by using any or all of the following methods:

1. The application of prolonged (about 10–20 minutes) cold packs to the adaptively shortened muscle. The packs must extend over the whole length of the muscle. This method encourages inhibition of the muscle which will relax more, making it possible to lengthen it more easily.

2. The use of 'hold, relax' techniques in which the adaptively shortened muscle is put into as elongated a position as is comfortable and then made to contract statically – hence the term 'hold'. As the contraction is held for a prolonged time it begins to weaken. When this occurs the patient is instructed to relax while the physiotherapist supports the joint or joints involved. When relaxation has occurred the physiotherapist further elongates the muscle passively. If successful she will find that the muscle will allow itself to be elongated more as it has relaxed sufficiently to allow an increase in length.

There are various theories as to why this should work. Some authorities say that the muscle relaxes more because of fatigue and others consider that the Golgi tendon organs which lie at the musculotendinous junction are stimulated by the contracting muscle pulling on the tendon. As was stated earlier these organs have an inhibitory influence on the motoneurone pools of their own muscle and may therefore help to induce this excessive relaxation (autogenic inhibition).

Cold packs may be applied at the same time as 'hold, relax' techniques.

'Hold, relax' is most suitable for use when the adaptively shortened group are opposed by completely flail antagonists.

3. A modification of the above is the 'slow reversal, hold, relax' technique. In this case the procedure is as for 'hold, relax' but after the relaxation stage has occurred the patient is stimulated to use the antagonist to the adaptively shortened muscle concentrically. In other words the adaptively shortened muscle is made to contract statically by a 'hold'. It is then commanded to relax and the reverse movement is brought about by active concentric activity of its antagonist. This technique is most useful when there is some activity available in the antagonist. The phenomenon of reciprocal inhibition is added to the phenomenon of autogenic inhibition in this case.

The above techniques are only of value when movement limitation is due to changes in length of muscle. They do not help if the limitation is due to ligamentous or bony changes.

Some workers claim to have used the above techniques to relax spastic muscle groups. The author does not use this particular technique for fear of facilitating spastic patterning. The student should, however, keep an open mind in all such matters and decide for herself which methods she will use, noting the results and accepting those which give good results while rejecting those which do not.

PREVENTION OF INJURY

This has been largely dealt with on p.98, since much of the damage which can occur in these cases is due to sensory loss.

The patient must be made aware of the dangers, if possible, and if he cannot change his position himself he must be frequently turned. He must be kept scrupulously clean and have his skin toughened and protected against the possibility of pressure sores.

If any area shows signs of breaking down it may be stimulated by ice massage to improve the local circulation, or by heat or mild doses of ultraviolet light. The use of heat has its dangers since sensory loss may make the patient endure a temperature that is too hot for safety. Cold is therefore the method of choice.

The use of ripple mattresses, sheepskins, protective rings and constant changes of position should effectively prevent the onset of sores. If they do develop they are very detrimental to the patient's general condition and must be treated as a serious problem.

CIRCULATORY PROBLEMS

Many patients show disturbances of circulation. Some of these are due to lack of movement and some are due to disturbance in some part of the autonomic system.

In the lower motoneurone problem the loss of 'muscle pump' activity will cause slowing of the circulation through the affected area and, in addition, the peripheral autonomic nerve fibres may also be involved.

These problems can be helped by encouraging activity in other parts of the body. This will speed up circulation generally.

Whirlpool baths for the affected areas may also be used. These will promote circulation to the skin over the affected muscle groups. Contrast baths may also prove valuable. They may stimulate such blood vessel activity as is available.

The central autonomic problem is well described in Chapter 8. Essentially the patient has to adapt gradually to change of position which puts greater demands upon the problem of maintenance of blood pressure.

In cases of causalgia, in which there is disuse due to pain, similar methods may be used to those advocated for the lower motoneurone problem. Wax baths may also help here, but on the other hand they may cause onset of pain and so should be used with reservation.

Many patients who have hemiplegic symptoms have problems in the posturing of the shoulder girdle. This can cause pressure and kinking of the axillary vessels giving rise to oedema which is further encouraged by lack of use and the dependent position. In this case the weight of the limb may have to be relieved by sling support to reduce pressure on the axillary vessels. This is unfortunate since it discourages movement of the limb. However, the sling need not be retained all the time and other treatments for oedema may be given which involve movement. As soon as the posturing of the patient improves the sling should be discarded.

RESPIRATORY PROBLEMS

Many patients show respiratory problems. These range from those which are due to paralysis of the muscles of respiration to those which are due to restriction of exercise because of the patient's disability.

Patients who have paralysis of the respiratory muscles will obviously need the help of a ventilator and will be in an intensive therapy unit. They may also require to have assisted coughing or may even need suction to help to remove secretions.

Only the local peripheral problems will totally escape from respiratory difficulties. The head injury case may well require tracheostomy, suction and to be ventilated (IPPV).

The patient with a central nervous system disorder of the progressive variety will be inclined to develop respiratory distress as the disease progresses. The muscles supporting the thoracic inlet may be hypotonic and will allow respiratory movements to have a suction effect on the chest wall in this area, thus diminishing the amount of air the thorax can house. Such patients may also have deglutition problems and it is possible for food to be inhaled.

Even the less handicapped patient may show weakness of respiratory movements and will need some help.

Breathing exercises should be incorporated into the treatment of all the heavily handicapped patients. They may be facilitated in lower motoneurone cases by using appropriate arm patterns and by giving repeated contractions to the muscles of inspiration. Both inspiratory and expiratory phases should be emphasised to get maximum respiratory excursion.

The central problem requires a more relaxed approach but respiration must not be forgotten. It is particularly important to the rigidity case and to patients with multiple problems like multiple sclerosis.

The advanced case of multiple sclerosis and also the patient with weakness in the thoracic inlet and deglutition group (omohyoid, mylohyoid, digastricus, thyrohyoid and sternothyroid) may be helped by giving head and neck patterns of a resisted nature, stabilisation of the head and neck and combining these with respiration.

PROBLEMS OF SPEECH

These problems are properly left to the speech therapist who is the specialist. The physiotherapist may be able to endorse the work of the speech therapist if the two team members can discuss matters with each other.

It is possible to stimulate movement of the tongue by using a spatula and moving the tongue with it, encouraging the patient to participate. Ice frozen on to the spatula may also help as the cold is a stimulus. As the water forms from the melting ice it acts as a lubricant to the tongue and mouth.

Activity of buccinator can also be encouraged by pressure from the spatula against the inside of the cheek. This may help to train the patient to keep the cheek against the teeth and therefore prevent collection of saliva. This can be very useful when treating facial palsy as the stretch stimulus can be used by pressing the cheek outwards while commanding the patient to pull in.

Speech in the severely handicapped is not easily available unless there is control of head position and the physiotherapist may be required to help in this way.

Deglutition is also difficult without head control and may be impossible if the patient is recumbent. The patient who has swallowing difficulties should be fed, if possible, in an upright position.

To speak, we also have to be able to swallow as otherwise we spit as we speak. The swallowing muscles may be stimulated by stroking or brushing over the anterior aspect of the under-surface of the chin and neck and by icing the tongue and lips.

EXERCISE TOLERANCE

This becomes lost if respiration and circulation are impaired but it may also be lost due to disuse. The wheelchair patient never fully uses himself unless encouraged to do so. If possible he should be encouraged to indulge in as active a type of exercise as possible to maintain good exercise tolerance.

Other patients should be given activities in their programme which tax them to their limits so that they maintain good general health. The only exception to this would be, perhaps, the patient who has had a cerebrovascular accident or one with cardiac complications.

Care must be taken to see that the patient and relatives understand that to be overweight is detrimental. The less exercise the patient is able to indulge in, the lighter should be the diet. Overeating is a common problem to the handicapped patient.

PAIN

This, as has been stated before, is a problem most associated with irritative lesions. Relief of the irritation leads to relief of the pain. Pain may also be the result of faulty posturing or of faulty muscle synergy leading to inflamed bursae, etc.

Pain relieving methods include: gentle heat to encourage relaxation; cold, which often helps when heat fails; soothing massage techniques associated with correction of malposturing; and the use of movement activities which help to reduce the discomforts of constant joint positioning.

Many patients who have loss of synergy in the shoulder have severe shoulder pain which spreads down the arm. The hemiplegic patient is particularly prone to this. The pain can often be relieved by the application of a cold pack over the shoulder area incorporating pectoralis major, deltoid and the scapula. If this is followed by rhythmical traction versus compression stimuli the patient frequently reports relief of pain. The explanation for this is obscure but it may be that the cold helps to relax the painful muscle spasm which will be superimposed upon the patient's other symptoms and the compression alternately with traction may stimulate more normal muscle synergy and therefore joint protection.

If the pain is part of a neuritis the position of the vertebral column and shoulder girdle is important.

Cervical traction may be advised as a measure to relieve pressure on the nerve roots and therefore act as a relief to irritation.

The pain of causalgia is another difficult problem and all pain relieving methods may be attempted. Heat is not always successful and may be dangerous if the patient's ability to appreciate degrees of heat is impaired.

Thalamic pain is not very responsive to physiotherapy and drugs may be the only thing to help the patient.

Drug therapy is used widely in the relief of pain which cannot

otherwise be helped and even surgical interference may be a
as a method of blocking sensory input of a painful nature.

LOSS OF CONSCIOUSNESS

Patients showing loss of consciousness require special care in an
intensive therapy unit. Attention must be paid to the accompanying
respiratory problems and the physiotherapist may be called in to help
in these matters.

As was indicated in Chapter 4 there are various levels of unconsciousness and much care must be taken to talk to the patient and not
about him in case he is receptive to some stimuli.

EPILEPSY

Fits of this nature are usually held in check by the administration of
phenobarbitone and allied drugs. The physiotherapist must know
whether her patient is prone to these attacks so that she is not completely unprepared should one occur during a treatment session.

If the fit is of a minor nature it may pass almost unnoticed, but if it is
of a more major type then care must be taken to prevent the patient
from injuring herself and other people. Such patients should not be
left unattended nor should they be treated in areas where they could
come to any severe injury should they have an attack. Pool therapy
may well be unwise for these patients on two counts. First, there
is a danger of inhalation of water and possible drowning. Second,
the shimmering effect of light on the water may well trigger off an
attack.

Epilepsy can be triggered off by light wave bands giving visual
stimulation and for this reason some patients show the onset of an
attack if they sit watching television for long. This is particularly
likely to happen if they are too close to it and in a darkened room.

The flickering light coming through trees and from the road upon
which there are multiple areas of shade and light may also be a
contributory factor and patients who are travelling as passengers are
advised to close their eyes when the light fluctuates in this way. Short
wave diathermy has been known to have a similar effect and care
should be taken if such treatment is contemplated for any patient
known to have epilepsy.

It is as well for the physiotherapist to know this since patients often
complain of feeling unwell or of having a mild attack when watching
television. The physiotherapist may be able to help by explaining the
cause.

INCONTINENCE OF URINE AND BACK PRESSURE

As was explained in Chapter 4 many of the more severely handicapped patients show these symptoms. Catheterisation is the standard method of dealing with this, but unfortunately it often leads to urinary infections which have to be controlled by antibiotics.

Back pressure into the kidneys can be relieved periodically by allowing the patient to adopt the upright position for periods during the day. If the patient is unable to stand he may be supported on a tilting couch which can be wound up into the upright position. The patient may have to be secured by strapping into position, but provided adequate padding is given, there is no danger of skin pressure.

The method of procedure can be useful for the patient suffering from multiple sclerosis who has reached the bedfast stage, and who is in danger not only of having urinary problems but also of going into a flexion position. The weight-bearing stimulus through the feet encourages extension and counteracts the flexion, while the urinary complications are minimised.

The patient may be held in this position in the gymnasium (which is a change from the ward) where he may have free use of any movements available in the arms and where he can make social contact with other patients. This may seem to be of small value but values must be related to the situation of the patient. If left, he would be curled up into flexion at this stage, have kidney failure, pressure sores and be unable to make any social contacts; the remaining weeks would be spent in more discomfort than necessary.

FUNCTIONAL INDEPENDENCE

At some stage in his rehabilitation the patient will require help towards functional independence. Exactly when this is encouraged will depend upon the type of condition and the method of management being used.

To be manageable at home the patient should be able to move himself up and down and about his own bed. He should be able to transfer himself from his bed to a chair of any kind and if he is a wheelchair patient, he should be able to manoeuvre the wheelchair about the house and transfer from wheelchair to toilet seat and into the bath etc. All these things should be possible with minimal assistance from relatives. In some cases special hoists have to be supplied to patients to help them to be independent and aids have to be given to make some functions possible. It is, however, most important that aids are only supplied as a last resort or as an intermediate measure from which the patient will progress.

The physiotherapist and occupational therapist are involved in functional independence and should work in close conjunction with each other.

Such activities as dressing and washing must be related to the patient's ability to balance in various positions and to carry out fine movements of the hands. Although the occupational therapist is very involved with this aspect the physiotherapist must also take an interest since she is probably responsible for the balance training and will know when the patient can be expected to use hand skills.

For the housewife kitchen training is dealt with as a rule by the occupational therapist who is concerned with any adaptation required for the patient's own kitchen. However, the physiotherapist may well be able to help by giving the patient the necessary skills of movement so that she may use her kitchen either as it is or with its adaptations.

Home visits may be necessary and should be made ideally by the occupational therapist and the physiotherapist together. Much of the patient's treatment programme can be adjusted to suit the particular home problems and the physiotherapist gains much by seeing the difficulties likely to be faced by the patient.

In some cases functional independence cannot be achieved without some kind of aid such as a weight-relieving or weight-bearing caliper, a pair of sticks, elbow crutches, or a wheelchair. The patient must be correctly assessed for these appliances and must also be adequately instructed in their use.

The education of relatives is important. When the patient is sent home the relatives have an all-powerful position and can make or break the patient's progress. They need help to understand the problems faced by the patient and to know how best they can help him. If they smother him with help they may make him relinquish his independence and then he will be wholly dependent and become a burden. If they offer too little help life may become too difficult for the patient and he will give up trying. Thus the relatives have a considerable responsibility when the patient finally goes home.

Finally, the need to get out and to see other people is very great and relatives and patient alike must appreciate that confinement to four walls eventually imprisons the mind. Herein lies a great problem. Handicapped people often rely upon others to help them to get out and if they do not get away from home they become fractious and difficult since their horizons become narrowed. The opening of day centres for severely handicapped patients helps a great deal. Patients who have been away from home for a day meet their relatives in the evening with refreshed minds and have something to offer as a social contact. Naturally it is hoped that most patients will be able to work but those who cannot must not be forgotten and it is for these patients that day centres are of most value.

BIBLIOGRAPHY

Bobath, B. (1967). 'The very early treatment of cerebral palsy.' *Developmental Medicine and Child Neurology*, **9**, 4.

Bobath, B. (1978). *Adult Hemiplegia: Evaluation and Treatment*, 2nd edition. William Heinemann Medical Books Limited, London.

Bobath, K. (1966). *Motor Deficit in Patients with Cerebral Palsy*. William Heinemann Medical Books Limited, London.

Buller, A. J. (1968). 'Spinal reflex action.' *Physiotherapy*, **54**, 6.

Campbell, E. J. M., Dickinson, C. J. and Slater, J. D. H. (1981). *Clinical Physiology*, 5th edition. Blackwell Scientific Publications Limited, Oxford.

Carr, P. and Shepherd, R. (1980). *Early Care of the Stroke Patient*. William Heinemann Medical Books Limited, London.

Carr, P. (1980). *Physiotherapy in Disorders of the Brain*. William Heinemann Medical Books Limited, London.

Gesell, A. (1971). *The First Five Years of Life*. Harper and Row, New York.

Goff, B. (1969). 'Appropriate afferent stimulation.' *Physiotherapy*, **55**, 1.

Haymaker, W. and Woodhall, B. (1953). *Peripheral Nerve Injuries*. W. B. Saunders.

Holle, B. (1977). *Motor Development in Children: Normal and Retarded*. Blackwell Scientific Publications Limited, Oxford.

Illingworth, J. S. (1965). 'Sequence of development in the child.' *Physiotherapy*, **51**, 6.

Illingworth, J. A. (1979). *The Normal Child*, 7th edition. Churchill Livingstone, Edinburgh.

Knox, J. A. C. (1968). 'Neuromuscular transmission.' *Physiotherapy*, **54**, 6.

Knott, M. and Voss, D. (1969). *Proprioceptive Neuromuscular Facilitation Patterns and Techniques*, 2nd edition. Harper and Row, New York.

Lance, J. W. and McLeod, J. G. (1975). *A Physiological Approach to Clinical Neurology*, 2nd edition. Butterworths, London.

Lane, R. J. (1969). 'Physiotherapy in the treatment of balance problems.' *Physiotherapy*, **55**, 10.

Matthews, P. B. (1968). 'Receptors in muscle.' *Physiotherapy*, **54**, 6.

Sheridan, M. (1975). *Children's Developmental Progress from Birth to Five Years. The Stycar Sequences*, 2nd edition. NFER Publishing Company.

ACKNOWLEDGEMENTS

The author expresses her thanks to everyone who has helped her in the preparation of these chapters. She is particularly grateful to Margaret Knott of Vallejo, California and Dr and Mrs Karel Bobath of the Western Cerebral

Palsy Centre, London who originally stimulated her interest in this field of work.

She also thanks the staff of the Audiovisual Department of the Coventry (Lanchester) Polytechnic who have been most helpful in providing the new illustrations. She is also grateful to the parents of the children shown in the illustrations.

Finally, she thanks all the patients she has treated and her students – they are the best teachers of all.

Chapter 8

Spinal Cord Lesions – 1

by B. GOFF, M.C.S.P., O.N.C., DIP.T.P.

In the developing embryo up to the third month of fetal life the spinal cord occupies the whole length of the neural canal. The rate of growth of the vertebral column is greater than that of the spinal cord so that at birth the lower end of the cord lies opposite the third lumbar vertebra. The growth rate of the vertebral column continues to exceed that of the cord so that finally the lowest limit of the cord in the adult lies opposite the disc between the first and second lumbar vertebrae. One consequence of this disparity of bone and cord levels is that when injury to vertebrae causes cord damage it is at a lower segmental level than is the bone damage. For example, at thoracic ten vertebral level, cord damage would be to the first, second, third and fourth lumbar cord segments (Fig. 8/1). Damage to bone below lumbar two would cause damage to nerve roots within the neural canal but not to the spinal cord. Such damage is known as a cauda equina lesion.

Table 1. Examples of anatomical relationships of spinal cord and bony spinous processes in adults

Cord Segments	Vertebral Bodies	Spinous processes
C8	Lower C6 Upper C7	C6
T6	Lower T3 Upper T4	T3
T12 L1	T9	T8
L5	T11	T10
Sacral Segments	T12 and L1	T12 L1

With minor exceptions each pair of spinal nerves supplies an area of skin with cutaneous nerves and autonomic motor nerves, certain muscles or parts of muscles and certain portions of bones.

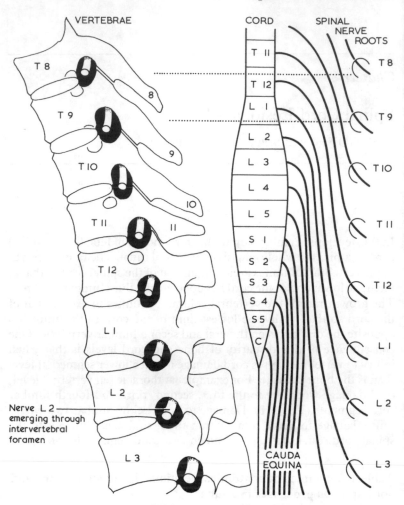

Fig. 8/1 Scheme to show relative nerve root, cord and bone levels of the lower segments of the spinal cord

The term *myotome* is used to indicate the muscles supplied by one pair of spinal nerves via the anterior root. The motor fibres arise from the anterior horn cells of one portion or segment of the cord, hence the term 'segmental innervation'.

Table 2. Simplified summary of motor segmental control of limb movements (myotomes)

LOWER LIMB

Hip	Adduction ⎫ Flexion ⎭	L2 ⎫ L3 ⎪	⎫ ⎬ L2 to L5
	Abduction ⎫ Extension ⎭	L4 ⎪ L5 ⎭	⎭
Knee	Extension	L3 and L4 ⎫ ⎬ L3 to S1	
	Flexion	L5 and S1 ⎭	
Ankle	Dorsiflexion	L4 and L5 ⎫ ⎬ L4 to S2	
	Plantar flexion	S1 and S2 ⎭	
Foot	Inversion Eversion	L4 L5 and S1	

Note that four segments of the cord control the hip movements overlapping with four segments which control the knee movements, the latter being one segment lower. Drop one segment and the next four segments control ankle movements.

UPPER LIMB

Shoulder	Abduction ⎫ Extension ⎭	C5
	Adduction ⎫ Flexion ⎭	C6 C7
Elbow	Flexion Extension	C5 and C6 C7 and C8
Forearm	Supination Pronation	C6 C6
Wrist	Flexion Extension	C6 and C7 C6 and C7

Fingers

Proximal interphalangeal	Flexion ⎤	C7
Metacarpophalangeal	Extension ⎦	C8
Distal interphalangeal	Flexion	C8
Metacarpophalangeal	⎧ Abduction ⎫	
	⎨ Flexion ⎬	
	⎩ Adduction ⎬	T1
Interphalangeal	Extension	
Thumb	Opposition ⎭	

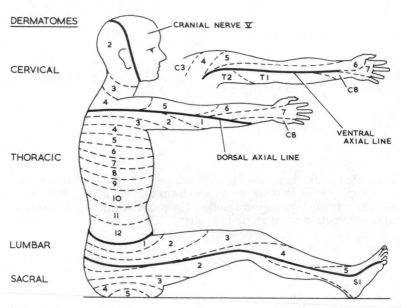

Fig. 8/2 Dermatomes of the body and segmental cutaneous distribution of upper limb

A *dermatome* is the term used to describe the area of skin whose sensory fibres pass to one segment of the cord via one sensory nerve root (Figs. 8/2 and 8/3). Similarly the term sclerotome is used for the area of the skeleton supplied via one spinal nerve root (Fig. 8/4).

Causes of Cord Lesions

1. The spinal cord can fail to develop, e.g. spina bifida and diastematomyelia.

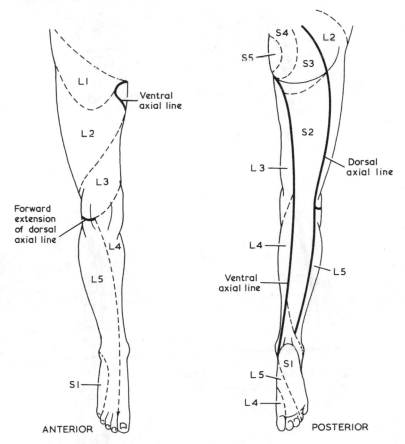

Fig. 8/3 Dermatomes of the lower limb

2. The cord may be crushed or lacerated as in fractures or fracture-dislocations of the vertebral column (Fig. 8/5).

3. The cord may be compressed as a result of bone disease, gross deformity of the vertebral column, oedema and inflammatory exudate and neoplasms.

4. The cord may, occasionally, be involved in inflammatory and degenerative lesions, e.g. in rheumatoid arthritis and osteoarthrosis.

5. The cord may be damaged as the result of inflammatory lesions which lead to an inadequate blood supply or conversely may cause a haemorrhage.

Trauma is most common in the cervical and the dorso-lumbar regions where mobility is greatest.

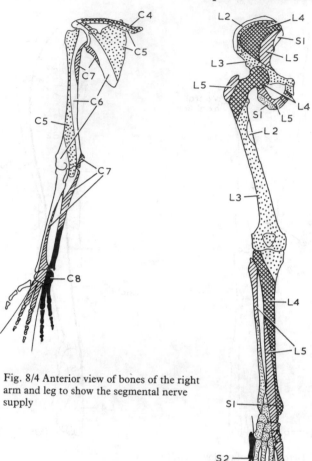

Fig. 8/4 Anterior view of bones of the right arm and leg to show the segmental nerve supply

The causes of spinal cord lesions produce various types of lesion. Sometimes the cord is completely destroyed for several centimetres, the damage may extend centrally to higher and lower segments, so-called 'coning', and possibly involve one or more nerve roots also. The cord may be only partially affected at one or more segments, the distribution being very variable but examples include a half lesion of one segment mainly affecting right or left halves of the cord, or certain tracts or cells. Accordingly the signs will vary not only with the level at which damage occurs but also depending upon its extent, severity and completeness.

Signs and Symptoms of Cord Lesions

The result of complete or partial destruction of a portion of the spinal cord can be considered in three parts.

1. Loss of function will occur of the cells destroyed at the level of the lesion.

2. There is loss of function of the fibres conveying impulses to the brain from below the level of the lesion. These are interrupted by the damage to the cord.

3. Tracts from cells in motor centres in the cerebrum, basal ganglia, cerebellum and brainstem are interrupted at the lesion causing loss of their modifying influence on spinal reflexes. The release symptoms of unmodified, exaggerated spinal reflexes only apply to the activity of undamaged segments of the cord caudal to the lesion. It should also be noted that some nerve roots may be permanently damaged within the neural canal or as they emerge from the intervertebral foramina.

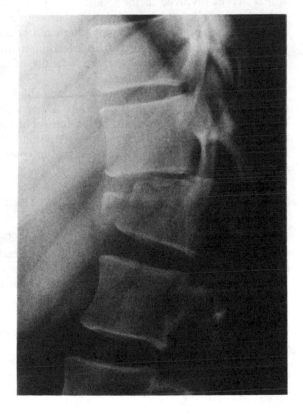

Fig. 8/5 Lateral radiograph of spine showing a fracture-dislocation of the thoracic 1 and lumbar 2 vertebrae, disrupting the neural canal

A variety of signs, symptoms, and functional disabilities result. The mode of onset, whether this is sudden or gradual influences the signs, as does the age of the patient. Treatment will accordingly vary with these factors.

SIGNS RESULTING FROM CELL DESTRUCTION

At the level of the lesion grey matter is destroyed. Destruction of lower motor neurone cells in the anterior horn results in permanent flaccid paralysis of the muscles they supply. Some muscles, partially innervated by spared motor neurones, will be weakened.

Cells in the posterior horn are interneurones and second order sensory cells. When these are destroyed incoming impulses at the level will fail to be transmitted further. Not only does this result in loss of sensation but it interrupts also the afferent arm of reflex arcs with resultant loss of reflex activity at the affected site. A similar result follows the destruction of cells in the posterior root ganglia of any spinal nerves involved in the lesion.

In the thoracic and upper two lumbar segments the cells in the lateral horn are preganglionic sympathetic motor cells. Destruction of these results in vasomotor disturbance leading to impaired circulation and nutrition. Also as a result there is failure of regulation of blood pressure and body temperature.

Similarly, in sacral segments the cells in the lateral horn are pre-ganglionic parasympathetic motor cells. Destruction of these in low level lesions destroys or impairs reflex control of the tone in the walls and sphincter of the urinary bladder. Automatic bladder control is thus almost impossible to train as a flaccid or spastic bladder persists after the initial stages.

SIGNS RESULTING FROM INTERRUPTION OF WHITE FIBRE TRACTS

It is thought that when white fibres are destroyed within the central nervous system they do not regenerate, so permanent interruption of nerve conduction occurs.

The ascending tracts convey impulses to the sensorium and also to many other centres in the brain. Interruption of these not only results in loss of all modes of sensation below the level of destruction but also produces a profound effect on centres controlling automatic postural reactions.

The descending tracts convey impulses from the pyramidal, extrapyramidal and cerebellar upper motor systems mainly via the cortico-spinal, reticulo-spinal, rubro-spinal and vestibulo-spinal tracts. Interruption of these tracts produces release symptoms because the undamaged motor cells below the level of the lesion are now free to respond, with no modification, to all incoming afferent stimuli. Spinal reflex action is apparent once spinal shock has worn off.

Stimuli which will produce flexor withdrawal, or crossed extensor reflexes include not only potentially harmful ones such as a pin-prick but also a sudden change in temperature, a pressure sore, bladder infection, sudden noise, or even the movement of bedclothes. All muscles respond to stretch so, after a flexor withdrawal has occurred and gravity tends to pull the limb down again, a second flexor spasm sometimes occurs elicited by the resulting stretch as the flexors relax. In some cases flexor spasticity is very difficult to prevent and every care must be taken to try to avoid reinforcement and exaggeration of this by such factors as are listed above.

SIGNS RESULTING FROM CELL AND FIBRE IRRITATION

Some cells and fibres may not be completely destroyed but inflammatory reaction and, later, scar tissue sometimes cause irritation which, especially in the case of sensory cells and fibres, is very troublesome. 'Girdle' pains and 'phantom limbs' are examples of this.

SIGNS RESULTING FROM INVOLVEMENT OF NERVE ROOTS

In most cases several nerve roots at the level of cord damage are also involved. This adds to the severity of the signs from damage at the level of the lesion.

In a minority of cases it appears that many nerve roots are damaged even below the bone damage, possibly from traction on the whole spinal cord at the time of the injury. This may explain the absence of spinal reflex activity which persists permanently in a minority of cases.

VISCERAL SIGNS

In complete lesions and in some partial ones control of external sphincters of bowel and bladder is lost so double incontinence occurs. There is also loss of sexual function.

FUNCTION LOSS

Control of active movement is impossible in complete lesions. In partial lesions spasticity is usually present so even if some control of limb movement is spared this is of a mass primitive type. Control of postural stability is absent or so masked by flexor or extensor mass patterns of movements that normal use of the limbs for stance, locomotion or manipulative skills is impossible.

Postural and equilibrium reactions are lost and absence of protective pain makes joint and skin damage a serious possibility.

Respiratory function and removal of secretions from the respiratory tract are impaired in all high level lesions.

Secondary Complications

CHEST COMPLICATIONS

In high level lesions where the intercostal muscles are paralysed, vital capacity and ventilation are reduced, and paralysis of the abdominal muscles makes coughing ineffective or impossible. Secretions collect in the lungs and cannot be removed by the patient's own efforts.

VISCERAL COMPLICATIONS

Bladder infection, retention or a high residual urine are likely complications.

CIRCULATORY COMPLICATIONS

Vasomotor paralysis, loss of movement and use of the affected parts all impair circulation. Deep vein thrombosis occurs in trunk or leg vessels of some patients.

Oedema and trophic changes frequently occur in the hands of tetraplegic patients. Because of interruption of nerve pathways from the vasomotor centre in the medulla oblongata the regulation of peripheral resistance and therefore of blood pressure is not adequate. Sudden changes of position from the horizontal to the vertical, result in pooling of blood in the abdomen and legs with the consequence that syncope and vertigo are frequent complications: this is most severe and persistent in high level lesions.

LOSS OF JOINT RANGE AND SOFT TISSUE RANGE

Joint range becomes limited and soft tissue contractures soon prevent good functional positioning unless treatment is vigilantly carried out regularly.

DEFORMITY

This may be defined as a malalignment of body segments which impairs or prevents function. It is related to loss of joint and soft tissue range. Impaired circulation, deposition of calcium salts in soft tissue around joints, persistent pull of spastic muscles or unopposed pull of spared muscles whose antagonists are flaccid all contribute to the risk of deformity. Certain muscle groups are stronger than their antagonists or more likely to be involved in spastic reflex actions and the force of gravity mitigates against some joint positions.

JOINT AND SKIN DAMAGE

Unrelieved pressure quickly impairs the circulation on weight-bearing surfaces. The loss of protective pain is devastating in its effect and because he is unaware of it the patient does not move to relieve pressure. Sunburn, extremes of temperature, scratches and strain on ligaments can all readily cause skin or joint damage. Prominent nails in shoes and failure to dry skin carefully after washing are other examples of how easily skin damage can occur. Poor circulation reduces the resistance to infection so abrasions or small pressure sores easily become infected. Careless handling of paralysed and insensitive parts can also contribute to joint or soft tissue damage or fractures.

CALCIFICATION OF SOFT TISSUE

In some cases calcium salts are laid down in soft tissue around joints (Fig. 8/6). The reasons for this are not fully understood but some disturbance of local circulation or trauma are possible causes.

SPASTICITY

The uncontrolled activity of lower motor neurones in undamaged segments of the spinal cord below the level of the lesion produces a

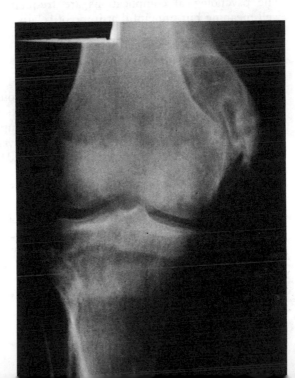

Fig. 8/6 Radiograph of knee joint showing calcified soft tissues

number of problems. The result may be severe flexor spasticity which predisposes to pressure sores, contractures, deformity and greatly reduced function. Even in partial lesions, with some control of movement of the trunk and limbs, spasticity prevents normal postural reactions and normal use of the part.

PSYCHOLOGICAL FACTORS

This is discussed finally not because it is the least important but because all other signs, symptoms and complications revolve around the degree of acceptance by the patient of his disability. The sudden complete loss of function, dependence on others and uncertainty about the future inevitably have a profound effect on the mental and emotional state of the patient. Even in patients whose lesion is at a low cord level or where the onset is gradual psychological problems may arise.

In the case of some tetraplegic patients the dependence, which lasts for many weeks and may be permanent, includes not only total care of bladder and bowel function, turning and all personal hygiene but also feeding with fluids and solid food.

Concern about dependants, relatives and friends, future occupation and indeed all domestic and social affairs can cause great distress to all but the very young.

The emotional state fluctuates: after an initial depression a period of reactionary optimism usually occurs followed later by the most difficult period of more penetrating realisation of the predicament. The psychological complications are frequently aggravated by a well-meaning but unhelpful attitude of relatives and friends.

The Influence of Mode of Onset

The rate and mode of onset influences the type of signs and symptoms which develop. A sudden interruption of the spinal cord, by violent trauma, haemorrhage or acute infection results not only in loss of function of the damaged segments but also, temporarily, of all function of the undamaged segments below the level of injury. This is known as 'spinal shock' and presumably is caused by lack of excitatory impulses from the brain since the segments above the lesion do not suffer in the same way (Fulton and McCouch, 1937). The signs are of complete loss of function of neurones and tracts. Thus there is complete loss of all forms of sensation of parts supplied from the level of the lesion and below it, together with flaccid paralysis of all skeletal muscles at and below the level of the cord injury. All reflex activity is lost. Visceral signs are of retention of urine and faeces and unless the patient is catheterised back pressure will occur and the kidneys will be damaged.

This state of complete non-function of the cord below the level of injury wears off gradually. Visceral signs change to overflow incontinence in a matter of days as some tone returns to the bladder wall. Spinal reflex activity returns gradually to the undamaged portion below the injured segments. The stretch reflex becomes apparent in muscles supplied from this portion of the cord presenting as spasticity of muscles. The time for this to develop is very variable as is the severity of flexor or extensor spasticity. In a minority of cases the flaccidity of all muscles below the level of the lesion remains permanent. The reason for this is not fully understood but one theory is that so many nerve roots are damaged at the time of the injury that conduction of nerve impulses along them is permanently interrupted.

Some injuries, being less severe than those described above, do not cause spinal shock. The signs are then similar to those described above as appearing when the spinal shock gradually wears off.

Cord lesions caused by pressure from the results of deformity or neoplasia and by degenerative lesions such as multiple sclerosis or syringomyelia also show no spinal shock. Instead a gradual development of impaired function presents as a variety of symptoms and signs. Loss of sensation is partial and may only include cutaneous or kinaesthetic sensation because interrupted impulses resulting in such loss normally travel in different tracts in the cord.

The motor signs are very variable but the most common sign is that caused by interruption of some fibres of the corticospinal tracts. This produces a spastic state of muscles similar to that in the leg of a patient with spastic hemiplegia.

The plantar response is extensor, ankle clonus occurs on slight stretch of the calf and gradually control of learned patterns of movement with selective control of individual joints is lost. Instead of the limbs taking part automatically in postural reactions to changing stimuli, only limited patterns of total movements are available.

Normal functions such as rising from sitting and normal gait are difficult or impossible. At first the extensor thrust pattern predominates, there being a combination of extension, adduction and medial rotation at hip, extension at knee, plantar flexion at ankle and inversion at the subtalar joint. Later, as the control from the brain is further reduced by more extensive cord involvement, the predominant pattern is of total flexor withdrawal of the leg or legs. It should be noted that these two patterns are produced by superficial muscles passing over two joints and the postural reactions of deeper muscles passing over only one joint are not elicited.

The reasons for this failure of normal postural reaction are complex. The spaastic total patterns prevent normal stimuli occurring in the deep pressure-bearing area of the heel or in the structures composing joints, thus abnormal afferent input elicits mass movement of withdrawal or thrust instead of postural stability for weight-bearing. There may also be interruption of some tracts of the spinal cord from the extrapyramidal and cerebellar centres, thus further reducing modification of spinal reflexes. If existing nerve pathways for postural reflexes are not used, synaptic resistance increases and the normal responses become less and less easy to elicit. Expressed differently this means that if spasticity is not relieved or reduced it becomes more severe. The flexor withdrawal reflex being the most primitive protective reflex is the most persistent and vicious reflex, once it is released from modification.

Circulatory disturbance occurs, which aggravates the sensory and motor disability. Secondary complications also produce further loss of function unless prevented by adequate treatment. Examples of this are contractures of soft tissue especially of the strong flexors of the hip and knee, the adductors of the hip and the calf muscles.

PRINCIPLES OF TREATMENT COMMON TO ALL SPINAL CORD LESIONS

Early Stage in Cases with Sudden Onset

The first principle is to save the patient's life. This is endangered from respiratory complications especially where the lesion is high in the cord. Secretions cannot be removed by coughing; therefore bronchial obstruction threatens to reduce further the vital capacity and ventilation which is already lowered by paralysis of intercostal and abdominal musnles. Intensive care is essential; a tracheostomy may be needed as well as artificial ventilation (IPPV). Secretions are removed by appropriate physiotherapy and suction.

Another basic need is to prevent further damage to the spinal cord while the vertebral column remains unstable. Means to achieve this include careful positioning and its maintenance by the use of pillows or special beds and, in cervical spine injuries, the use of skull traction.

The development of pressure sores, the loss of range in joints and soft tissue and circulatory complications can be discouraged by careful nursing procedures, turning and moving the patient at regular intervals. Physiotherapy plays an important part through passive movements and careful handling.

From the commencement of treatment and throughout the whole

rehabilitation programme the patient must be helped to accept his disability. A positive attitude must be encouraged and every means taken to help him achieve as much independence as possible. It should be pointed out that many occupations and sporting activities can be enjoyed. A paraplegic woman can run a home, bear children and bring them up. Insemination is possible by some males with spinal cord injuries; medical advice should be sought on this subject if required.

Stage When Weight-Bearing Through the Spine is Permitted

A work habit of regular hours five or six days a week is established once weight-bearing through the spine is permitted, usually at eight to twelve weeks after a spinal injury. Social activities during the evenings, at weekends and in competitive meetings such as paraplegic sporting contests all help to give a cheerful atmosphere to a spinal injuries unit.

Once weight is allowed through the spine emphasis is on activity to gain independence. This is achieved by nursing, physiotherapy and occupational therapy: adjustment to sitting and standing positions in wheelchairs and in splintage must be acquired; balance and posture training are taught. Care of their own skin and joints in insensitive areas must be taught by example and instruction.

Transfers from bed to chair, chair to lavatory, chair to floor and back must be learned and practised assiduously. Locomotion is achieved in a wheelchair or in some cases by the use of leg calipers and crutches. Resettlement at home and in a suitable occupation is the most important and all-pervading essential. The efforts of the patient, the whole medical and paramedical team together with the local welfare authorities and the patient's relatives must be coordinated to this end. The medical director of a specialised spinal injuries unit has an inspiring example of how to achieve such an objective in the person of the late Sir Ludwig Guttmann.

A final principle of increasing importance as more patients are successfully resettled out of hospital care is that of follow-up and after-care. Bringing patients back into hospital for regular review only partly achieves continued support. A system of domiciliary visiting by a specially trained nurse or therapist is helpful and this is now established for the wide area covered by the Midland Spinal Injuries Unit.

TEAM WORK

As is evident from the foregoing section, team work is essential. Consultation among and cooperation of the activities of all members of the team are imperative. All personnel concerned in any way with treatment and resettlement must understand the objectives at all stages. Each must have some knowledge of the role of the other members of the team. Often treatment involves nurses and therapists working together and the timing of turns and other procedures needs careful coordinating. This is necessary not only to avoid overlap but also to avoid too much disturbance of the patient or disruption of the programme of one or other team members. Ideally patients with spinal injuries should be treated in special centres with facilities for their total care at all stages of rehabilitation. In some instances it is also helpful if cases of progressive lesions of the spinal cord can be accommodated in a spinal injuries unit.

A list of the personnel concerned in the care of such patients is given below. It should be noted that the ambulance or first-aid team head the list as unskilled handling of a person with a suspected spinal cord injury can cause increased neurological damage.

Team Members

The team includes the following:
Ambulance and first-aid personnel.
Medical personnel including physicians, neurologists, orthopaedic surgeons, urologists, plastic surgeons, and radiologists. The medical director of a spinal injuries unit not only heads the team of consultants and registrars but coordinates the efforts of all personnel concerned in the well-being of the patients. Prognosis is his responsibility, as is the difficult task of deciding when to explain this to the patient and his relatives. When the patient is ready to go home the general practitioner plays a part in the ultimate stages of patient care.
Nursing personnel include the chief nursing officer, nurses at all levels of seniority and nursing aides and orderlies, both in hospital and the community.
Occupational therapists and physiotherapists whose efforts are often combined both have a vital role in rehabilitation of paraplegic and tetraplegic patients, both in hospital and the community.
Splint fitters and makers play an important part in preparing patients for standing and ambulation.
Welfare personnel include the social worker who provides an essential link between home and hospital. Her responsibility includes the arrangement of necessary social adjustments such as arranging for financial benefits and for alterations to the house. Local Authorities and the Disablement Resettlement Officer (DRO) of the Department of Health and Social Security are contacted by the social worker.

Physiotherapists, occupational therapists, nurses and the social worker usually cooperate in selecting and ordering such aids as splintage, urinals, wheelchairs, motorised vehicles, and also in advising on alterations to the home.

The DRO contacts employers and attempts to re-establish in suitable employment all patients who were wage earners previous to their illness or injury.

Personnel in training centres and industrial rehabilitation centres must also be included among those concerned with resettlement.

RELATIVES AND THE PATIENT

Lastly, but of vital importance, the relatives must be included as they have the task of support at all times. Eventually it is they and the patient himself who share the responsibility for the success or otherwise of restoring him to an independent life in the community. In the case of the most severely disabled patients the relatives may be able to undertake nursing care at home after suitable instruction and with the necessary equipment, e.g. a turning bed. The services of district nurses and health visitors may be required.

PROCEDURES

Surgery, nursing, physiotherapy and occupational therapy for patients varies in detail with the diversity of symptoms and signs at the different levels of cord injury. They also differ in accordance with the severity of interruption of cord activity. For this reason examples of therapy will be discussed in sub-sections. Certain procedures are common in all cases and are discussed as follows.

Surgery

Some surgeons favour open reduction of the fracture-dislocation for a very few cases. Indications for surgery include severe pain associated with massive haematoma, displacement of vertebrae which is unlikely to reduce spontaneously, and a history and x-ray evidence suggesting that surgery would relieve pressure and might thereby reverse some neurological signs. A further indication for surgery is the need to obtain stability of the vertebral column in cases where the paralysis of muscles and excessive weight of the patient cause mechanical difficulty. Surgery merely to attempt to relieve cord pressure is useless if there are signs of complete destruction of several segments of the cord. Such destruction is permanent and relief of pressure cannot obtain any improvement of neurological function. Contra-indications to surgery include signs of irreversible cord damage to a complete cross-section of the cord, sepsis, expectation of respiratory complications following general anaesthesia, and weakening of spared back muscles by surgical incisions.

Positioning

The principal aim of careful positioning is to hold the spine in such a position that further cord damage is prevented. This principle should be observed by the personnel who convey the patient from the scene of the accident to a hospital. It should continue to govern the subsequent procedures until the spine is considered sufficiently stable to allow trunk movement and weight to be taken through it in a vertical position. This is not usually until eight to twelve weeks after injury. Such positions must be maintained during all x-ray examinations, throughout all nursing and therapeutic procedures such as washing, attendance to bowel and bladder functions, clearing secretions from the chest and necessary change in position or passive movements of the limbs.

Secondary aims of careful positioning are to prevent circulatory complications, prevent deformity and damage to skin, joints, or soft tissue. Prevention of compression of veins especially in the calf and prevention of pressure on bony prominences help to achieve these aims.

Details of positions and methods to maintain them vary according to several factors. The level of the lesion is one factor; skull traction and support for the neck by sandbags, a cervical collar or special head rest is used for patients with cervical cord lesions. In the case of patients with a dorsal or lumbar vertebral level of lesion, support for the neck is not essential but the lower parts of the spine must be prevented from moving and the lumbar lordosis maintained. This is usually achieved by the placing of pillows. It is vital for all team members to be meticulous about positioning and in each case they must know which method is used and why it has been selected.

Another consideration in choosing a method of positioning is the number of persons available to turn the patient at regular intervals. A method which has been proved to be effective is the use of firm pillows and small mattress sections carefully placed under head, trunk and legs and to separate the legs and support the feet. A minimum of three trained persons is needed to execute each turn to a different position while maintaining the immobility of the spine. Details of this method may be found in standard nursing textbooks (see p.210).

Special beds have been designed to achieve maintenance of appropriate positions and to allow automatic and/or continual turning. The Rota-Rest bed is an example; its mechanism, electrically operated, turns the bed slowly through one hundred and thirty degrees, thus pressure on any point is never prolonged. A beneficial effect is also obtained on the lungs and possibly the kidneys. When the motor is switched off the bed remains stationary in any desired position so that nursing or physiotherapy procedures can be attended to. One great advantage of this type of bed is that a team is not needed for turning, therefore it is suitable for use both where there is a staff shortage and in the home for tetraplegic patients who cannot turn themselves even in the chronic stage.

Turning

Turning the patient in rotation from right side lying to supine, to left side lying and back to supine position is necessary during the early stage of bed rest. At first the turns are at two-hourly intervals throughout each twenty-four hours but gradually this may be reduced to three- or four-hourly turns providing there are no signs of threatened skin breakdown on pressure-bearing points such as the sacrum or the femoral trochanters. During the turn the position of the spine must be maintained and special instruction and training must be given to all personnel on the ward who at any time help to form the turning team. The senior nurse present must direct the team and ensure that the turn is correctly done; she also gives commands so that the timing of the turn is coordinated. During the turn linen may be changed, the undersheet straightened and meticulous care taken to ensure that no crumbs or other abrasive material are left in the bed. The skin must be inspected to detect any signs of threatening pressure sores. Care must be taken not to disturb the catheter, if present, or other intubation such as a naso-oesophageal tube or tracheostomy tube. Details of care of a tracheostomy tube and treatment for respiratory complications will be discussed later but it should be noted that physiotherapy techniques to help clear secretions and to assist coughing are frequently needed prior to, and after, turning.

The nursing and physiotherapy staff should work in close cooperation at all times but in the early stages of care of the cervical cord cases this is particularly necessary, not only to avoid too many disturbances for the patient, and to make the contribution of each team member more effective, but also because they often act as a substitute for each other. Physiotherapists frequently act as members of the turning or lifting team; and all personnel working on a spinal unit should be taught how to make the patient cough to help clear secretions.

Another important feature of the turn is that the limbs are re-positioned at each turn. This not only ensures relief of pressure on bony points but helps maintenance of circulation and joint and soft tissue mobility. It is a disadvantage of the use of the automatically turning bed that the limb joints are not moved as it turns. Physiotherapy care for patients on these beds needs to be more frequent for this reason. Special types of bed in spinal injuries units include water beds, low air loss beds and automatic turning beds.

Chest Care

Respiratory complications occur in patients with spinal cord lesions for many reasons, for example, pre-existing chronic respiratory disorder, lowered resistance to infection, paralysis of muscles of inspiration or those needed for effective coughing. An added factor is paradoxical respiration caused by paralysis of intercostal muscles. Details of physiotherapy will be found on p.186, but any case of spinal cord injury or dysfunction from other causes may require treatment to prevent internal secretional obstruction and to improve the ventilation of the lungs. All cases should have respiratory function tests carried out regularly and the results should be recorded. Vital capacity measurements with a spirometer, peak flow measurements using a Wright's peak flow meter or a Vitalograph machine are routine procedures in most spinal injuries units.

Care of the Urinary Bladder and the Bowels

As the paraplegic or tetraplegic patient has double incontinence the care of the kidneys, urinary bladder and excretion of urine and faeces is as urgent and essential as care of the chest, skin and circulation. Ultimate responsibility for this is borne by the medical director but the task of catheterisation in the early days of spinal shock and later of training an automatic bladder function, falls to the medical and nursing staff. The physiotherapist needs to be fully aware of the care to avoid retention of urine, or infection of the bladder and also how to avoid damage to urinals by careless handling, positioning or application of splintage.

In later stages of treatment the activities of the patient are largely carried out by or in the presence of the therapist and she must appreciate that the insensitivity of the patient's skin prevents his awareness of the leakage of urine or faeces, or the twisting and trapping of any part of his urinal; she must teach him, therefore, by the example of her careful handling and observation and by instruction how to avoid such accidents. Tact is needed to help the patient 1) to accept the distressing complication of double incontinence, 2) to be responsible ultimately for his own care of bladder and bowel function and 3) to help him to realise how vital is such care not only to his social acceptability but also to his general well-being.

Retention of urine or a bladder infection not only have a direct effect on kidneys and general health but also greatly increase the severity of spasticity of the limbs. Obviously the care of these matters is more difficult or even impossible for the tetraplegic patient, but the responsibility can still be his as he can request attention if needed and should be encouraged to take such responsibility for himself.

Transfers

Certain fundamental points relating to transfers apply equally whether the patient can achieve them himself or has to depend on others to lift him (p. 180). All members of the team concerned in any way with patient care should know how to lift patients alone or with help, and how he should lift himself, if possible, without damage to skin or joints. The physiotherapist can help instruct other personnel such as orderlies and nursing aides in this important procedure.

Assessment and Documentation of Records

The capabilities of the patient, his control of movement, the extent of motor and sensory loss and also later his ability to compensate for motor loss must be assessed at regular intervals. Joint range and the presence of any deformity likely to impair function should also be considered. The examination of the patient and tests for functional ability including the respiratory function tests are carried out by several members of the team: doctors, physiotherapists and occupational therapists all share this responsibility. Charts of function achievement specially prepared for paraplegic and tetraplegic patients are helpful.

ACHIEVEMENT CHART
NAME
AGE

PHYSIOTHERAPY AND OCCUPATIONAL THERAPY
CLINICAL DIAGNOSIS
CORD LEVEL

Weight and Pulley (Shoulder Extensors ....lbs...........lbs...........lbs...........lbs
and Adductors)
Springs fixed to bed head (Triceps) ....lbs...........lbs...........lbs...........lbs

		A	Date	Ach	Date	Comments
Balance	i. Long sitting					
	ii. High sitting					
Wheelchair management	i. Propulsion					
	ii. Brakes					
	iii. Pressure relief					
Transfers	Bed ....Chair					
	Toilet ....Chair					
	Floor ....Chair					
	Bath ....Chair					
	Easy Chair........Chair					
	Car ....Chair					
Turning	i. Mat					
	ii. Bed					

A.D.L. (Women)	i. Feeding					
	ii. Drinking					
	iii. Teeth					
	iv. Washing and Drying					
	v. Make-up					
	vi. Hair					
Housecraft	i. Kitchen					
	ii. Housework					
	iii. Laundry					
	iv. Ironing					
Standing Walking	a. Bars					
	i. 4pt.					
	ii. Swing-to					
	iii. Swing-thro'					
	b. Crutches					
	i. 4pt.					
	ii. Swing-to					
	iii. Swing-thro'					
With crutches	i. Transfers					
	ii. Stairs					
	iii. Kerbs					
	iv. Uneven surfaces					

		A	Date	Ach	Date	Comments
Dressing and undressing	i. Top half ii. Bottom half iii. Shoes & Stockings					
A.D.L. (Men)	i. Feeding ii. Drinking iii. Teeth iv. Washing & Drying v. Shaving vi. Hair vii. Emptying Urinal					
Communication	i. Writing ii. Typing					
Sport	i. Archery ii. Table Tennis iii. Swimming iv. Others					
Motorised transport	i. Normal ii. Hand Controls					

A=Attempted   Ach=Achieve

Nurses measure and chart such things as body temperature, pulse and respiratory rate, arterial blood pressure, fluid intake and output.

All records must be carefully dated and filed and be freely available to other team members. Regular consultation between all team members at case conferences are needed and are greatly enhanced by well kept records.

REFERENCE

Fulton, J. F. and McCrouch, G. P. (1937). 'Spinal shock.' *Journal of Nervous and Mental Diseases*, **86**, 125.

BIBLIOGRAPHY

See p. 210.

Chapter 9

Spinal Cord Lesions – 2

by B. GOFF, M.C.S.P., O.N.C., DIP.T.P.

Both the degree of potential independence a patient can achieve and the necessary physiotherapy vary according to the level and severity of damage to the spinal cord. Treatment will be discussed in sections.

COMPLETE LESIONS

LOW PARAPLEGIA

If a fracture of the ninth thoracic vertebra causes damage to the spinal cord the segments involved will be in the region of the twelfth thoracic and first and second lumbar cord segments. The roots of the twelfth thoracic and first lumbar nerves may also be damaged as may nerve roots of thoracic nine, ten and eleven as they also lie within the neural canal at the level of the fracture (see Fig. 8/1, p. 150).

Severe damage to the cord at this level is a frequent consequence of fracture-dislocation of the spine and results in permanent neurological dysfunction. This level of lesion has been selected as typical of a complete low level paraplegia. 'Complete' is taken to mean a lesion in which no voluntary control of muscles returns and in which the complete sensory loss is permanent. In some such cases there is clinical evidence that motor centres in the mid-brain may have some influence over the spinal reflex activity of the undamaged cord segments below the lesion. This implies that there may be nerve conduction via some upper motor pathways although those necessary for willed movement are interrupted.

As onset is sudden, spinal shock occurs and persists for several weeks. Medical and nursing care is described in Chapter 8. Physiotherapy will now be described, giving details of the most important techniques at various stages of rehabilitation.

Treatment in the Early Stage

The aims of physiotherapy are to help prevent the complication of deep vein thrombosis; to help maintain a good circulation to the lower limbs, thus lessening the risk of pressure sores and to maintain range of joints and soft tissue. As soon as is allowed, strengthening exercises are given for the upper limbs; the exact time for this after injury depends on the stability or otherwise of the spine and whether there are any fractures of the clavicle or ribs. Activity also helps to achieve another aim which is to aid the patient's psychological adjustment to his disability.

Only cases with pre-existing chronic chest disorders or trauma to the chest at the time of injury are likely to need intensive physiotherapy to maintain or improve respiratory function.

During all treatments the principle of preserving the correct position of the spine and its immobility must be observed. Care is taken not to disturb the catheter. Vigilant observation of skin colour and temperature is necessary and signs of any circulatory abnormality such as oedema must be noted and reported, as should any sign of return of muscle tone to the leg muscles.

METHODS

Passive movements to the legs: These are carried out at least twice daily in the first three to six weeks and possibly reduced to once a day later if good circulation and range are being maintained. As hip extension to neutral is not possible in the lowermost limb with the patient in side lying it may be necessary to visit the patient several times so that each leg can be treated when it is uppermost.

Sensitive handling is needed because damage can occur to soft tissue around joints especially during the stage of spinal shock. It is also necessary later to guard against eliciting spinal reflexes. The physiotherapist must learn to feel when the limit of joint and soft tissue range is approached. Movements should be in normal patterns, performed slowly and eventually in full range at least twice at each handling. During the first few weeks pain at the site of the lesion may limit slightly the range obtained on passive movement.

Maintenance of the length of some structures which pass over more than one joint is especially important to prevent deformity which would later hamper good function such as long sitting, standing, or crutch walking. Overstretching of soft tissue is harmful, but functional length must be maintained in the following structures: muscles, tendons, ligaments, and fascia. For long sitting, length is needed in the hamstrings. For standing, full hip and knee extension and length of calf and fascia sufficient to allow at least 90° at the ankle with knee straight and the foot flat on the floor are required. Toes should not be allowed to curl or claw so that shoes can be put on easily and do not cause pressure sores.

To improve circulation passive leg movements are repeated for at least three minutes to each leg and for this purpose need not be in full range. The legs are moved one at a time and care is taken not to allow sufficient hip flexion to cause movement of the lumbar spine. If there is any sign of oedema careful measurement of girth of the calf is made, recorded and subsequently repeated for comparison. The prothrombin time is taken and the leg movements stopped until the doctor gives permission to recommence them. After treatment the pillows supporting the legs and feet are replaced correctly.

The exact number of treatments needed each day depends upon such factors as the method of nursing and turning the patient, his age and the probability of circulatory complications. When the automatic turning bed is used, limb movements by physiotherapists are needed more frequently than for patients who are turned manually as in the latter case leg positions are changed at each two-, three- or four-hourly turn.

When spinal shock wears off, muscle tone returns to the leg muscles and very careful nursing and handling during physiotherapy are needed to prevent reinforcement of spasticity. The physiotherapist's hands should be smooth and warm and care taken not to elicit either a flexor withdrawal or an extensor thrust (Fig. 9/1). Pressure through the heel and the long axis of the limb together with slow smooth movements tend to elicit a postural response of all deep muscles acting on the knee and ankle. These then work in combination to stabilise the

Fig. 9/1 Position of contacts when handling leg with spasticity

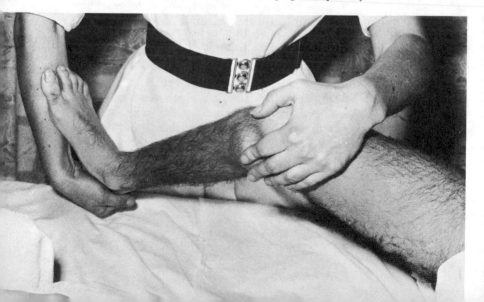

joint as they do in normal weight-bearing and total spastic movements are inhibited.

Exercises: Six to eight weeks after onset some increasing activity of upper limbs is usually allowed. Exercises are given to strengthen the arm and upper trunk muscles and to maintain full range of movement in preparation for transfers, use of wheelchair and crutch walking. Any suitable method of graded resisted exercises is used and progressed as the muscles strengthen. Strong grip, elbow extension, shoulder adduction and extension and depression of the shoulder girdle are needed for activities.

Instability of the spine or pain in the back may delay the start of greater activity but at eight to twelve weeks after injury the patient is usually allowed to commence taking weight vertically through the spine. During the rest period a wheelchair is ordered and it is ready by the time the patient gets up. Full length band-topped calipers, hinged at the knee, are measured for and supplied, either at the end of the bed stage or early in the weight-bearing stage.

Residual neurological defects are now apparent and must be assessed and recorded. The level of cutaneous and kinaesthetic loss is from thoracic eleven or twelve downwards including the skin of the lower trunk, buttocks and legs and joint sensation of pelvis and legs. The lower portions of the trunk muscles, the hip flexors and adductors are often found to remain flaccid when spinal shock wears off. This is because the lower motor neurone cells at thoracic twelve and lumbar one and two cord segmental levels are destroyed by the damage to the cord.

The nerve roots of thoracic nine to twelve spinal nerves are also likely to be damaged at the level of the spinal injury where they lie within the neural canal.

The remainder of the leg muscles usually show spasticity because the lower part of the cord is not damaged but is partially or completely isolated from the influence of the brain and shows only spinal reflex activity.

The severity of spasticity varies with the efficiency of early treatment, with the position of the patient and in response to incoming stimuli from the skin, deep structures of the legs and from the urinary bladder. If involuntary spasms occur the risk of pressure sores is increased. Sores, bladder infection, and contractures in soft tissue all increase stimuli likely to elicit spasms and aggravate spasticity. A vicious cycle may result as increased spasticity and uncontrolled spasms predispose to a greater risk of contractures, sores, bladder dysfunction and later, when the patient is allowed up, to poor posture and function (Fig. 9/2). It is affected by psychological stress and is

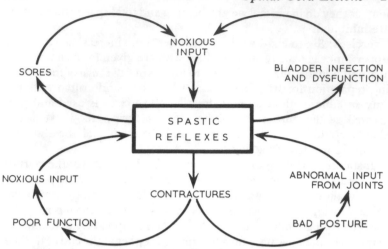

Fig. 9/2 Vicious cycles

much more troublesome in some patients than in others. Although so many factors influence spasticity an attempt should be made to evaluate its severity. Techniques to try to relieve spasticity and to prevent its reinforcement will be discussed on pp. 191–4. It must be remembered that there is a great risk of dominance by the flexor withdrawal reflex in complete cord lesions unless adequate treatment is given to prevent this.

Stage When Weight-Bearing Through the Spine is Permitted

Treatment is rapidly progressed to increasing activity by the patient. The nursing staff are usually responsible for sitting the patient up in bed with the back supported by a back rest. Physiotherapy is given with the patient sitting up in bed to commence balance training and lifts to relieve pressure.

When the patient is allowed to sit out in a wheelchair the aims of treatment are as follows:

READJUSTMENT OF POSTURAL SENSE AND EQUILIBRIUM REACTIONS

The patient must learn to retain a good posture and to maintain balance in many positions without the support of a back rest or his arms (Fig. 9/3). The physiotherapist must appreciate that until the patient sits up for the first time with no support or contact with a

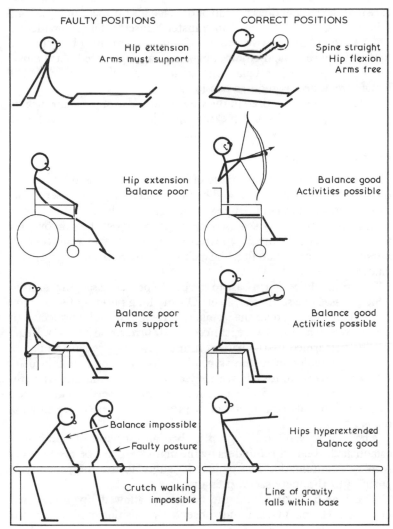

Fig. 9/3 Correct and faulty positions

supporting surface for his head, trunk or arms he cannot fully realise the consequence of the sensory loss in the lower part of his body.

Posture correction and balance is trained with the patient sitting on a pillow on a low plinth. The feet should be supported on the floor or a low platform so that the thighs are fully supported and the hips, knees and ankles are at a right angle. The physiotherapist should take great care that the patient does not fall or damage his buttocks or legs. Until he is strong and has learned to transfer himself safely the patient is lifted to the plinth by two people. Use of a mirror may be helpful at first and any suitable method of balance training is used. Arm movements are given when balance is good and activities including ball games are added as soon as possible.

Balance is also practised in the wheelchair. Use of the chair, negotiation of slopes, curbs and picking up objects from the floor are all taught.

CARE OF SKIN AND JOINTS

This must be taught by example of careful handling and by instruction. All insensitive parts should be protected by vigilant observation, avoidance of extremes of temperature, careful positioning and inspection. A hand mirror is used by the patient to inspect the skin over the sacrum and ischial tuberosities. He is instructed to report to the nursing staff immediately he suspects that there is any sign of skin damage.

There should be a firm base to the bed to prevent a sagging mattress which causes creases in the sheet. During long periods of sitting in a wheelchair the skin over the ischial tuberosities must be protected by using a wooden-based, sheepskin covered, firm sorbo cushion. Regular lifts performed by the patient himself, relieve pressure and allow return of circulation to the skin. The lifts must be maintained for fifteen to thirty seconds and are needed every fifteen minutes when the patient first sits up. Some patients eventually need to lift at less frequent intervals but the relief of pressure soon becomes an automatic action.

The patient can turn himself in bed and a habit of doing so is established. Regular reminders by the night staff may be needed until turning is automatic. The patient is taught to use the prone lying position to eliminate sacral pressure.

The length of time that the patient is allowed up is gradually increased. He must be taught to observe the position of his legs and to lift them carefully when moving.

SELF-CARE

The patient must be able to wash, dress, attend to his own urinal, maintain joint range in the legs by doing his own passive movements and apply his calipers. These activities are taught by several members of the team but balance in the long sitting position must be achieved to facilitate good function.

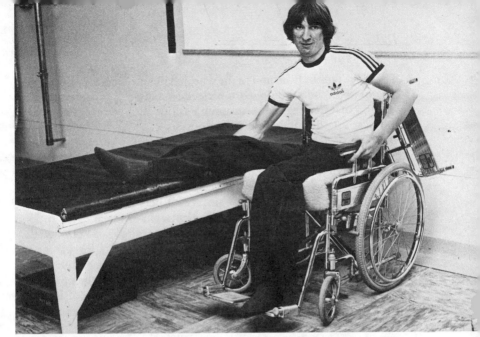

Fig. 9/4 Preparation to transfer from chair to plinth. Chair arm is removed; the chair is alongside the plinth; the near leg lifted to the plinth

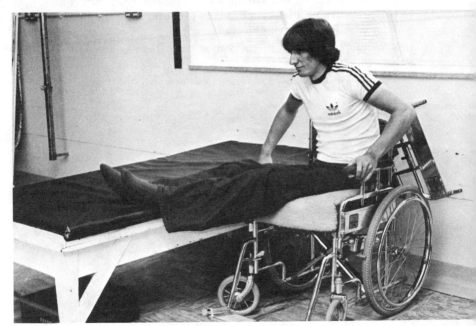

Fig. 9/5 The far leg has been lifted to the plinth; the arms are ready to lift

TRANSFERS (Figs. 9/4 to 9/7)

These are taught from and to the wheelchair and the bed, plinth, bath, lavatory seat, and motorised vehicle. Also taught is safe transfer from and to a mat for treatment sessions. Various methods are tried out and the best for the individual is finally selected.

In teaching safe transfers the principles include correct positioning of the chair, ensuring that the brakes are fully on and lifting the legs with the hands on to the plinth, bed or floor from the footplates of the chair. During these manoeuvres care must be taken not to knock the legs or drag them along a hard surface. When the legs are positioned correctly the trunk is lifted so that the buttocks are clear of the support and will not be dragged or knocked as the transfer is completed.

In transferring from a wheelchair to a plinth the approach can be from the side or one end. In the former case the chair is placed slightly obliquely alongside the plinth, the arm of the chair on the near side is removed and if necessary a pillow placed over the top of the large wheel of the chair; the brakes are applied securely. Next the legs are lifted and placed on the plinth, the far leg is sometimes crossed over the other. Then the near-side hand is placed on the plinth sufficiently centrally to allow room for the buttocks to be placed on the plinth also, the other hand is placed on the far side-arm of the chair. A good high lift of the trunk follows and it is swung over onto the plinth and the long-sitting position is thus obtained.

Whatever method of transfer is used there is a risk of the chair

Fig. 9/6 A high lift is necessary to clear the chair wheel, as the trunk is lifted to the plinth

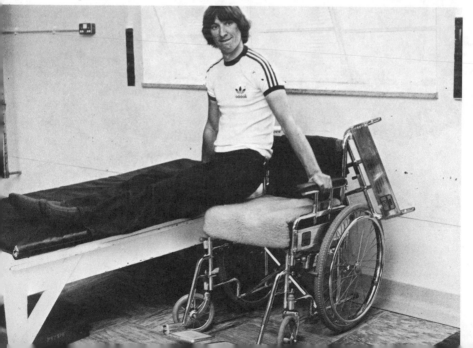

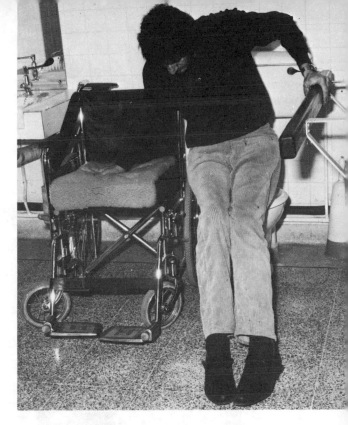

Fig. 9/7 Transfer from a wheelchair to lavatory

moving if the tyres are worn or the floor slippery. The patient soon learns to be cautious and to position the chair correctly to avoid slipping between the chair and the plinth (Fig. 9/4).

A PROGRAMME OF RESISTED EXERCISES (Figs. 9/8 and 9/9)

This is arranged for all spared muscles. Mat work, transfers, use of weight and pulley circuits including the use of a Westminster pulley circuit and also proprioceptive neuromuscular facilitation (PNF) techniques of manually resisted trunk and limb patterns of movement are all useful. Rookwood Hospital, Cardiff and Oswestry, use a Gym-pac System for resisted exercises (see p.210).

SPORT

This is now included, e.g. swimming, team ball games in wheelchairs, archery and field events. These achieve many objectives, for example, they provide strong exercise, balance training, stimulation of increased exercise tolerance and an opportunity for social activities in the evenings and at weekends in competition with other patients.

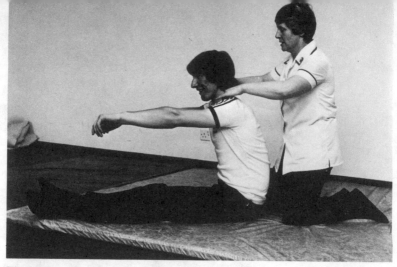

Fig. 9/8 Balance training

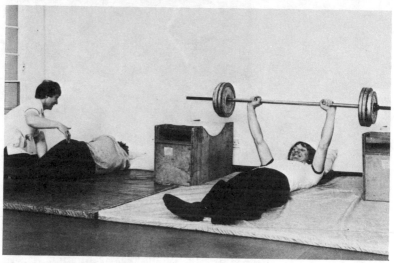

Fig. 9/9 Rolling and weight lifting

STANCE AND GAIT

These are trained as soon as sitting balance is good. Standing balance in leg calipers is taught in parallel bars. The posture is very important as the weight must be over the feet to keep upright without the control of muscular power in gluteal muscles and hamstrings. The patient must learn to pay attention to sensation in the upper trunk and compensate for loss of equilibrium reactions in the legs and lower trunk. The hips must be slightly hyperextended and the dorsal spine straight. Many patients can maintain good balance for short periods without the support of both arms. This skill is essential for a good 'swing-to' or 'swing-through' gait.

To get to standing from the wheelchair the patient first extends the knees passively and locks the knee hinges in extension. Some patients need to place the leg on a support to achieve this, others manage by a 'high kick' type of lift or by extending the leg out in front of the chair with the foot on the floor. When both knees are locked in extension, and the chair correctly placed with the brakes on, the buttocks are lifted forward to the front of the chair seat, the hands grip the parallel bars or wall bars and a lift up and forward takes the body into the standing position. Care is needed to see that the feet do not slip forwards.

In the early stages of training, weak patients, or those with short arms, may need assistance and the physiotherapist stands in front of the patient, between the bars, placing her feet in front of the patient's shoes and if necessary gripping the top of trousers or slacks to assist the action of standing.

Gait is trained at first in parallel bars progressing to one crutch and one bar as the patient gains confidence and proficiency. Finally, two crutches are used and steps, slopes, curbs, rough surfaces and stairs are negotiated if possible. The four point gait is the most elegant and takes least room in a crowded place. However the swing-to or swing-through gait is quicker and most young patients with strong arms can achieve this method of crutch walking. Elbow crutches with swivel tops are used so that the patient can stand and rest his forearm on the upturned arm support and have his hand free to open doors. 'Canadian' type ring top crutches with the ring above the elbow have been found useful. The hand can be used to open doors, and the crutch remains on the arm (Fig. 9/10). Some spinal units use rigid walking frames instead of crutches.

When the patient is proficient in crutch walking he learns to get up from the chair to standing, place the crutches correctly for use, turn and walk away from the chair. This activity needs careful planning, strong arms and upper trunk and good equilibrium reactions to gain balance once upright. The exact method is usually worked out by each patient to suit his or her particular abilities. The physiotherapist uses her experience to help each patient learn this activity. A demonstration by more experienced patient, such as one back in hospital for review, can be most helpful.

One method of standing up from the wheelchair with no other support than the chair will be described. The turn can be to either side to suit the individual's abilities but will be described as for turning to

the left. The chair is placed with the back against a wall or firm
support and the brakes secured. The calipers are locked in extension
and the right leg lifted across the left. The shoulders and trunk are
twisted to the left so that the left hand is placed behind the patient's
trunk on the right chair arm and the right across in front of the trunk
on to the left arm of the chair. A good high lift follows with a twist of
the pelvis to bring the patient to standing facing the chair. He then

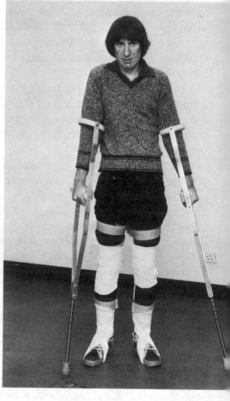

Fig. 9/10 Patient standing with the
aid of Canadian crutches and back
splints

achieves balance in standing so that he can release one arm to reach
and place his crutches ready to back away from the chair and walk.

Other methods may be possible, each patient should be encouraged
to find the most suitable method for his ability. The crutches must be
placed near or leaning against the chair so that they are within reach
when stance is achieved. Patients should be encouraged to discuss
their achievements and difficulties during treatment sessions, and
group activities are of great psychological value.

Overcoming physical difficulties can be a source of great fun and the sense of achievement is similar to that of learning any new skill. To create a happy atmosphere but one of hard work should be the objective of every physiotherapist working in a spinal unit.

TRANSPORT

This should be encouraged in either a car supplied by the Department of Health and Social Security to a disabled driver or in a specially adapted car of his own. Transfers to and from these and lifting a transit chair into and out of the car must be taught and arrangements made for driving instruction.

ASSESSMENT OF THE PATIENT'S ABILITY

Function charts are useful to record this. Regular reassessments are helpful, not only to note progress but to stimulate the patient's interest and to help to wean him from dependence on physiotherapy or nursing staff. Detailed sensory charts are completed by the medical staff or may be the responsibility of physiotherapists. Tests of voluntary power are only appropriate for muscles completely or partially denervated by loss of lower motor neurones at the level of the lesion. Power in spastic muscles cannot be graded on a voluntary power scale but the severity of spasticity should be evaluated and recorded.

During the time of increasing activity the social worker and the occupational therapist will discuss possible occupational training which may be needed, also any necessary alterations to the home.

Every encouragement should be given to include relatives in the rehabilitation of patients from an early stage. For example they are shown by the physiotherapist how to help the patient care for his skin and how to maintain full joint and soft tissue range.

As can be seen by the variety and extent of the new skills the patient must learn, there should be very little time for inactivity. A full day's programme five or six days a week is helpful in maintaining a work habit and is of immense psychological value. He should be responsible for his own timekeeping as this helps to restore self-respect and leads to independence.

Before the patient is finally discharged he is usually allowed home for weekends. This allows for gradual adjustment to a new life style, and on his return any problems encountered can be discussed. Time spent at home is eventually increased to periods of a week or longer before final discharge.

Follow-up after discharge by frequent reviews is needed to provide continuing support when the patient returns to the community.

At each review the following must be checked: the range of joints and soft tissue, the health of the bladder and of the skin, also the state

of splints, crutches and the wheelchair. Any problems which
have occurred can be discussed and all help given to maintain full
independence.

HIGH PARAPLEGIA

A cord lesion in the upper thoracic segments occurs with severe bone
damage of the upper thoracic vertebrae, the cord level being one or
two segments lower than the bone level. A cord lesion at thoracic three
and four segments is taken to illustrate a case of typical high complete
paraplegia.

The sensory loss will be from about the nipple line downwards so
only the upper back and shoulder, the head and upper limbs will have
normal sensation. Autonomic involvement will include extensive
vasomotor paralysis leading to postural hypotension, which is a great
problem when the patient first sits upright. The motor involvement
includes a lower motor neurone lesion with flaccid paralysis of several
pairs of intercostal muscles and spastic paralysis of the lower trunk
muscles, the abdominals and all leg muscles. The spasticity is of the
type found in complete cord lesions, there being only spinal reflex
activity. The spasticity gradually becomes apparent as spinal shock
disappears several weeks or months after onset.

All bladder reflexes are absent at first but as tone returns in the wall
and sphincters of the bladder it is often possible to establish a good
automatic bladder emptying. The reflex centres of control of bladder
and bowel are in the lumbar and sacral cord segments so these escape
destruction. There is no voluntary control of the external sphincters
so double incontinence occurs.

Treatment in the Early Stage

This is as for a low lesion but greater range of hip movement may be
permitted. Additional problems may arise from respiratory complications, the chest wall and abdominal muscles being flaccid. Paradoxical
chest movements may occur and coughing is ineffective. Physiotherapy is needed to prevent obstruction by internal secretions. This
should be carried out at regular intervals throughout the day and,
when necessary, during the night.

The combined resources of medical, nursing and physiotherapy
personnel are needed if serious respiratory complications develop.
Once secretions have collected in the upper respiratory tract the
physiotherapist is able to assist coughing by careful placing of her
hands or hands and one forearm and by giving firm pressure on the

upper abdomen and lower parts of the chest in time with the patient's effort to give a forced expiration. This procedure needs experienced care both to be effective and to avoid damaging the chest cage or the contents of the abdominal cavity. Figures 9/11 and 9/12 show the position of the hands for assisted coughing.

Auscultation and chest x-rays are used to locate areas especially involved in the collection of secretions or atelectasis but the physiotherapist learns from experience to palpate the chest to locate abnormalities of air entry.

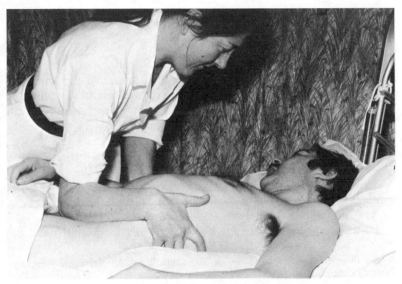

Fig. 9/11 The position of the hands and forearm for assisted coughing

Fig. 9/12 The position of the hands for assisted coughing

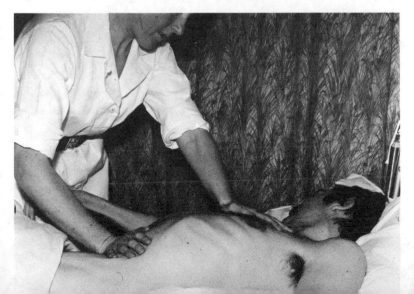

Respiratory function tests are carried out each week or daily if thought necessary. Vital capacity is estimated by the use of a spirometer and the effective force of expiration by estimating the peak flow in litres per minute by the use of a peak flow meter.

Cooperation with nursing staff is essential for good treatment of respiratory complications. Secretions collect in the lower side of the chest and after each change of position these must be cleared. Timing must coincide with turns and the nurse and physiotherapist often work together to use chest care and suction techniques.

Treatment When Weight-Bearing Through the Spine is Permitted

This is as for low lesions with the following additional points:

1. To avoid or control postural hypotension when the patient is placed in sitting, he should be instructed to take several deep breaths and, if necessary, he should be lowered to the lying position. A tilt table is sometimes used to gain gradual adjustment to the upright position (see p.199).

2. Balance training, posture training, transfers and self-care are all taught but progress will not be as rapid as for low lesions, and care should be taken to see that the patient does not fall. For example, while reaching footplates or the floor with one hand, the other arm can be hooked behind the handle of the chair back.

Patience and persistence are needed by both the therapist and the

Fig. 9/13 (*left*) Standing frame. Lowest strap is placed behind feet; centre strap in front of knees; highest strap is fixed behind and below buttocks

Fig. 9/14 (*right*) The wheelchair is placed ready for the lift to standing, the feet being placed in front of the lowest strap

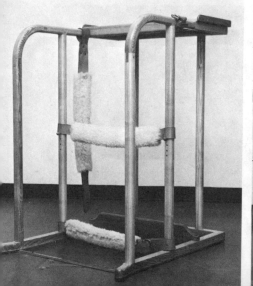
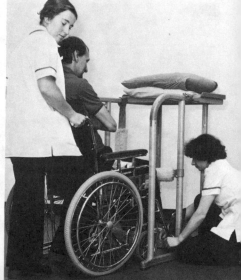

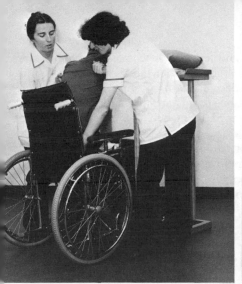
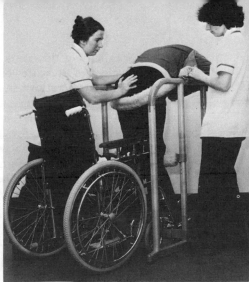

Fig. 9/15 (*left*) The patient is lifted to lean standing

Fig. 9/16 (*right*) The toe strap being fixed

patient and always the aim of gaining independence must be the weaning from reliance on the medical team.

3. A standing frame may be used; the construction of which, together with the use of sheepskin covered straps, enables a patient to stand without using leg supports (Figs. 9/13 to 9/18). Balance training is given, the kidneys benefit, spasticity in the legs is reduced and the patient derives psychological benefit from the periods of standing.

Fig. 9/17 (*left*) The patient can stand alone supported in the frame. Balance training, ball games etc can be carried out

Fig. 9/18 (*right*) Rear view of the patient in the standing frame

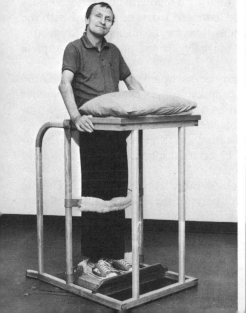
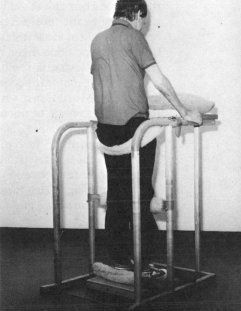

4. Spasticity of the trunk and legs may become a problem if the complications of pressure sores or a bladder infection occurs. Kuhn (1950) stated 'alterations in dominance of postural and protective reflexes may occur but extensor spasms are the natural outcome of complete transection of the cord in man if complications can be avoided'.

Resettlement can be difficult for high level paraplegics and very few are able to return to their former occupation. The use of a wheelchair is essential for locomotion because crutch walking is only possible over short distances and in ideal conditions. Every effort should be made to return the patient to the community. Baroness Masham (1971) has said 'They do not want pity but opportunity'.

INCOMPLETE LESIONS

LOW LEVEL

A partial lesion at lumbar one cord level results in an incomplete paraplegia. Spinal shock may not occur, or if it does, lasts only a few days or weeks. Muscle tone returns very quickly to those muscles supplied from the undamaged segments of the cord below the lesion. The reflex activity in the legs, elicited by handling the legs during nursing procedures or even spontaneously by contact with the bed clothes, is often mistaken for return of voluntary power in leg muscles. This situation can raise false hope in the patient and his relatives who must be warned not to mistake reflex movement for recovery. No psychological harm is done from the caution if subsequently the patient does gain some control of movement.

Various syndromes result from a partial cord lesion at the twelfth thoracic and first and second lumbar cord segments. Posterior sensory tracts may be the most severely damaged tissue of the cord with the result that loss of kinaesthetic sense may be the main disability factor. Cutaneous sensation may be partially spared or almost complete cutaneous anaesthesia result.

Autonomic motor function may be disrupted producing circulatory defects in the legs. Usually reflex and voluntary control of the bladder reflexes and control of micturition are disturbed, the degree of dysfunction being variable. The bladder wall may be flaccid or spastic and each contribute to complications such as retention of urine or infection of the urinary tract. The external sphincter is usually flaccid so there is incontinence of urine.

The motor signs also vary considerably from case to case. The hip flexors and adductors and lower parts of the abdominal muscles are usually flaccid because the lower motor neurones in the anterior horn of grey matter are destroyed at the level of the lesion. All the other leg muscles are usually spastic but there may be some control of movement in total spastic patterns of flexor withdrawal or extensor thrust. The lack of control of isolated movements and the release of primitive spinal reflex mass movement is caused by interruption of some fibres in the cortico-spinal tracts.

The hypertonicity is of the spastic type similar to that in the stage of residual signs of spastic hemiplegia caused by a cerebrovascular accident (see also Chapter 11). The extensor thrust pattern usually predominates unless the patient is inactive, gets severe bladder complications or pressure sores in which circumstances a flexor withdrawal reflex becomes dominant. If the hip flexors and abdominal muscles are weakened or denervated completely the flexor withdrawal is not as strong as it is if these muscles are innervated and therefore play a part in the withdrawal reflex. Sometimes upper motor tracts from the basal ganglia, reticular formation and the vestibular nuclei are still partially intact and so release of tonic reflexes influences the spinal reflexes. An example of this is observable if the patient has a much stronger extensor thrust in the supine position than in side lying or prone lying which indicates some release of the tonic labyrinthine reflexes.

As stated above a vicious cycle can develop if spasticity is allowed to increase the risk of sores and contractures (see Fig. 9/2, p.176).

Treatment in the Early Stage

The aims and methods of treatment are as described for a complete lesion. As muscle tone returns very quickly, positioning in bed may become difficult to maintain and if flexor spasms occur the trunk position is disturbed. Should this occur the instability of the spine may allow further displacement at the fracture site endangering the cord anew. For this reason surgery may be contemplated to ensure stability and possibly also with the hope of relieving some pressure on the cord with relief of neurological damage.

Because the cord lesion is only partial the neurological signs may change rapidly as inflammation subsides. The physiotherapist must be especially observant as she performs passive movements to the legs. Any change in muscle tone, sign of voluntary control of movement or of return of sensation should be recorded and reported to the medical director. Prognosis depends on the extent and rate of recovery of neurological function in the first weeks after onset.

If there is sensory sparing the patient should be encouraged to think of the movements of the legs as the physiotherapist performs these.

Similarly, if some voluntary control of movement returns at this stage he is encouraged to try to assist leg movements as the physiotherapist performs them.

An explanation of spasticity should be attempted by the physiotherapist to the patient. This often proves difficult and the difficulty in controlling a spastic limb with imperfect voluntary movement is more frustrating to some patients than is the acceptance of a completely paralysed one.

Even during the early stage of bed rest the physiotherapist must try to elicit a postural response of support and stability rather than a mass movement of the leg. Quick movements must be avoided and the placing of skin contacts selected with great care. Methods of handling suitable for a spastic paralysis are discussed in Chapter 7. These should be used and those found most effective selected.

Another important consideration is that strong muscle work in the unaffected parts may cause overflow to the lower segments of the cord. This may elicit spasms or reinforce spasticity so the programme of muscle strengthening for the arms may have to be modified.

The time needed for healing of the spinal injury is as for a complete lesion.

Stage When Weight-Bearing Through the Spine is Permitted

This is similar to that described for a complete low paraplegia: only the difference of treatment which may be needed will be discussed.

If not previously completed a full assessment of sensory loss and motor ability must now be carried out. Some attempt must be made to grade the severity and distribution of spasticity. This is not easy as the factors influencing spasticity are many and vary from time to time. The testing position influences the dominance of flexor or extensor reflexes as will the combinations of position or movement requested or imposed by the examiner. Most favourable and least favourable conditions should be estimated and noted as a guide to planning treatment and for comparison with subsequent findings.

In estimating joint range and range of soft tissues the influence of spasticity must not be overlooked as this can so easily mask true joint and soft tissue range. An example of this is the apparent tightness in the calf and apparent lack of control and power in the dorsiflexors of the ankle if the movement of dorsiflexion or control of this movement by the patient is attempted while the knee is held passively extended. If the spasticity of the calf is reduced by appropriate procedures the foot can usually be brought to a right angle with the knee straight and the patient may even be able to control this combination of positions of knee and ankle voluntarily.

The patient must learn self-care and postural control and must practise all activities needed in preparation for transfers, stance and gait. The principles involved are those discussed for a complete paraplegia and methods are similar. However, modifications must be made in teaching activities according to the individual differences of each patient's abilities, symptoms and signs.

Where sensory loss is complete, care of skin, joints, and teaching postural adjustments are tackled in the ways described above. Even when some control of movement is spared, spasticity usually complicates all activities. The methods used to reduce spasticity and teach transfers, stance and gait must be selected with great care and frequent adjustments made to achieve the best possible function. The physiotherapist must learn from experience to be aware which positions, stimuli and techniques are helpful and which elicit an undesirable result. Reinforcement of spasticity by strong resisted arm and trunk exercises must be avoided and yet the patient must be encouraged to be active. The patient must be aware that in his efforts to gain independence he must learn to manage his spastic limbs in such a way that he does not elicit spasms so defeating the purpose.

It is impossible to give techniques suitable for each case and every physiotherapist must utilise those techniques which she can use successfully. However, certain basic principles should be considered and these will be discussed briefly.

The flexor withdrawal and the extensor thrust are both mass movements and neither is suitable to support the weight of the body or useful for activities, such as standing from sitting, standing or walking.

Every consideration must be given to providing afferent stimuli which produce a stabilising co-contraction of the deep muscles whose activity results in providing a mobile but stable postural background. If this can be achieved the patient will be able to realise his potential for independence.

Preparation must be planned for good postures of sitting, prone kneeling, kneeling and standing (Fig. 9/3, p. 177). The patient must learn to elicit a postural response rather than a spastic total movement. For example the spasticity of the calf is often a great nuisance, prevents a good stance and makes walking almost impossible. The length of the soleus is the key to the situation and a slow maintained lengthening must be achieved by the physiotherapist and by the patient before standing is attempted. Even if long leg calipers are needed and even if an attempt is made to control the extensor thrust by ankle control on the caliper a reduction of spasticity prior to standing will be of great benefit. If no caliper is needed the patient should sit in a good position with the heels firmly on the floor and some weight through the tibiae should be provided by pressure on the knees. The pressure should be maintained for five minutes or until the calf relaxes.

Insufficient hip flexion to get the weight of the trunk well over the feet is another fault of sitting posture. This is likely if the extensor thrust is strong and is also contributed to by too much decline in the angle of the back of the chair (Fig. 9/3, p. 177). The patient must learn to lean well forward, keeping the spine straight and head posture good.

When the correct starting position is achieved the patient is instructed and helped if necessary to stand, pushing the heels down, the hips forward and the shoulders up and back. The physiotherapist should help to keep the patient stable by pressure down through the legs by pressure on the iliac crests. Once a good standing position is achieved the trunk should be moved, keeping an upright posture, so that the weight is transferred from side to side, from before backwards and in a turning motion rocking over the feet. At all times the aim is to keep good pressure on the heels and avoid a sudden stretch of the ball of the foot which elicits a thrust pattern.

When the patient is sitting in a wheelchair or on a stool and in long sitting the correct posture must always be attempted. Figure 9/3 illustrates good and bad postures.

A position which has been found useful for patients with spasticity is a modified cross sitting. The hips are flexed, laterally rotated and abducted, the knees flexed and the soles of the feet are in contact. This must be accompanied by a posture of erect spine, not a rounded spine and only in a sitting position so that it is not a flexor-withdrawal pattern of legs and trunk.

Standing with or without calipers with the support of parallel bars or a standing frame is helpful to reduce spasticity providing a good normal alignment of feet, legs and trunk can be achieved (Figs. 9/3, 9/17 and 9/18). Some patients may not need long calipers but may find a below knee splint useful to control the ankle position.

The patient must be aware that a sudden stretch on the ball of the foot may elicit an extensor thrust and throw him backwards off balance.

Most patients with incomplete low paraplegia can walk well eventually but need the use of crutches, sticks or a 'fender' aid. They learn to negotiate stairs and obstacles but many need a wheelchair for long distances.

Resettlement problems are similar to those of patients with complete lesions and all the members of the team assist in solving difficulties. Follow-up is essential for these patients and at review a careful reassessment must be made especially of the spasticity and problems it may create. Length of soft tissues must be assessed to ensure that contractures are not developing. Good function, once achieved, is the best way to prevent deterioration.

HIGH LEVEL

Incomplete paraplegia may result from a cord lesion at any level below the first thoracic. Treatment for a high partial lesion is as discussed for a low one with added consideration of respiratory complications. When weight is allowed through the spine, postural hypotension and lack of trunk stability make progress slower than for a low partial lesion. Each patient needs individual consideration after a careful assessment so that appropriate treatment is given. Resettlement may be difficult unless the disability is minimal.

COMPLETE TETRAPLEGIA

A cord lesion above the first thoracic cord segment involves some paralysis of the hand and arm muscles, sensory loss in the hands and possibly the arms and impaired circulation to the arms. As all four limbs are involved as well as the trunk such cases are known as tetraplegic patients.

The precise level of the lesion decides the degree of involvement of the arms and a physiotherapist working in a spinal injuries unit must be familiar with the segmental innervation of skin and muscles of the arm. The distribution of paralysis is not always symmetrical; one hand, wrist or elbow may be spared more control than the other. The principal nerve roots and cord segments which control each joint movement are summarised in Table 2, p. 151.

It should be noted that a cord lesion at cervical seven or just below this leaves some control of elbow extension and wrist extension. One just below this leaves some control of flexion of the proximal interphalangeal joints of the fingers and some control of the thumb may be spared also. A higher level of lesion destroying the seventh and eighth cervical cord segments leaves elbow flexion intact but no elbow extension. High cord lesions occur with little or no control of any arm movement except some abduction, extension, and lateral rotation at the shoulder joint if the fifth cervical cord segment is spared.

The function possible when the patient is allowed up in a chair varies enormously according to the precise muscle power which is spared. Lower motor neurones in the injured segments are destroyed so a flaccid paralysis occurs of the muscles supplied by these segments. The loss of function is aggravated by loss of cutaneous and kinaesthetic sensation in the hands. Even when sensation and muscle power exist in the upper part of the arm an insensitive, powerless hand at the distal end of the limb makes motivation and use of the limb very unlikely.

An added problem is the loss of autonomic motor supply to the blood vessels, sweat glands and hair follicles of the denervated dermatomes. Trophic changes occur, the skin of the hand becoming dry and scaly and in severe cases changes in circulation and in bone health occur, similar to those in Sudeck's atrophy.

In very high cervical cord lesions the spinal cord segments supplying the lower part of the arm and hand may be intact but isolated from the high centres in the brain. A spastic paralysis can be observed in some patients with this type of lesion after the spinal shock wears off.

Paralysis of intercostal muscles and abdominal muscles produces effects on respiration similar to those already described as obtaining in high thoracic cord lesions and in very high levels of lesion the diaphragm may be weakened also.

The patient with a fracture-dislocation of the cervical spine needs extremely careful handling and the attention available at the time of injury may have a profound influence on the final outcome. While the neck is still unstable slight movement may increase cord damage. The patient should not be lifted from the stretcher except under the supervision of the surgeon. X-ray examination is carried out with the patient still on the stretcher unless the surgeon is present to direct the lift to an x-ray table. When the x-ray is available the surgeon will decide on the type of support needed. Skull traction is frequently used and special head and neck support also.

Treatment in Early Stages

The principles of nursing care and physiotherapy are observed. Intensive therapy is an urgent necessity to save the patient's life. Unless there is pre-existing chronic chest disease or an infection of the respiratory tract occurs a tracheostomy should not be necessary. The secretions are cleared from the chest by regular physiotherapy consisting of gentle vibrations and shaking, timed to follow immediately before and after a turn to change the patient's position. Cooperation with nursing staff is essential, the nurse usually clearing secretions from the throat by the use of suction apparatus and an endotracheal tube. Sips of a drink made from diluted unsweetened fresh lemon juice are helpful. Inhalations or the introduction of a small quantity of fluid into the endotracheal tube, e.g. a solution of bicarbonate of soda, may help to reduce the viscosity of secretions.

Assisted coughing is attempted but in the early stages this needs to be gently and cautiously performed to avoid any damage to the ribs or abdominal contents. While spinal shock is present there is no tone at all in the abdominal muscles and similarly the tone is low in the walls of the gut. In these circumstances a firm compression of the abdominal wall is likely to cause damage to the gut and so produce further complications. The risk of a paralytic ileus must not be overlooked.

Respiratory function tests are carried out as described for high paraplegics. Passive movements must be performed as described for paraplegia and movements to the upper limbs must be included. The length of biceps must be maintained so that the hand can be brought flat on a supporting surface with the forearm pronated, the elbow extended and the shoulder adducted and extended. This combination of positions of the segments of the arm is necessary to prop up the trunk during certain activities when the patient is allowed up. It is also needed for self-care and feeding. Similarly, a functional length must be maintained in the long finger flexors; these must not be over-stretched because if wrist extension is actively possible the hand may be able to grip objects by a 'tenodesis' action. This is a passive flexion of the joints of the fingers produced by active hyperextension of the wrist. If the long finger flexor tendons are overstretched such an action is not possible.

Circulation to the hand is frequently very poor and the maintenance of range in the joints of the hands is then very difficult. A roll of sorbo rubber is placed in the hand to try to preserve a good position. One method of trying to control oedema in the hand is by the use of inflatable plastic splints. These are placed around the hands and forearms, care being taken to see that the whole hand is encircled; the splints are inflated until a comfortable gentle squeeze is experienced on the fingers of the physiotherapist when she places them within the grip of the splint. These splints are left on for up to twenty minutes once or twice a day. Ideally, a pump should be connected to the valve of the splint so that an intermittent pumping action is obtained. Care is needed to ensure that the pressure is not too high, for the patient cannot guard against this as the hands have no sensation. In some units the hands are bandaged in the 'boxing glove splint' devised by Professor J. I. P. James and developed by Dr Cheshire and Glenys Rowe (Bromley, 1980; Cheshire and Rowe, 1970). Even later when the hands are left free by day, the bandaging is continued at night.

The length of soft tissue must be preserved. Elbow extension is difficult to maintain if the elbow flexors are active and the extensors flaccid or very weak. The patient bends his arms and cannot then extend them. A splint or padded board to which the extended arm is bandaged is useful but must be carefully applied and removed to allow repeated rapid passive movements to be given to help maintain the circulation to the hand.

In a very high cervical lesion the biceps may be spastic which also causes a problem and often leads to contractures at the elbow. The posterior fibres of deltoid become tight unless full length is maintained by passive movement.

During all treatment the **stability of the neck** must be maintained. If the patient is on skull traction this must be maintained during the turns. The patient must have treatment for the chest and arms and great care is needed to give it adequately while preserving the correct neck posture. Vigorous shoulder or shoulder girdle movements must be avoided. Careless handling or neglect of arm movements may cause a periarthritis.

Some patients suffer pain which may arise in the neck or in the shoulder joint. The exact cause of this is debatable but one theory is that it is caused by irritation of nerve roots from the cervical segments of the cord. Every possible means should be used to maintain both a good a range of movement as is feasible as well as the health of the skin, bone, ligaments and muscles in the forearm and hand. Thus, whatever muscle power is spared the best possible use can be made of it.

The psychological problems for the patient and relatives are very great. A realistic outlook must be taken by the physiotherapist who must not get emotionally involved in the patient's problems. It is wrong to raise false hope; it is equally wrong to offer no hope at all. While the patient is in bed the long hours of inactivity are almost overwhelming for some, but the realisation of the extent and permanence of their disability is gradual. Once the patient is allowed to sit up in a chair as much activity as is possible and tolerable will help him to have a more positive and objective outlook.

Stage When Weight-Bearing is Permitted Through the Spine

As for other levels of cord lesion the degree of stability of the vertebral column decides when weight may be taken through it. In the case of cervical cord lesions a sorbo collar to support the neck is sometimes needed when the patient is first propped up against the support of a back rest.

POSTURAL HYPOTENSION

This is an almost inevitable complication of cervical cord lesions although as tone returns to trunk and leg muscles some adjustment occurs. The use of an abdominal binder or support of some kind assists the control of this problem and also allows a measure of stability to the trunk.

A semi-reclining chair with a high back is used for patients with a high cervical lesion. Later the patient may be able to tolerate a more vertical trunk position in sitting and a lower chair back.

A tilting table of some kind is very useful, especially one with a mechanical device to tilt it. The patient is lifted on to the table which is covered with a suitable soft mattress or foam rubber pad, a pillow is placed under the head and one over the hips. Straps secure the patient to the table at the knee and the hip and it is then raised at the head end until it is almost vertical. Two attendants must be present to help to keep the patient firmly and correctly positioned and to ensure that the table can be swiftly lowered to the horizontal position should the patient suffer from syncope. The upright position is only maintained for a very short period at first. The time is gradually increased as the patient's tolerance of the vertical position improves. Later, the patient can be supported in a standing frame or in parallel bars if leg splints of some kind are used.

CHEST PHYSIOTHERAPY

This can be more vigorous than in the early stages. If necessary more vigorous assistance can be given while the patient is breathing out. This is done when the patient is in supine or side lying. Positioning of the hands and forearm for assisted coughing for a tetraplegic patient is shown in Figures 9/11 and 9/12, p. 187. Correct timing is essential to achieve a good result. A specimen of sputum should be collected for pathological examination if a chest infection occurs, and regular treatment given as often as is necessary.

ADJUSTMENT OF POSTURE AND BALANCE

This must be taught. Extreme patience and encouragement are needed on the part of the physiotherapist and she must be vigilant in her care to ensure that the patient does not fall or become very frightened of doing so. Although substitution by sight for lost kinaesthetic sense is encouraged, the use of a mirror is distasteful to some patients.

These patients must be helped to be more aware of subtle changes of position of the head than is usual and to compensate quickly if their balance and stability are threatened. Slight head movements and arm movements may correct the alignment of body segments sufficiently to maintain a sitting position or the arms may be used in a saving reaction.

A good position of the legs with the feet on the floor under the knees, a right angle at ankle, knee and hip and the legs in slight abduction gives a measure of stability to the trunk even though the patient has no control of movement and has no sensation below neck level.

Balance is practised in long sitting and in the wheelchair once the patient has gained sufficient confidence and adjustment of vasomotor function to allow this.

SELF-CARE OF THE SKIN

This is taught even if the patient cannot actually do it for himself. The responsibility is his for seeing that he is lifted at frequent intervals. He must request the nursing staff or other therapists who are with him to lift him so that the circulation can return adequately to areas taking his weight. One method of lifting a seated paralysed patient to relieve the weight on the ischial tuberosities is as follows:

The patient folds his arms, the lifter stands behind with her arms under the patient's shoulders and hands gripped over the patient's forearms (Figs. 9/19 and 9/20). It is then possible to give a sufficiently high lift to allow the return of circulation to the buttock region. The lift must last for at least fifteen seconds. It is repeated as frequently as

Fig. 9/19 (*left*) Preparation to lift a patient in order to relieve pressure. Note the physiotherapist's grip under the axillae and over the folded arms of the patient

Fig. 9/20 (*right*) The actual lift to relieve the pressure

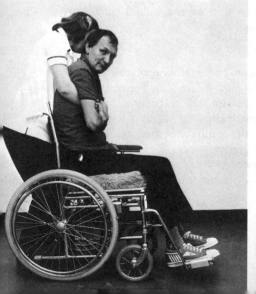 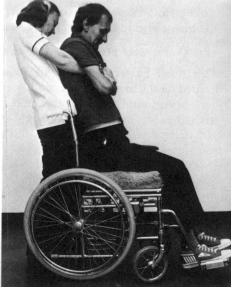

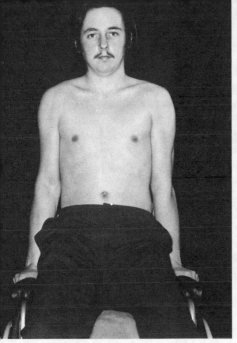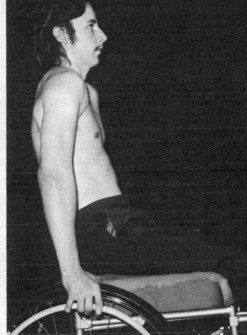

Fig. 9/21 (*left*) Patient lifting himself to relieve pressure by pushing up from the arms of the chair

Fig. 9/22 (*right*) Patient lifting himself to relieve pressure by pushing up from the wheels of the chair

necessary to keep the skin in a healthy condition. Later the patient is taught to relieve pressure himself by lifting upwards or by rolling onto one buttock and then onto the other (Figs. 9/21, 9/22 and 9/23).

As described previously the use of a firm base to a firm foam cushion, which is covered in sheepskin, helps to prevent pressure sores.

Training in the care of the hands is included. Gloves or special palm mittens are worn while wheeling the chair. Cigarette holders must be used if the patient smokes. Hot plates and mugs must not be placed in

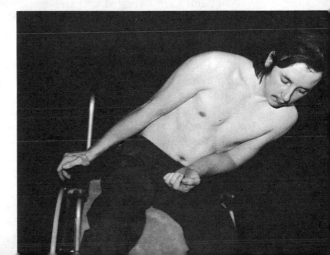

Fig. 9/23 A low cervical tetraplegic rolling sideways to relieve pressure

the hand or rested on the legs. Gloves must be worn in cold weather and for activities such as gardening.

The patient is responsible for requesting that the skin is inspected daily and that the urinal is not causing friction.

FUNCTIONAL ABILITY

There is a great difference in functional ability of a patient with voluntary control of elbow extension and one who has none.

A patient with control of an active triceps can support himself firmly on one or both arms, lift safely to relieve pressure on his seat and wheel his chair strongly even with no active control of the hand.

If triceps is active some use is usually possible also in the wrist extensors as these share the same segmental supply from cervical seven nerve root. With gadgets strapped to the hand, feeding, shaving, smoking, attention to personal hygiene and hair grooming are possible.

The patient, without active elbow extension, is much more disabled; he must rely on the force of gravity to extend his elbows so cannot keep them stable in any position except possibly a vertical position with the hand on a firm surface directly below the shoulder. The shoulder adductors are weak also, so the arm cannot be firmly pressed over the hand.

Activities are commenced as soon as the patient has adjusted to sitting up. Mat work is very valuable. The patient must be lifted on to the mat carefully and mat activities such as rolling, balance training in long sitting and modified cross sitting are taught (see Figs. 9/8 and 9/9).

Some patients, particularly those with active elbow extension and radial wrist extension achieve a remarkable degree of control of activities. Some can hook their thumbs into their trouser pockets and sit up using the shoulder adductors and extensors and in the same way raise the trunk. Others get to forearm support and then to arm support.

Ball games are arranged and archery, swimming, and table tennis are possible, with adapted apparatus if needed.

Morale is aided by helping each patient to take a pride in his or her own appearance. A wig should be provided for a patient who has had to have the scalp shaved during the period on skull traction. Girls are helped to make up the face and men to shave with special electrically operated razors.

A full programme of physiotherapy, occupational therapy, bladder training, skin care, and personal hygiene is arranged. The patient must be responsible for getting himself to the correct place on time for treatment. Even those with no control of the elbow joints can have an electrically driven chair supplied so that they can be responsible for their own locomotion.

The problem of spasticity has not been discussed but it is an ever-present threat of becoming a severe complication unless sores, contractures and bladder infection can be avoided.

Standing with leg support in some form of splint such as plaster of Paris shells or a specially designed standing frame is to be encouraged. The patient gains a psychological uplift from a period of standing which may not be understood by those of us who have never had to lie flat or sit immobile throughout days, weeks and years. Physiological benefits of standing include better drainage of the kidneys, some beneficial stimuli to keep the leg bones strong, a position which maintains length of hip flexors, knee flexors and calf and a means of reducing spasticity. In many cases standing improves the activity of postural muscles of the neck and upper trunk. The patients can have some apparatus supplied so that they can stand for a period daily at home when they are discharged from the spinal unit.

Occupational therapy is essential for tetraplegic patients. In the acute stage with the patient absolutely helpless in bed, tape-recorded books and a suck-blow page turner for the patient's use are most valuable. These are supplied by the occupational therapist who teaches the use of the page turner. Later, when the patient is sitting up, simple gadgets can usually be supplied for page turning, feeding and use of an electric typewriter.

For the more disabled patients with very high lesions more complex aids may be found useful.

Art therapy is very valuable when it is available. Gadgets to hold pencils or brushes can be used by some patients or special dental devices used to paint with the mouth.

Apparatus controlled by the mouth by pneumatic control can be supplied to enable a patient to switch on and off lights, electric fires, radio or television sets. It can also be used to control a telephone, page turner or electric typewriter. This is known as the Patient Operated Selector Mechanism (POSM or POSSUM).

Other apparatus designed for a tetraplegic patient include a ball-bearing feeding device, an opponens splint and flexor hinge splints.

Reconstructive surgery for the hand is sometimes considered but great care is needed to ensure that no ability is lost by attempts to improve hand skill.

Motorised transport can be controlled by a tetraplegic patient who has active use of the elbows and wrists but the patient has to be lifted into and out of the car. This is facilitated by the use of a sliding board.

Resettlement presents many difficulties and the relatives must be thoroughly trained to care for the patient at home. This is the responsibility of all members of the team and should begin as soon as is practicable (p. 164).

Follow-up and frequent review is necessary and domiciliary visits from experienced nurses, occupational therapists, or physiotherapists are of great value.

Although the patients need a personal attendant the prognosis is more favourable for tetraplegics who return to the community than for those forced by circumstances to remain in institutional care. The future is grim for those young patients who must depend entirely on others to be fed and for all personal care and who have no family able and willing to do so.

Even those patients who can achieve some degree of self-care need adapted buildings, accommodation and some supervision, if they are to live away from home or institution.

INCOMPLETE TETRAPLEGIA

Because the cervical spine is relatively mobile and also vulnerable, injury is common and frequently produces a partial cord lesion.

As discussed previously, partial lesions present with great variation and the precise treatment needed depends on the clinical symptoms.

Treatment in the Early Stage

Even in mild cases the principles of treatment for patients with a cord lesion should be observed. If mobility at the site of injury is permitted the neurological damage may increase. Nursing care should be meticulous and an explanation is needed to gain the patient's cooperation in maintaining a good position even if he can control some movement of the trunk and limbs.

In cases with more severe involvement the treatment will be as described for complete lesions. Range of joints and soft tissue length must be maintained in the legs and hands and signs of sensory or motor recovery must be reported and recorded. Spinal shock will wear off rapidly in partial lesions. When muscle tone returns to the trunk and legs, spasticity will be apparent and extreme care must be taken to try to avoid eliciting flexor or extensor spasms. As soon as possible an assessment is made of spared motor and sensory function but care must be taken not to raise false hope by mistaking spinal reflex activity for voluntary control of movement.

Treatment When Weight-Bearing is Allowed Through the Spine

This follows the principles for all cord lesions. The individual needs of each patient must be carefully considered.

In all but the most mild cases some residual flaccid paralysis of the hands will make manipulative skills difficult or impossible. This factor with the added problem of imperfect control of the spastic trunk and lower limbs, leads to a very frustrating situation. The use of crutches or sticks may be almost impossible for a patient with weak or insensitive hands. The spasticity of the legs can be reduced by the patient's own handling if he has normal use of his arms, but this is usually impossible for incomplete tetraplegics.

As for all partial lesions, assessment of the individual abilities and difficulties of each patient is essential.

A plan of treatment must be made and cooperation is needed with occupational therapists and the social worker to try to help each patient to realise his potential for rehabilitation.

FEMALE PATIENTS WITH CORD LESIONS

Treatment for female patients is as described above but some added problems arise. One example is the relative shortness of arms and heavier pelvis and legs of a woman compared to that of a man. These factors make transfers difficult for all but the most slender and youthful females.

Another problem is the difficult situation of double incontinence; no really satisfactory urinal is available. Bladder training is therefore of vital importance to the female patient. Nurses are responsible for attempting to establish a regular automatic reflex emptying of the bladder. Fluid intake is carefully regulated both in quantity and times when it is taken. The patient must understand the aim of the training and if possible learn to express the bladder manually to ensure good emptying. Menstruation brings special problems and may upset the automatic bladder function. Young patients often achieve a remarkable success in bladder training. The physiotherapist should understand the aim of training.

In spite of these physical difficulties women show great determination and courage and many paraplegics achieve complete independence.

CHILDREN WITH COMPLETE CORD LESIONS

Children with cord lesions present a challenge but no greater problems than adults, if care is taken to prevent deformity.

Because growth is retarded when normal use of a part is prevented, the lower limbs of a child with paraplegia are relatively short. This factor is an advantage as transfers and gait are facilitated if the arms are long and the lower part of the body lighter than normal.

Many children show great adaptability to physical defects and are very rewarding to train in new skills. They become almost recklessly proficient in the use of wheelchairs, take to swimming eagerly, learn swing-through gait and develop speed and expertise in this rapidly. Many children can get up from the floor unaided, gain balance in standing, place the crutches for use and walk off. Calipers are needed for these activities but do not need to be hinged at the knee for very young children.

Regular, frequent review is needed, however, to ensure that good function is preserving good joint range and length of soft tissue.

As the child grows, new splints are needed and the older child needs hinged calipers to enable him to sit correctly on a stool or chair.

Bladder training is as essential as it is for adults, and regular checks are made by the urologist to see that kidney function is good. Parents should be instructed in the care of skin, bladder, use of splints and shown how to give passive movements to preserve joint and soft tissue range.

If possible, normal schooling should be arranged but the school authorities must be instructed in precautions against skin damage from extremes of temperature or from abrasion.

CHILDREN WITH PARTIAL CORD LESIONS

Partial cord lesions may be caused by trauma, developmental errors, infection or severe bone disease.

Treatment follows the principles of treatment for the cause and should be appropriate for the individual neurological symptoms.

Assessment should be attempted but in very young infants the examiner needs a knowledge of the normal motor behaviour and experience of handling young children with neurological defects.

Prognosis is made by the medical personnel but is aided by a concise report of examinations and observations by the physiotherapist. The habitual posture or response may be difficult to assess in a short examination session and the physiotherapist who handles the child for a longer time and more often, should be able to give a valuable account of her observations. Methodical examination and simple, clear, well-documented, dated reports are required.

Treatment for the neurological symptoms varies according to the precise clinical defects of muscle control and sensory loss.

A careful plan of treatment is facilitated by good assessment. Methods should be selected which are appropriate to the age of the child and the exact defects, and which are found, by subsequent assessment, to be proving helpful.

The problem of deformity is increased if some muscles are active and the antagonists, flaccid or very weak. This problem arises whether the active muscles are under control of the will or are merely activated by spinal reflex activity. In the former case a difficult decision may face the medical director of the case because surgical intervention is irreversible and the possible beneficial use of innervated muscles may be permanently prevented. Splintage must be chosen with care and its measurement, fitting and application must be meticulous to gain the maximum benefit without the risk of skin damage.

The problem of incontinence usually arises and is one of the most distressing factors for both parents and child.

Further discussion and details of treatment are given in Chapter 19.

CORD LESIONS NOT CAUSED BY TRAUMA

Vascular accidents, neurofibromas, transverse myelitis, disease of bone such as tuberculosis and degenerative lesions, for example multiple sclerosis are among other causes of cord lesions. When these involve the upper lumbar cord segments the neurological symptoms are similar to those in an incomplete traumatic cord lesion.

Some lesions, for example transverse myelitis, occur suddenly and show signs of spinal shock. Other lesions are usually of gradual onset. The former are treated almost identically to patients with traumatic lesions except for the medical care which will include chemotherapy to control infection, or surgery to decompress lesions caused by abscesses or neurofibromata.

Other lesions may necessitate rest in bed to control bone disease in which case the treatment is similar to that for traumatic cases. Where the onset is very gradual the patient will probably not require in-patient treatment.

Physiotherapy in all cases follows the principles discussed for traumatic lesions of the spinal cord. A careful assessment must be made of the abilities of each patient and the causes of disability must be considered in planning suitable treatment. The precise regime is decided by the nature and extent of the signs and symptoms.

CAUDA EQUINA LESIONS

A lesion of the spine below the second lumbar vertebra may cause damage to the roots of spinal nerves passing from the lower segments of the cord within the neural canal until they emerge at the corresponding intervertebral foramina.

As the nerve roots contain only nerve fibres, these may regenerate and conduction of nerve impulses along them will be restored. However, dense scar tissue sometimes prevents good recovery of function and if regeneration does occur it takes up to two years for nerve axons to grow to the most distal muscles and skin.

Treatment of the initial injury follows the principles for fractures of the spine and treatment for neurological symptoms must be appropriate for severe and extensive lower motor neurone lesions.

The latter is similar to that needed for polyneuritis and details are given in the section on polyneuritis.

If the tip of the lowest segment of the spinal cord is involved the lesion is known as a combined conus and cauda equina lesion. In these cases some partial or complete loss of control of the external sphincters may create problems of incontinence which are permanent.

Loss of skin sensation over the buttocks may also occur and be permanent, thus appropriate training is needed in skin care.

REMINDERS FOR PATIENTS WITH SPINAL INJURY, AND FOR THEIR ATTENDANTS

Care in Bed

1. See there are no creases in the bottom sheet.
2. Use a firm mattress on a firm support so that the mattress does not sag.
3. Turn regularly as instructed by the nurses.
4. Do not use hot water bottles.
5. Inspect the skin each night and morning. Use a hand mirror to see posterior parts. If any redness occurs investigate and take necessary measures to prevent breakdown of skin.
6. Inspect skin of legs when calipers are removed.
7. If sheets are wet these must be changed at once.

Care While Dressing

1. Do not use safety pins.
2. Do not wear tight clothing, trousers, stockings or shoes. Avoid holes in socks.
3. Keep finger and toe nails short and smooth.
4. Check temperature of bath or washing water with a thermometer to avoid scalds. Water must be below 36.5°C (98°F).
5. Check inside shoes before putting them on to ensure there are no nails or other harmful objects inside. Inspect feet when shoes have been removed.
6. Be careful not to have sharp objects in trouser pockets.

Transfers

1. Always move the legs carefully, lift them and do not drag them along, place down carefully.
2. Always lift high enough to avoid dragging buttocks over hard surfaces.
3. See the brakes are on and the wheelchair secure.
4. Do not sit on hard surfaces, use a cushion or rubber seat in the bath and lavatory.

Care When in the Wheelchair

1. Lift every fifteen minutes for fifteen seconds.
2. High cervical lesions must be lifted every thirty minutes.
3. Do not sit too near a fire or radiator.
4. Tetraplegics should wear gloves when wheeling chair.
5. Take care while smoking not to drop hot ash or cigarette ends; tetraplegics should use a cigarette holder.
6. Avoid exposing the legs to extremes of temperature, e.g. wrap up in a rug if outdoors in cold weather.
7. Do not expose insensitive skin to strong sunlight.
8. Do not rest hot plates or mugs on your legs. Tetraplegics should use insulated mugs.

Care in Motorised Transport

1. Transfer with care.
2. Use a cushion.
3. Do not use a car heater.
4. Wrap up legs if weather is cold.

REFERENCES

Bromley, I. (1980). *Tetraplegia and Paraplegia: A Guide for Physiotherapists*, 2nd edition. Churchill Livingstone, Edinburgh.

Cheshire, D. S. E. and Rowe, G. (1970). 'The prevention of deformity in the severely paralysed hand'. *Paraplegia*, 8, 1, 48–56.

Kuhn, R. A. (1950). 'Alteration in dominance of postural and protective reflexes.' *Brain*, 73, 1.

Masham, Baroness (1971). Included in Report of the Annual Congress. *Physiotherapy*, 57, 11.

EQUIPMENT NOTE

The address for the Gympac System of resisted exercises mentioned on p.181 is:

Gympac Systems Limited
Unit 5. Ty Verlon Industrial Estate
Cardiff Road
Barry. South Glamorgan.

BIBLIOGRAPHY

Bromley, Ida (1980). *Tetraplegia and Paraplegia: A Guide for Physiotherapists*, 2nd edition. Churchill Livingstone, Edinburgh.

Burke, David C. and Murray, D. Duncan (1975). *A Handbook of Spinal Cord Medicine*. Macmillan Publishers, London.

Fallon, Bernadette (1976). *'so you're paralysed'*. Spinal Injuries Association, London.

Ford, Jack R. and Duckworth, Bridget (1974). *Physical Management for the Quadraplegic Patient*. F. A. Davis and Co, Philadelphia, Pennsylvania.

Guttmann, L. (1976). *Spinal Cord Injuries*, 2nd edition. Blackwell Scientific Publications Limited, Oxford.

Harris, Philip (Ed.) (1970). *Spinal Injuries*. Proceedings of a Symposium at the Royal College of Surgeons of Edinburgh, 1963. Morrison and Gibb.

Roaf, R. and Hodkinson, L. (1977). *The Paralysed Patient*. Blackwell Scientific Publications Limited, Oxford.

Rogers, Michael A. (1978). *Paraplegia: A Handbook of Practical Care and Advice*. Faber and Faber, London and Boston.

Rossier, A. (1973). *Rehabilitation of Spinal Cord Patients*. Documenta Geigy Acta Clinica, Basel.

Walsh, J. J. (1964). *Understanding Paraplegia*. Tavistock Publications, London.

Journals

Paraplegia – the official journal of the International Medical Society of Paraplegia. Obtainable from Churchill Livingstone, Edinburgh. Published bi-monthly.

ACKNOWLEDGEMENTS

The author thanks her colleagues at the Robert Jones and Agnes Hunt Orthopaedic Hospital, Oswestry for their help in the revision of these chapters. She particularly thanks the patients who allowed their photographs to be taken and used in these chapters. She also thanks the photographer at the Orthopaedic Hospital for his help, and finally she thanks the Salop Area Health Authority for permission to publish the photographs.

Chapter 10

Hemiplegia – 1

by J. M. TODD, M.C.S.P. and
P. M. DAVIES, M.C.S.P., DIP.PHYS.ED.

Lesions which result in hemiplegia occur in the brain or upper segments of the spinal cord and can affect any age group. The characteristic feature of hemiplegia is the loss of voluntary movement with alteration of muscle tone and sensation throughout one side of the body.

Causes

Hemiplegia in infants is caused by birth injury, congenital malformations, specific fevers, or space-occupying lesions. The above lesions affect an immature brain, and the additional management and handling required come under the umbrella of cerebral palsy (see Chapter 20).

In young adults hemiplegia may be brought about by trauma, vascular causes (e.g. thrombosis, haemorrhage or embolism), or space-occupying lesions (e.g. tumour or abscess).

In the middle-aged or elderly hemiplegia is caused by cerebral thrombosis, cerebral haemorrhage, or space-occupying lesions. Cerebrovascular accidents resulting in hemiplegia occur most frequently in later life because of degenerative changes in blood vessels and raised blood pressure.

ANATOMY AND PATHOLOGY

The two internal carotid and the two vertebral arteries carry the blood supply to the brain. A linkage between these arteries at the base of the brain is called the circle of Willis. The main vessels arising from the circle are the anterior, middle and posterior cerebral arteries, each responsible for supplying important regions in the cortex, basal ganglia and upper brainstem.

Collateral circulation may be sufficient to compensate for a slowly forming occlusion of any one of the main vessels supplying the brain, but a sudden, complete occlusion or lesion of one of the terminal branches of the circle of Willis usually produces clinical signs.

Hemiplegia due to vascular lesions commonly has its origin in a thrombotic or embolic process originating in the internal carotid arteries in the neck. A similar clinical picture may arise from occlusion of any of the major branches of the circle of Willis. Branches of the middle cerebral artery supply not only a major part of the main motor and sensory areas, including the speech area, but also the internal capsule. The internal capsule, closely related to the basal ganglia, has a concentration of fibres coming from many parts of the cortex, and occlusion of even a small vessel supplying this section can cause considerable damage. The anterior cerebral artery supplies the more medial parts of the anterior hemisphere, and near its origin has an important role in areas concerned with the maintenance of consciousness as well as higher intellectual functions.

Where haemorrhage causes localised destruction of brain tissue, there is additional damage to surrounding areas as a result of pressure from reactionary swelling. Both thrombosis and embolism obstruct the blood supply and cause infarction of brain tissue as a result of anoxia. Once brain cells or fibres are damaged they are gradually removed by neuroglial phagocytic cells, leaving either a cystic space or a fibrous scar.

The Normal Postural Reflex Mechanism

To assess and treat the problems of the hemiplegic patient the factors underlying normal movement must be understood. The normal postural reflex mechanism which provides a background for movement has two types of automatic reaction: righting reactions and equilibrium reactions.

Righting reactions allow the normal position of the head in space and in relation to the body, and normal alignment of trunk and limbs. They give the rotation within the body axis which is necessary for most activities (see p.31).

Equilibrium reactions maintain and regain balance. More complex than the righting reactions, they may be either visible movements or invisible changes of tone against gravity. Basic patterns of movement evolve from the righting reactions of early childhood, which later become integrated with the equilibrium reactions (see p.32).

The brain is continuously receiving sensory impulses from the periphery, informing it of the body's activities. All movement is in response to these sensory stimuli and is monitored by proprioceptors (in muscles and joints), extroceptors (in skin and subcutaneous tissue) and telereceptors (the eyes and ears). Without sensation human beings do not know how to move or how to react to various situations, but in the conscious state intention may govern these reactions (see p.28).

Normal function of the body depends on the efficiency of the central nervous system as an organ of integration. Every skilled movement depends on:

NORMAL POSTURAL TONE

Postural tone, which is variable, provides the background on which movement is based, and is controlled at a subcortical level. It must be high enough to resist gravity yet still permit movement. Hypertonicity is loss of dynamic tone, giving stability without mobility. Hypotonicity precludes the stable posture necessary for movement. With each movement posture changes, and cannot be separated from it.

NORMAL RECIPROCAL INNERVATION

Reciprocal innervation allows graded action between agonists and antagonists. Proximally the interaction results in a degree of co-contraction which provides fixation and stability. Distally, skilled movements are made possible by a greater degree of reciprocal inhibition.

NORMAL PATTERNS OF MOVEMENT

Movement takes place in patterns that are common to all but there are slight variations in the way different people perform the same activity. Normally, the brain is not aware of individual muscles, only of patterns of movement produced by the interaction of groups of muscles.

DIFFICULTIES ASSOCIATED WITH HEMIPLEGIA

When treating the hemiplegic patient it must be remembered that the problem is loss not only of motor power but also of normal movement patterns, with abnormal tone, abnormal sensation and the presence of stereotyped associated reactions.

Weakness

The inability to initiate movement is due to disturbed tone and reciprocal innervation and not to actual muscle weakness.

Alteration in Tone

After the onset of hemiplegia the abnormal quality of postural tone appears initially as hypotonus, but at a very early stage increased tone may become apparent in certain groups, e.g. finger flexors or retractors of the scapula, so that a mixture of flaccidity and spasticity is present. Tone usually changes and increases as the patient becomes more active. The basic tone may change gradually for 18 months or longer. When hypotonicity is present the tone is too low to initiate movement. There is a lack of resistance to passive movement and the patient is unable to hold a limb in any position. When hypertonus develops there is resistance to passive movement and active movement is difficult or impossible. The increase in tone is usually more marked in certain patterns involving the anti-gravity groups of muscles, i.e. the flexor groups in the arm and the extensor groups in the leg.

Reflex activity and alterations in posture may also affect the distribution of tone, e.g. there may be resistance to extension of the arm when it is held by the side but resistance to flexion if held above the head. If marked co-contraction is present, resistance to all passive movement may be felt (see Chapter 7).

Perceptual and Sensory Disturbance

There may be disturbance of awareness of parts of the body in relation to each other or their position in space. Loss of sensation impairs the patient's ability to move and balance normally. In many cases, the deficit can be attributed to inattention towards the affected side rather than actual loss of feeling. Impairment of sensation can be improved with treatment, and there would seem to be many exceptions to the traditional belief that sensory deficit precludes functional recovery and that the loss is greater in the arm than the leg (see Chapter 6).

Loss of Isolated Movement

Although many patients with hemiplegia appear able to move all parts of their bodies, they may be unable to move one part in isolation without other muscles acting simultaneously in a stereotyped pattern of movement, e.g. they may only be able to grip while the elbow flexes and the shoulder adducts, or stand up with the hip and knee extended and the foot plantar flexed. Similarly dorsiflexion of the foot may only be possible when the hip and knee flex.

Loss of Balance Reactions

With every movement, posture must be adjusted to maintain balance, but with altered tone present the required reactions are impaired or absent.

Associated Reactions

Associated movements occur in the normal person during strenuous activity, but with hypertonicity they appear as associated reactions in abnormal stereotyped patterns which inhibit function.

Speech

Speech may or may not be affected, but speech difficulty is usually associated with right-sided hemiplegia. It is sometimes purely a sensory-motor problem, where correct articulation is hampered by loss of voluntary control, or in other cases there is difficulty in inter-preting the written or spoken word, and in expressing ideas. Often there is a combination of varying degrees of affliction. Everyone who is in contact with the patient must be aware of and understand his individual difficulties.

APPROACH TO TREATMENT

The Unilateral Approach

It is generally accepted today that patients who have suffered a stroke need not spend the rest of their lives in bed, but most traditional methods of treatment are directed towards gaining independence by strengthening and training the sound side to compensate for the affected side. Many disadvantages are inherent in such methods:

1. The resultant one-sidedness accentuates the lack of sensation and awareness.

2. Relying on a tetrapod or stick for balance not only increases spasticity and abnormal associated reactions, but prevents use of the unaffected hand for functional tasks (the hand being solely involved in maintaining the patient in an upright position).

3. One-sidedness requires increased effort to perform any function, making movement tiring and difficult. Consequently, spasticity increases and movement becomes more abnormal in a self-perpetuating manner.

4. Progressive spasticity in the lower limb demands increasingly complex appliances which are difficult, if not impossible, for the patient to apply himself, and which may ultimately fail to control the position of the foot.

5. Increased tone in the upper limb leads to a distressingly obvious deformity which hinders mobility and everyday activities including washing and dressing.

The Bilateral or Symmetrical Approach

Preferable methods stress the need to re-educate movement throughout the body, realising that as the quality of movement improves function will automatically improve. They aim to normalise tone and to facilitate normal movement, thus providing the sensorimotor experience on which all learning is based. If the patient is allowed to move in an abnormal manner with abnormal muscle tone, such experience of movement will be all he knows and correction afterwards will be more difficult. Everyone, regardless of age, should be treated in a way which gives the opportunity to develop maximum potential. Even if dramatic motor recovery is not achieved they will be better able to function and live more normally. For those who have not reached complete independence at least they will feel safer and move more freely, and therefore will be easier to help.

All treatment should be directed towards obtaining symmetry with normal balance reactions throughout the body. The affected side should be bombarded with every form of stimulation possible to make the patient aware of himself as a whole person again. Re-education of bilateral righting and equilibrium reactions in the head and trunk are vital if independent balance is to be regained.

From the beginning, the patient must be discouraged from using the good arm to assist every movement as this reduces stimulation of the normal postural reflex mechanism and could prevent return of control on the affected side.

The patient should never struggle to perform an activity which is too advanced for him. Any movement he is unable to manage himself should be assisted to make the action smooth and easy without being passive. Excess effort induces abnormal tone and unwanted associated reactions. Assistance should be gradually lessened until he performs the movement unaided. Repetition re-establishes a memory of the feeling of normal movement.

When and if movement returns to the limbs it will be in abnormal patterns. It is most important to make the patient very aware of unwanted abnormal movements or associated reactions; such stereotyped patterns must be firmly corrected at once to prevent them becoming established habits. It is vital to teach him to inhibit such reactions himself, e.g. he must learn to stop the arm flexing up or the leg shooting into extension each time he does anything.

If everyone in contact with the patient reinforces the approach from the start, hours of physiotherapy time will be saved, easier and quicker learning is facilitated and the final result will be far more satisfactory. Because it is an overall management of the patient, he is never 'too ill to treat'.

INSTRUCTION FOR NURSES AND RELATIVES

Careful instruction and involvement of nurses and relatives is of paramount importance and will eliminate or minimise many of the complications associated with hemiplegia.

For the Nurses

POSITION OF THE BED IN THE WARD (Fig. 10/1)

The patient benefits if the position of his bed in the ward or room makes him look *across* his affected side at general activity or items of interest, e.g. television (Fig. 10/1). Similarly, with the locker on his affected side, he has to reach across the midline for a glass of water, tissues, etc.

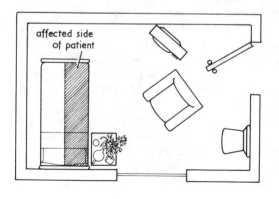

affected side
of patient

Fig. 10/1 Position of the bed in ward

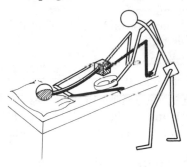
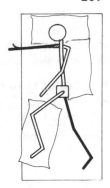

Fig. 10/2 (*left*) Presentation of bedpan by nurse. (The right side of the patient is affected and is shown in black)

Fig. 10/3 (*right*) Position of patient lying on the affected side

NURSING PROCEDURES (Fig. 10/2)

Great therapeutic value can be incorporated in routine procedures by encouraging the patient's participation. While bathing him in bed, the nurse can focus his attention on each part of the body by naming it, and asking for his help to facilitate washing, e.g. rolling on to his side with her aid, and holding up the affected arm with the sound hand; or rolling actively as she is making the bed. When bedpans, medicines or food are brought to the patient, the approach should be from his affected side, thereby increasing his awareness of it (Fig. 10/2).

POSITIONING THE PATIENT IN BED

The bed must have a firm mattress on a solid base and the height should be adjustable. It will need to be lowered to enable easy and correct transfer of the patient into a chair. Five or six pillows will be required to maintain the correct alignment of the head, trunk and limbs. The patient's position should be changed frequently to avoid chest complications, pressure sores and discomfort. Two- to three-hourly turning is advisable in the early stages while the patient is confined to bed. Even when he is out of bed during the day and more active, correct positioning at night must continue.

POSITION LYING ON THE AFFECTED SIDE (Fig. 10/3)

1. The head is forward with the trunk straight and in line.

2. The underneath shoulder is protracted with the forearm supinated.

3. The underneath leg is extended at the hip and slightly flexed at the knee.

4. The upper leg is in front on one pillow.

5. Nothing should be placed in the hand or under the sole of the foot because this stimulates undesirable reflex activity, i.e. flexion in the hand and extensor thrust in the leg.

POSITION LYING ON THE SOUND SIDE (Fig. 10/4)

1. Patient is in full side lying, not just a quarter turn.

2. The head is forward with the trunk straight and in line. If necessary a pillow under the waist will elongate the affected side further.

3. The affected shoulder should be protracted with the arm forward on a pillow.

4. The upper leg is in front on one pillow. (The foot must be fully supported by the pillow and not hang over the end in inversion.)

5. A pillow is behind the back.

6. Nothing should be placed in the hand or under the sole of the foot.

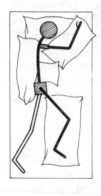 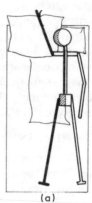 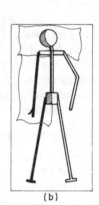

(a)   (b)

Fig. 10/4 (*left*) Position of patient lying on sound side

Fig. 10/5 (*right*) (a) Position in supine with the arm elevated. (b) Position in supine with the arm at the side on a pillow

POSITION IN SUPINE (Fig. 10/5)

1. The head is rotated towards the affected side and flexed to the good side.

2. The trunk is elongated on the affected side.

3. The affected shoulder is protracted on a pillow with the arm elevated or straight by the side.

4. A pillow is placed under the hip to prevent retraction of the pelvis and lateral rotation of the leg.

5. Nothing should be placed in the hand or under the sole of the foot.

In the supine position there will be the greatest increase in abnormal tone because of the influence of reflex activity, and this position should be avoided whenever possible.

SITTING IN BED (Fig. 10/6)

Sitting in bed for meals is not desirable, but may be necessary to fit in with staffing and ward routine. The half-lying position should never be used, as there is increased flexion of the trunk with extension in the legs and greater risk of pressure sores.

1. The patient should be as upright as possible with the head and trunk in line and his weight evenly distributed on both buttocks.

2. The affected arm is protracted at the shoulder, both hands are clasped together and placed forward on a bed-table.

3. The legs are straight and not laterally rotated.

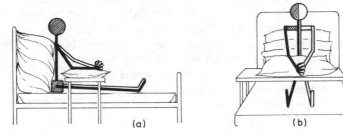

Fig. 10/6 Sitting in bed (a) side view and (b) front view

TRANSFERRING FROM BED TO CHAIR (Fig. 10/7)

Much damage can be done to the patient's shoulder as well as to the nurse's or therapist's back during this manoeuvre if it is performed incorrectly. It can also be a very frightening time for the patient if he is suddenly transferred without any explanation or chance to move himself. The following is an easy, safe, therapeutic way of transferring a patient from bed to chair.

The chair is placed in position on the affected side and the patient is rolled or assisted on to his affected side. The helper places one hand under the patient's affected shoulder, swings his legs over the edge of the bed with her other hand, and brings the patient to the sitting position. During this phase elongation of the trunk occurs, and if a pause is needed to rearrange clothes, etc., the patient can be propped on the affected elbow and take weight through it (Fig. 10/7a).

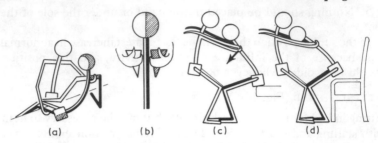

(a)   (b)   (c)   (d)

Fig. 10/7 Transferring from bed to chair. (a) Bringing the patient from lying to sitting over the side of the bed. (b) Starting position for transfer, from behind patient. (c) Starting position for transfer from side. (d) Pivot round to chair – seat well back in chair

The patient is moved to the edge of the bed by rocking or wriggling from side to side. The assistant's arms are placed under the patient's shoulders with her hands over the scapulae while her legs wedge the patient's feet and knees (Fig. 10/7b and c). The patient's arms are placed round the helper's waist or on her shoulders, but he must not grip his hands together. If he does he will pull on the assistant's neck so that she takes his weight instead of him bearing weight through his legs. His trunk is then pulled well forward and he is brought to standing by pressure forward and down on the shoulders, so that his weight goes equally through both legs. No attempt is made to lift him up at all. The assistant's weight counter-balances the patient's, and with shoulders and knees fixed he is pivoted round to sit on the chair (Fig. 10/7c and d).

Transferring in such a way emphasises the hemiplegic side and encourages weight-bearing and weight transference to that side.

TRANSFERRING MORE ACTIVELY

A stool or chair placed well in front of the patient will enable him to come forward more easily, until, with his clasped hands on the chair, his head is over his feet. The assistant holds his trochanters and helps him to lift his buttocks and turn them to sit well back in the chair, on the bed or toilet (Fig. 10/8).

Once he has learned to transfer in this way he can progress to transferring on his own. The same movement sequence is used, only now without the support of the stool. His clasped hands are stretched out in front of him (Fig. 10/9).

Transferring will then be a preparation for standing up from sitting, i.e. the patient will have learned to bring his weight sufficiently far forward over his feet to enable him to come to standing without pushing back into extension.

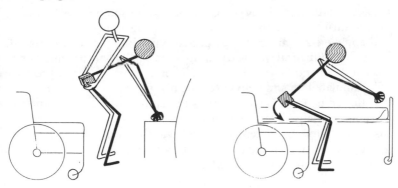

Fig. 10/8 (*left*) Transferring more actively with assistance

Fig. 10/9 (*right*) Transferring more actively on his own

SITTING IN A CHAIR (Fig. 10/10)

A better sitting posture can be obtained in an upright chair.

1. The chair should be of sufficient height to allow the patient's hips, knees and ankles to be at approximately right angles when he sits well back in the chair.

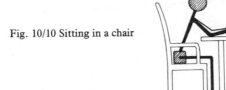

Fig. 10/10 Sitting in a chair

2. His head and trunk are in line with the bodyweight evenly distributed over both buttocks. His hands are clasped and placed well forward on a table in front of him.

For the Relatives

Within the first few days the physiotherapist should meet the patient's relatives and explain his difficulties and how they can help to overcome them. They enjoy being involved, and having something concrete to do while visiting, and often have more time to spend with the patient than either nurses or therapists.

When visiting the hemiplegic patient, relatives tend to sit on his unaffected side as his head is usually looking that way, and it is easier to gain his attention. They should sit on his affected side and be shown how to turn his head towards them by placing a hand over his cheek and applying a firm prolonged pressure until the head stays round. They should then strive to attract his attention by encouraging him to look at them and talk to them, etc. Their conversation and presence will stimulate him and help to restore his state of awareness. Holding his affected hand will give sensory stimulation and bring awareness of the limb. Initially, interested relatives can encourage the patient to do his self-assisted arm exercises and later, they can encourage other appropriate activities such as correcting posture and assisting in the therapeutic performance of self-care activities.

Chapter 11

Hemiplegia – 2

by J. M. TODD, M.C.S.P. and
P. M. DAVIES, M.C.S.P., DIP.PHYS.ED.

Treatment must commence immediately after the onset of hemiplegia. Progress will be more rapid if the patient is treated two or three
times a day in the early stages, even if only for ten minutes at a time.

The patient's ability and tolerance are directly related to the site and
severity of the lesion and his physical condition prior to the illness
rather than to the length of time since the incident. Treatment must
progress accordingly.

Most patients will sit out of bed within a few days and it is important
for them to move from the ward or bedroom so that they are stimulated by the change of surroundings. Shaving, wearing make-up,
dressing in everyday clothes all help to overcome the feeling of being
an invalid.

Rehabilitation in a hospital department has the advantage of invaluable contact with other people and patients with similar problems as
well as the stimulation of leaving home and dealing independently
with new situations. Many stroke patients never attend hospital and
are treated in their homes. The physiotherapist in attendance must
use all her ingenuity to provide a similar rehabilitation without special
apparatus and to overcome the limitations of space. However,
adequately instructed relatives and friends can provide a very effective
learning environment and are often able to give more reinforcement to
the concept.

The following outline of physiotherapy is not a fixed regime or
programme for all patients but suggestions for activities which will be
of benefit to many. Careful and continuous assessment must be made
as the problems arising from hemiplegia will be different for each
individual and may alter from day to day. Treatment must be carefully
selected and progressed.

For simplicity the activities have been divided into sections but the
therapist must be aware that one part of the body cannot be treated in

isolation, e.g. working on the leg in sitting or standing may adversely affect the trunk and arm if they are flexing and retracting with effort. Similarly attention must always be given to the trunk before normal movement of the limbs can be achieved.

ACTIVITIES IN LYING

Mobilising the Arm

Although most hemiplegics with severe paralysis will never regain full functional use of the affected arm, it is important that it should remain fully mobile. A stiff painful arm impedes balance and movement of the whole body, limits treatment and interferes with daily living. If full passive elevation of the arm is performed every day the complication need never arise.

ELONGATION OF THE TRUNK (Fig. 11/1)

The patient lies in half crook lying with his affected leg flexed and adducted. Place one hand on his pelvis, the other hand over his shoulder and elongate his trunk until his hip remains forward off the bed.

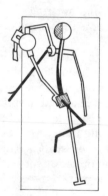
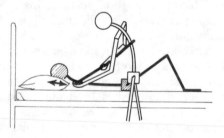

Fig. 11/1 (*left*) Elongation of the trunk

Fig. 11/2 (*above*) Mobilisation of the scapula

MOVEMENT OF THE SCAPULA (Fig. 11/2)

Place one hand over his scapula, the other supporting his arm. Protract his shoulder and slowly elevate and depress his scapula until spasticity releases and it moves freely. Ease his arm into lateral rotation while moving the scapula.

ELEVATION OF THE ARM (Fig. 11/3)

Maintaining lateral rotation at the shoulder, extend his elbow and lift his arm into elevation. Continue until full elevation is obtained with supination of the forearm, extension of the wrist and fingers and wide abduction of the thumb. Move his arm until it will stay in elevation without pulling down into flexion.

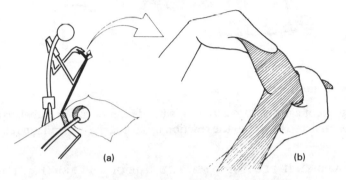

Fig. 11/13 (a) Elevation of the arm. (b) Close-up of hand grip

ABDUCTION OF THE ARM (Fig. 11/4)

From full elevation take his arm out to the side in abduction and up again maintaining the extension at the elbow, fingers and wrist with supination of the forearm.

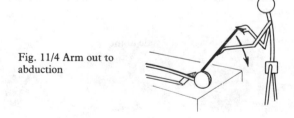

Fig. 11/4 Arm out to abduction

SELF-ASSISTED ARM MOVEMENTS (Fig. 11/5)

Teach the patient at an early stage to clasp his hands together, interlacing the fingers, and to lift them up into full elevation. The movement should begin with protraction of the shoulders and extension of the elbow. The patient must be encouraged to perform this activity frequently throughout the day and to continue this when he is sitting in a chair.

Fig. 11/5 Self-assisted arm movement

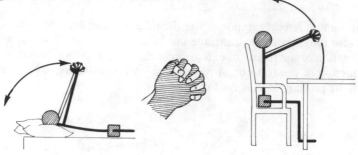

Moving the Leg

To prevent associated reactions his hands can be clasped in elevation or he can learn to inhibit the reaction by letting the arm remain relaxed at his side.

HIP AND KNEE FLEXION OVER THE SIDE OF THE BED (Fig. 11/6)

Place his leg over the side of the bed with his hip extended and hold his knee in flexion and his foot in full dorsiflexion until there is no resistance. Maintain the position of the foot and knee and guide the leg up on to the bed while he actively assists. Repeat the movement preventing any abnormal pattern occurring, e.g. extension of the knee or lateral rotation of the hip.

If the exercise is perfected the patient will be able to bring his leg through when walking and climb stairs in a normal manner, one foot after the other.

Fig. 11/6 Hip and knee flexion over the side of the bed

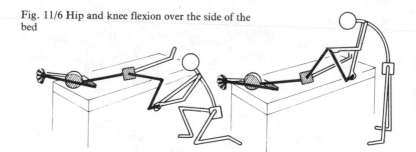

KNEE EXTENSION WITH DORSIFLEXION (Fig. 11/7)

Hold his foot in dorsiflexion, and move his leg from full flexion into extension without his toes pushing down and without rotation at the

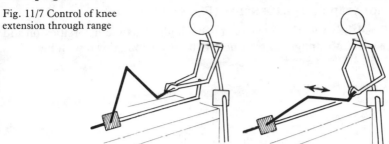

Fig. 11/7 Control of knee
extension through range

hip. The patient takes the weight of his limb, making it feel light
throughout.

HIP CONTROL WITH THE FOOT ON THE BED (Fig. 11/8)

In crook lying, the patient moves alternate knees smoothly into medial
and lateral rotation without his other leg moving and without tilting
his pelvis.

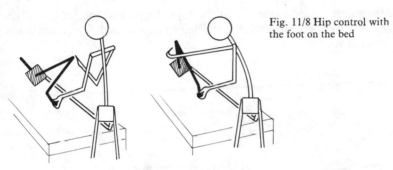

Fig. 11/8 Hip control with
the foot on the bed

HIP CONTROL WITH THE HIP IN EXTENSION (Fig. 11/9)

In half crook lying with his affected leg flexed and adducted the
patient lifts his affected hip forward off the bed and, maintaining hip
extension, moves his knee out and in.

Fig. 11/9 Hip control
with the hip in extension

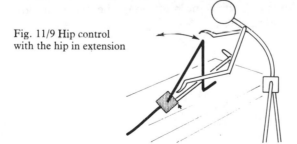

ISOLATED KNEE EXTENSION (Fig. 11/10)

Place the patient's foot against your thigh to maintain dorsiflexion and ask him to straighten his knee without pushing down with his foot.

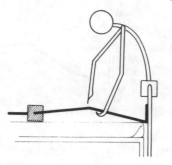

Fig. 11/10 Isolated knee extension

Bridging

BRIDGING WITH ROTATION OF THE PELVIS (Fig. 11/11)

Maintaining good extension at the hips the patient rotates his pelvis equally to either side while preventing any associated movement in his affected leg.

Fig. 11/11 Bridging with rotation of the pelvis

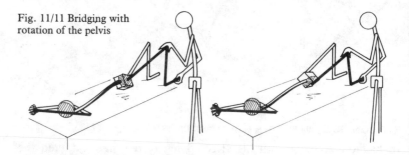

BRIDGING ON THE AFFECTED LEG (Fig. 11/12)

The patient bridges on both legs and lifts his sound foot off the bed while maintaining the same position of the pelvis and affected leg.

Progress to raising and lowering his hips several times.

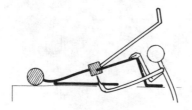

Fig. 11/12 Bridging on the affected leg

Rolling

Correct rolling brings awareness of the affected side, release of spasticity by rotation between the shoulder girdle and pelvis and facilitates
active movement in the trunk and limbs.

TO THE AFFECTED SIDE (Fig. 11/13)

Place his affected arm in abduction and ask him to lift his head and
bring his sound arm across to touch his other hand. Instruct him to lift
his sound leg across his affected leg without pushing off from the bed.

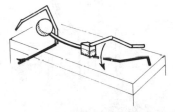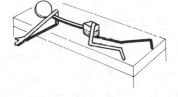

Fig. 11/13 Rolling to the affected side

TO THE SOUND SIDE (Fig. 11/14)

Guide the patient's affected leg over his other leg giving less and less
assistance until he can perform the action himself. He can clasp both
hands together and rotate his upper trunk by moving both arms to the
sound side.

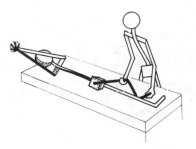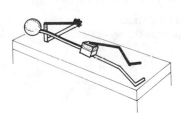

Fig. 11/14 Rolling to the sound side

ACTIVITIES IN SITTING

The patient should be moved into sitting as soon as possible even if he
is not fully conscious, to stimulate balance reactions.

WEIGHT TRANSFERENCE FROM SIDE TO SIDE; FEET
UNSUPPORTED (Figs. 11/15 and 11/16)

Sit on the patient's affected side and draw his body towards you so that
his bodyweight passes through one buttock only. Elongate his trunk
on that side and inhibit any flexion in his arm. His good leg is then free
to be raised in the air.

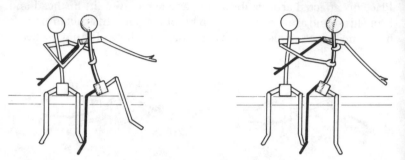

Fig. 11/15 (*left*) Weight transference in sitting to the affected side

Fig. 11/16 (*right*) Weight transference in sitting to the sound side

Shift his bodyweight over his sound side and place his head in
position if it does not right automatically. Facilitate side flexion of his
trunk on the affected side by giving pressure at his waist with your
hand and encourage him to lift his buttock clear of the bed.

Repeat the movement in a rhythmic manner until automatic head
and trunk righting occurs to both sides.

MOVING IN SITTING (Fig. 11/17)

The patient must move in sitting without using his hand. Teach him
to shuffle or walk on his buttocks forwards and backwards and later

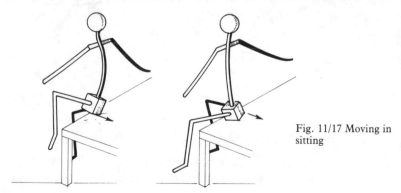

Fig. 11/17 Moving in
sitting

sideways. Help him by placing one hand under each hip or thigh and then rock and move him from side to side.

WEIGHT TRANSFERENCE THROUGH THE ARMS BEHIND
(Fig. 11/18)

Take both arms carefully behind the patient with his hands supported on yours. Facilitate extension by using a sharp push-pull action up through his arms until they support his weight. Progress by shifting his weight from one side to the other without his elbow bending.

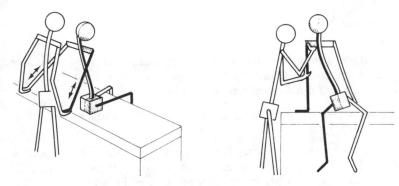

Fig. 11/18 (*left*) Weight transference through the arms behind

Fig. 11/19 (*right*) Weight transference through the arm sideways

WEIGHT TRANSFERENCE THROUGH THE ARM SIDEWAYS
(Fig. 11/19)

Practise a similar activity with his affected arm at the side. Place his hand flat on the bed or plinth and with one hand under his axilla and the other supporting his elbow, draw the patient towards you elongating his trunk at the same time.

INDEPENDENT MOVEMENT OF THE LEGS (Fig. 11/20)

To prepare for walking teach the patient to move his legs without moving his trunk. Lift one leg at a time asking him to make it feel light by taking the weight himself. He must maintain control while his leg is lowered on to the bed. Ask him to keep his trunk still and not to lean back throughout the activity.

INHIBITION OF EXTENSOR THRUST (Fig. 11/21)

Cross the patient's affected leg over the sound one and hold it in full flexion and lateral rotation with the foot and toes in full dorsiflexion

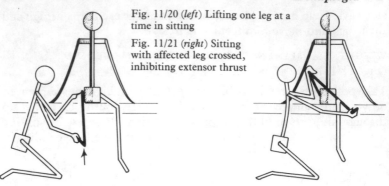

Fig. 11/20 (*left*) Lifting one leg at a time in sitting

Fig. 11/21 (*right*) Sitting with affected leg crossed, inhibiting extensor thrust

until it will stay in position on its own. Maintain inhibition at his foot and ask the patient to uncross his leg and lower it, making it feel light and to raise it once more across his other leg.

RAISING THE HIP IN SITTING WITH THE LEGS CROSSED (Fig. 11/22)

While one leg remains crossed make the patient transfer his weight on to the hip of his underneath leg and lift his other buttock off the bed. Facilitate flexion of his trunk with pressure at his waist.

Repeat the same activity to both sides.

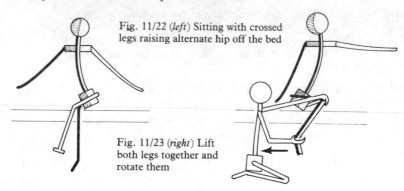

Fig. 11/22 (*left*) Sitting with crossed legs raising alternate hip off the bed

Fig. 11/23 (*right*) Lift both legs together and rotate them

BALANCE REACTIONS OF THE UPPER TRUNK AND HEAD (Fig. 11/23)

Facilitate increased balance reactions of his head, trunk and upper limbs by lifting both legs together and rotating them to either side. Alter the speed and position to obtain the required reactions in the rest of the body. The affected arm should assist balance in a similar way to the sound arm and not pull into flexion.

STANDING FROM A HIGH BED OR PLINTH TO THE GROUND
(Fig. 11/24)

The patient wriggles to the edge of the bed and puts his affected leg to the floor without his foot pushing down. If necessary mobilise his foot by pressing down over the front of his ankle to ensure that his heel is on the ground and that dorsiflexion is possible.

When his affected foot is on the floor practise isolated knee extension before bringing his hip forward to take full weight through the leg. The plinth will prevent his hip pushing back in a pattern of total extension.

Do not allow his affected knee to snap into extension as his sound leg is taken off the bed. Take the same precautions when lifting his sound buttock up first to return to the sitting position.

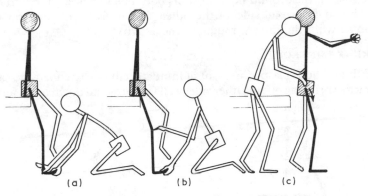

Fig. 11/24 Standing from sitting. (a) Affected leg on the ground with foot dorsiflexed. (b) Isolated knee extension. (c) Coming off on to the affected leg

STANDING FROM A CHAIR (Fig. 11/25)

Place the patient's feet together with his affected foot slightly behind the sound one to ensure good weight-bearing as he comes to standing. Make him lean forward until his head is vertically in front of his feet and to stand without pushing up with his hand. If his trunk and arm retract too much at first the patient can assist standing by pushing his arms out in front of him with hands clasped together. When returning to sitting his affected foot remains behind and his head is kept well forward while his bottom is placed far back in the chair. He must not put a hand down on the chair as this spoils the symmetry and alters the weight-bearing. Instead he should look behind and back up until he is correctly aligned with the chair.

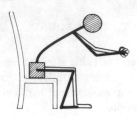 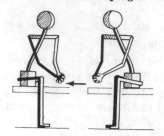

Fig. 11/25 (*left*) Standing from a chair

Fig. 11/26 (*right*) Moving the bottom from side to side in sitting

MOVING IN SITTING WITH THE FEET ON THE FLOOR (Fig. 11/26)

Practise a similar action when the patient moves in sitting. With his feet flat on the ground he can lift his bottom and place it forward or back and from one side to the other. His heels should remain in contact with the floor throughout the activity.

TRUNK CONTROL (Figs. 11/27 and 11/28)

With his hands clasped in front of him, and elbows extended, he can practise reaching out to either side, well forwards and down to his feet.

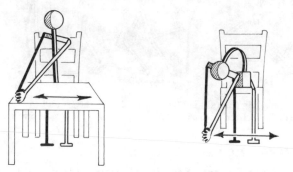

Fig. 11/27 (*left*) Reaching sideways and forwards

Fig. 11/28 (*right*) Reaching down to feet

ACTIVITIES IN STANDING

Correct weight-bearing at an early stage provides good afferent stimulation and is a most effective way of normalising tone. Preparation for walking can be carried out adequately in an area of one square yard. It is of no benefit to practise walking with a patient who is unable either to take weight on his affected leg or bring it forward in a reasonably normal manner. The same applies to someone who already walks with a poor gait pattern because repetition merely reinforces the experience of incorrect movements which in time may actually contribute to a reduction in ability. It is better to assess the difficulty carefully and practise relevant activities.

Weight-Bearing on the Affected Leg
(Preparation for the stance phase of gait)

1. Standing on the patient's affected side draw his weight towards you, giving as much support as he requires. Ask him to take steps forward with his sound leg. Prevent his knee from snapping back into extension by keeping his hip well forward.

2. In the same position ask the patient to place his sound foot lightly on and off a step in front of him (Fig. 11/29).

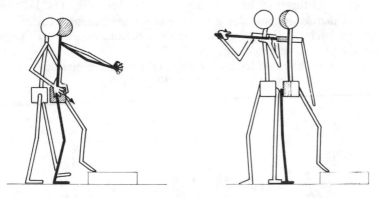

Fig. 11/29 (*left*) Placing the sound leg on a step

Fig. 11/30 (*right*) Stepping out to the side with the sound leg

3. Repeat the activity with the step placed well out to the side. Encourage the patient to keep his affected hip against your hip (Fig. 11/30).

4. Still preventing his knee from locking back ask the patient to draw large letters on the floor with his sound foot, ensuring weight-bearing on a mobile leg (Fig. 11/31).

5. Make the patient stand on his affected leg and lightly place his sound foot at right angles in front or behind the other foot, without transferring his weight on to it (Fig. 11/32). If the activity is performed accurately it helps him to gain control of the hip abductors and extensors.

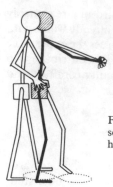

Fig. 11/31 (*left*) Making a figure-of-eight with the sound leg

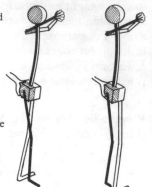

Fig. 11/32 (*right*) Placing the sound foot at right angles to the hemiplegic foot

6. Place the patient's affected leg on a 15cm (6in) step in front of him. With your hand pushing down on his knee and keeping his weight well forward, he steps up on to the step (Fig. 11/33).

7. Practise stepping down with his sound leg placing it further and further back, and tapping it on the floor behind keeping the weight forward on his affected leg (Fig. 11/34).

8. Put his affected leg on the step and help the patient to push up and step right over and back again (Fig. 11/35).

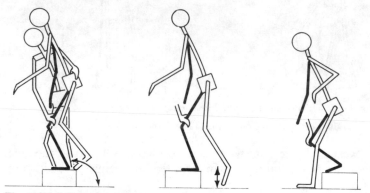

Fig. 11/33 (*left*) Stepping up on to a step with the affected leg on the step

Fig. 11/34 (*centre*) Putting the sound leg further and further back (Eros)

Fig. 11/35 (*right*) With the affected leg on the step, step up and over

Releasing the Knee and Moving the Hemiplegic Leg
(Preparation for the swing phase of gait)

1. The patient stands with his feet close together. Guide his pelvis

forward and down to release his knee on the affected side. Instruct him to straighten it again without pushing his whole side back. His heel must remain in contact with the floor, only possible if his pelvis drops forward (Fig. 11/36).

2. Practise the same activity in step standing with his affected leg behind, and the weight forward over his extended sound leg (Fig. 11/37).

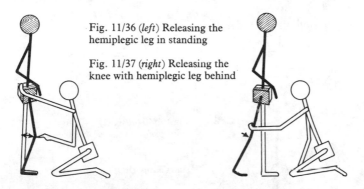

Fig. 11/36 (*left*) Releasing the hemiplegic leg in standing

Fig. 11/37 (*right*) Releasing the knee with hemiplegic leg behind

3. The patient stands with the weight on his sound leg. Facilitate small steps backward with the other foot by holding his toes dorsiflexed and instructing him not to push down. Do not allow him to hitch his hip back (Fig. 11/38).

4. Make the patient walk sideways along a line crossing one foot in front of the other. When his sound leg takes a step, keep his affected hip well forward so that his knee does not snap back into extension (Fig. 11/39).

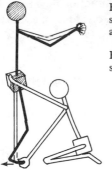

Fig. 11/38 (*left*) Taking small steps backwards with affected leg

Fig. 11/39 (*right*) Walking sideways behind a line

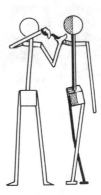

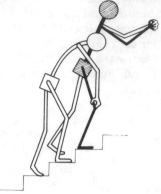

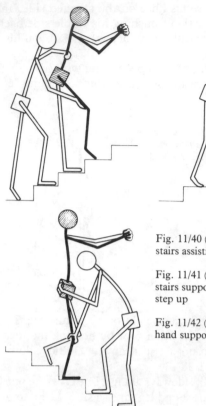

Fig. 11/40 (*above left*) Climbing stairs assisting the affected leg up

Fig. 11/41 (*above right*) Climbing stairs supporting the affected knee to step up

Fig. 11/42 (*left*) Descending stairs – hand supporting the affected knee

Stairs

Practise climbing stairs at an early stage, even before independent gait is achieved, as it is both therapeutic and functional. Teach him to perform the activity in a normal manner, i.e. one foot on each step and without the support of the hand-rail.

ASCENDING (Figs. 11/40 and 11/41)

In the early stages it may be necessary for you to lift his affected leg on to the step rather than allow him to struggle. Support his affected knee as he steps up with his sound leg and keep his weight well forward.

DESCENDING (Fig. 11/42)

Guide the pelvis well forward on his affected side as he puts the foot down, preventing the leg pulling into adduction. Your hand on his knee will give support as he steps down with his sound leg.

Activities on the Tilt Board (Figs. 11/43 and 11/44)

The tilt board is not essential for treatment but is most helpful when re-educating correct transference of weight.

1. Stand on the floor behind the patient and help him to step on to the tilt board with one foot on either side. His feet should be parallel to one another throughout the exercise. Tilt the board slowly from side to side, pausing at each extreme to correct the patient's position and make sure that his hip comes right over his foot, that his side lengthens and that his pelvis does not rotate (Fig. 11/43).

2. The patient turns on the board so that he is in step standing across it with his affected leg in front. Tilt the board slowly forward and back, stopping at the extreme of movement to check his position. Make sure that his weight is taken well forward over the front foot without the pelvis rotating. His feet must remain parallel (Fig. 11/44).

3. The same activity is performed with his affected leg behind.

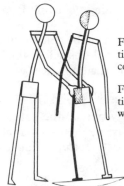
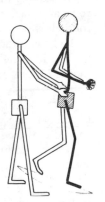

Fig. 11/43 (*left*) Stride standing on the tilt board – side lengthening as weight comes over affected side

Fig. 11/44 (*right*) Step standing on the tilt board – hemiplegic leg in front – weight over the front leg

Facilitation of Gait

Once the patient has sufficient tone and movement in his leg, walking can be assisted providing the therapist or relative is able to prevent abnormal patterns of movement and a reasonably normal gait can be facilitated. Hold his pelvis on either side from behind and make the action as smooth and rhythmic as possible. It is important to keep the affected hip well forward during the stance phase on that side so that the knee does not snap back into extension (Fig. 11/45). Press down on the pelvis during the swing phase to help him to release the knee instead of hitching the hip to bring the leg forward.

The arms may be held forward to help overcome any flexion and

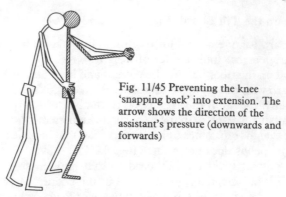

Fig. 11/45 Preventing the knee 'snapping back' into extension. The arrow shows the direction of the assistant's pressure (downwards and forwards)

retraction on the affected side or remain at his side without any associated increase of tone.

As walking improves less assistance is required and a normal reciprocal arm swing can be facilitated by lightly rotating the trunk from the pelvis or shoulders.

To be confident when walking the patient needs to be able to turn his head, to talk, and to step to one side to avoid obstacles which means he can regain his balance and save himself automatically.

USE OF A STICK

If balance and weight transference are properly trained the patient should not need to lean on a stick. Avoid the use of a tetrapod at all costs as it is clumsy, unsightly and prevents the patient from using his sound hand for more skilled tasks.

Activities on the Mat

To assist the patient getting down on to the mat stand behind him and ask him to step forward with the sound leg and kneel down on his affected leg. Support the affected hip with your knee to prevent him from collapsing as he brings the other knee down (Fig. 11/46).

1. In kneel standing support him from behind, with your arms over the front of his shoulders and your hands behind each side of his pelvis. Move his weight sideways over his affected leg, with his trunk lengthening on that side and his hip kept well forward. Repeat the movement to the sound side. The patient should practise holding the position with the weight fully over each side, with less and less assistance (Fig. 11/47).

2. Also in kneel standing make the patient take steps forward and

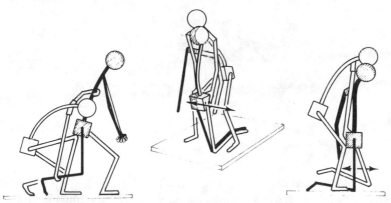

Fig. 11/46 (*left*) Assisting the patient to kneel down on the mat

Fig. 11/47 (*centre*) Kneel standing – transfer weight over affected leg – hip forward

Fig. 11/48 (*right*) Stepping forward with sound knee – affected hip stable

back with his sound knee, while keeping his affected hip stable (Fig. 11/48).

3. Assist the patient as he sits down to either side, and learns to balance in side sitting without using his hands to support him (Fig. 11/49).

4. Instruct the patient to step forward with his sound foot and practise activities balancing in half kneel standing. Make him tap lightly on the floor with his foot (Fig. 11/50).

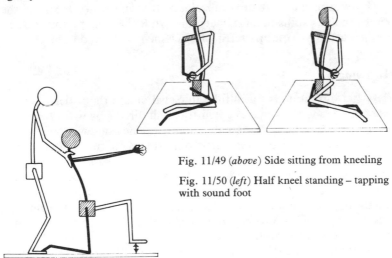

Fig. 11/49 (*above*) Side sitting from kneeling

Fig. 11/50 (*left*) Half kneel standing – tapping with sound foot

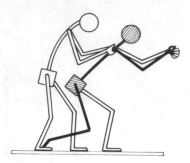

Fig. 11/51 Assisting the
patient to stand from
kneeling

5. The patient can get up from the floor by kneeling up on both knees, stepping forward with his sound foot, and standing up. Assist him at first from behind, putting your hands under his shoulders to guide him well forward as he pushes up to standing (Fig. 11/51).

It is worth mastering these activities as they will also enable the patient to get in and out of the bath without using aids and, even if complete independence is not attained, the assistance required will be much less strenuous.

ACTIVITIES FOR THE RECOVERING ARM

When the hemiplegic arm shows signs of recovery every effort must be made to encourage movement and restore function as much as possible.

There is usually difficulty in isolating movement to one part of the limb, and in stabilising proximal joints while the hand performs more skilled actions. Total patterns of movement tend to dominate.

In Lying

1. After inhibiting the arm fully in elevation ask the patient to let it stay there, and then move it slightly in all directions with the elbow extended. Gradually increase the range until he can lower it slowly to his side and lift it again, and take it out sideways to full abduction and up to vertical again (Fig. 11/52).

2. Ask the patient to touch his head (and lift his hand up again) without his elbow pulling down to his side. He can also place his hand on the opposite shoulder and lift it again. You can assist by maintaining extension of his fingers and thumb as he does so and by reminding him that his elbow must remain in the same position (Fig. 11/53).

3. While you hold his hand in extension and his forearm supinated,

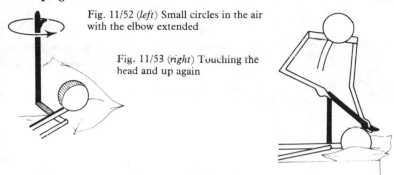

Fig. 11/52 (*left*) Small circles in the air with the elbow extended

Fig. 11/53 (*right*) Touching the head and up again

ask him to extend and flex his elbow; small movements without the shoulder participating (Fig. 11/54).

4. (a) Holding a pole with both his hands let him lower it and raise it slowly while maintaining elbow extension (Fig. 11/55).

(b) Practise walking his hands along the pole, while it is held in elevation.

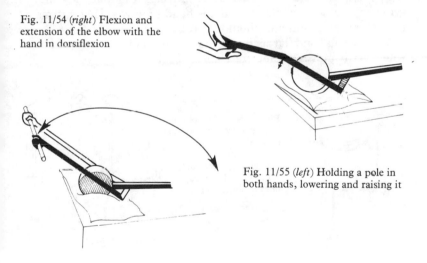

Fig. 11/54 (*right*) Flexion and extension of the elbow with the hand in dorsiflexion

Fig. 11/55 (*left*) Holding a pole in both hands, lowering and raising it

In Sitting

1. Practise protective extension sideways with his hand on your hand, giving small quick pushing movements up through the extended arm, until the arm can remain straight even when you let it go and the outstretched hand lands on the plinth (Fig. 11/56).

2. The patient holds a towel in his affected hand and allows you to

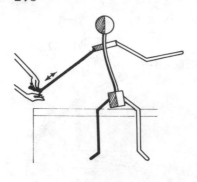

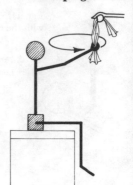

Fig. 11/56 (*left*) Protective extension sideways – hand outstretched

Fig. 11/57 (*right*) Holding a towel in the affected hand

swing it round freely without him letting go, or pulling into total flexion to maintain his grip (Fig. 11/57).

3. Hold the rolled towel vertically in front of him and ask him to grip and release it, while walking his hand upwards. He must maintain elbow extension and shoulder protraction (Fig. 11/58).

4. Place his hand flat against yours and ask him to follow your hand whenever it moves without resistance (Fig. 11/59).

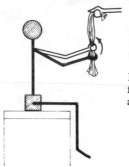

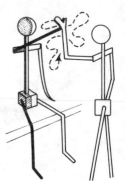

Fig. 11/58 (*left*) Holding rolled towel, vertically walk hand upwards

Fig. 11/59 (*right*) Place hand flat against the therapist's hand and move without resistance

In Standing

1. Lift the patient's arm into elevation and ask him to leave it there when it feels light. The movement will be easier if his weight is on his affected leg.

2. The patient places both his hands flat on a table in front of him.

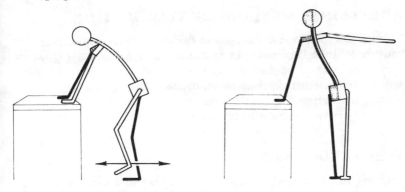

Fig. 11/60 (*left*) Weight-bearing through the extended arms

Fig. 11/61 (*right*) Weight-bearing on the affected arm while rotating the trunk away

Assist him to extend his elbows and maintain the elbow extension by keeping his shoulders forward. He then walks his feet away from the table and back again without changing the position of his arms (Fig. 11/60).

Ask him to turn his feet until he is sideways on to the table and reach out with his sound arm while his affected arm remains in position (Fig. 11/61).

3. The same activities can be practised with his arms outstretched and hands flat on a wall or mirror in front of him. He can also bend and straighten his elbows slightly without his hands sliding down (Fig. 11/62).

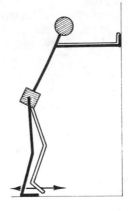

Fig. 11/62 Hands flat on the wall – lift sound leg

ADDITIONAL METHODS OF STIMULATION

Stimulation improves sensation and facilitates movement. Spasticity must be inhibited before any extra stimulation is given, and excitatory techniques should be graded very carefully because overstimulation will cause undesurable abnormal movements.

Weight-bearing is one of the most effective ways of bringing awareness and activity to the affected limbs.

Voice and Use of Words

The way in which you use your voice and choose words can help the patient to move correctly without excessive effort. The volume, inflection and speed of your instructions can increase or decrease tone. Choose words which give the patient the feeling of the movement required, and change the words until you find the one which evokes the required response from the individual.

Ice

(a) Plunging his hand into a bucket of melting ice brings intense awareness of the part and often improves movement. For the best results, crushed or shaved ice should be mixed with just sufficient water to allow his hand to be easily submerged.

(b) Stroking or teasing his hand or foot with a piece of ice will often evoke movement.

Pressure Tapping

With your fingers pressed together tap firmly over the dorsum and lateral aspect of the patient's foot to encourage dorsiflexion. Elbow and hip extension can also be facilitated by tapping.

Heel Banging

The patient sits in a chair or stool and you hold his foot in full dorsiflexion with toes extended. With one hand on his knee bang his heel on the floor to facilitate active dorsiflexion. In the same position rub his heel firmly backwards and forwards on the floor to make him aware of the heel.

Tickle or flick his toes upwards to gain isolated dorsiflexion and extension of the toes. A bottle-brush can be used in the same way to excite movement.

MANAGEMENT OF SOME COMPLICATIONS

If the methods of treatment described are carefully followed many complications and failures will be avoided.

The Painful Shoulder

Careful mobilisation of the shoulder after full release of spasticity around the scapula and in the trunk will soon free the shoulder and relieve pain.

A sling should never be worn as it reinforces the pattern of spasticity and enforces immobility – both of which contribute to the condition in the first place. Once the patient has learned to move his arm with the assistance of his other arm the problem ceases to exist.

The Swollen Hand

If the patient's hand suddenly becomes swollen the therapist must take immediate steps to relieve the situation. If the swelling persists the hand will become contracted and even if movement returns may never become fully functional.

A small cock-up splint made of plaster of Paris and firmly bandaged with a crêpe bandage should be worn continuously till the swelling subsides. The hand should be placed in the ice bucket twice daily, the arm positioned in elevation at all times and the patient encouraged to do his self-assisted arm movements. If treated in this way the swelling should subside within a few days.

Splinting

Splinting reduces sensory stimulation and diminishes the need for activity and consequently inhibits the return of voluntary control as well as preventing normal movement. It is far better to retrain dorsiflexion and correct weight-bearing than resort to early bracing. A caliper should only be used when all other methods of re-education have failed or when there is a risk of trauma to the ankle joint.

Foam rubber spreaders are useful for inhibition of flexion and adduction in the fingers and toes, to facilitate extension.

INTEGRATION OF THERAPIES

As well as the involvement of relatives and nursing staff, close co-operation with all therapists is necessary to avoid confusing the patient and to ensure that all preparation for function proceeds along similar lines.

Reinforcement of principles and repetition of specific movement sequences can take place in actual situations in combination with re-education of speech or perceptual abilities and during the activities concerned with daily living.

One of the advantages of this method of management is the ease with which the level of function is maintained because of the manner in which daily activities are performed, serving as a continuous 'treatment'. The way the patient moves in sitting, dresses himself, stands from sitting, walks and climbs stairs will help to reduce spasticity and maintain or even improve the standard he has reached.

BIBLIOGRAPHY

Affolter, F. and Stricker, E. (eds) (1980). *Perceptual Processes as Prerequisites for Complex Human Behavior*. Hans Huber Publishers, Bern.

Bach-y-Rita, P. (1980). *Recovery of Function: Theoretical Considerations for Brain Injury Rehabilitation*. Hans Huber Publishers, Bern.

Bobath, B. (1971). *Abnormal Postural Reflex Activity Caused by Brain Lesions*, 2nd edition. William Heinemann Medical Books Limited, London.

Brunnstrom, S. (1970). *Movement Therapy in Hemiplegia: A Neurophysiologic Approach*. Harper and Row, Publishers Inc., New York.

Jay, P. E. (1979). *Help Yourselves: A Handbook for Hemiplegics and their Families*, 3rd edition. Henry (Ian) Publications Limited, Hornchurch.

Johnstone, M. (1976). *The Stroke Patient: Principles of Rehabilitation*. Churchill Livingstone, Edinburgh.

Johnstone, M. (1978). *Restoration of Motor Function in the Stroke Patient: A physiotherapist's approach*. Churchill Livingstone, Edinburgh.

Luria, A. R. (1975). *The Man with a Shattered World*. Penguin Books, Harmondsworth.

See also Bibliography on pp. 147 and 265.

ACKNOWLEDGEMENTS

The authors gratefully acknowledge the work and teaching of Dr and Mrs Karel Bobath on which these two chapters have been based.

Chapter 12

Stroke Care in the Home

by F. W. FRAZER, B.A., M.C.S.P.

Various studies (Cochrane, 1970; Langton-Hewer, 1972; Brocklehurst et al, 1978) have demonstrated that the ratio of stroke patients
treated at home as opposed to being admitted to hospital is roughly
3:2. It has been suggested by Brocklehurst (1978) that social factors
are the most significant elements which influence the doctor in his
decision to treat the stroke patient at home. It has been claimed,
however, that many doctors lose interest in the stroke patient once the
acute phase of the illness has passed and that most patients in the
community receive very little, if any, long-term rehabilitation (Mulley, 1978). The provision of domiciliary care is described by Opit
(1977) as expensive in time, money and personnel. That this need not
be the case has been clearly demonstrated within the South Birmingham Health District where a three year study has shown that domiciliary physiotherapy is cost effective as well as achieving results which
compare favourably with the hospital service (Frazer, 1979). Table 1
shows the proportion, in a sample of 500 patients, of stroke patients
who were treated by the domiciliary physiotherapy service.

There are a number of approaches to the treatment of the stroke
patient, each with their enthusiastic advocates; this chapter borrows
aspects of different techniques which are usually selected empirically
and tailored to fit the needs of the individual patient and his family.
The methods used are similar to those employed in hospital and the
treatments in Chapters 10 and 11 can be applied equally well to the
treatment of the stroke patient in the home. Within the home there are
not the comprehensive facilities available in hospital; this factor along
with problems of space, equipment, old and infirm relatives and
unsuitable beds all create special challenges for the domiciliary
physiotherapist when treating the stroke patient at home.

Table 1. A sample of 500 patients treated at home, by diagnosis

CONDITION	0–64	65–69	70–74	75–79	80–84	85–89	90+	
Rheumatoid arthritis	5	7	5	4	7	1		29
Osteoarthritis	3	2	24	22	30	9	4	94
Cervical spondylitis	–	–	–	2	2	–	1	5
Frozen shoulder	–	–	1	–	2	1	1	5
Low back pain	–	3	2	1	1	2	1	10
Other pain	–	–	4	1	3	3	3	14
CVA (Stroke)	19	31	33	39	23	11	4	160
Parkinson's disease	–	2	4	3	–	–	–	9
Multiple sclerosis	6	3	1	–	–	–	–	10
Other CNS	7	5	1	2	–	1	1	17
Circulatory	1	2	–	2	2	1	2	10
Bronchitis	1	4	5	3	2	–	1	16
Other respiratory	2	2	3	–	–	–	–	7
Fractured femur	1	3	5	2	5	6	1	23
Other fractures	1	–	3	4	5	1	1	15
Hip operations	–	1	1	1	–	1	–	4
Other orthopaedic	3	1	–	3	7	2	4	20
Amputee	1	–	1	1	–	–	–	3
Other diseases	6	7	6	9	10	11	–	49
TOTAL	56	73	99	99	99	50	24	500

TREATMENT PLAN

Before treatment commences it is essential that a plan is prepared with a detailed assessment of the patient including physical dependency, communication problems, mental state, social background and medical diagnosis.

This initial record can be based on a number of different functional tests. No particular system of recording is wholly satisfactory and there is no general acceptance among physiotherapists as to which is most suitable. The ideal system needs to be easy to complete, simple, and reproducible by different physiotherapists on the same patient. The importance of accurate recording cannot be overstated as it will form the basis for any future research activity into the rehabilitation of the stroke patient.

As well as this initial assessment, there should be a continuous monitoring of progress, preferably by an independent physiotherapist, in order to obtain an unbiased assessment of the patient's achievement.

PROBLEMS ASSOCIATED WITH STROKE

These have been described in Chapters 10 and 11 and the same problems of hypotonia, spasticity, loss or disturbance of proprioception, perceptual and communication difficulties, visual and psychological problems will be present in the domiciliary stroke patient. In common with the hospital patient, many stroke victims suffer one or more of these problems in addition to the loss of motor function.

Although certain of these problems are regarded as the province of other specialties, the community physiotherapist needs to be capable of recognising *all* of the patient's problems and to be capable of providing basic advice and instruction on them.

PROBLEMS ASSOCIATED WITH DOMICILIARY TREATMENT

These can be considered under a number of headings which are not listed in any order of importance as the circumstances may alter from patient to patient: psychological, social, environment, equipment, communication, diagnosis, supporting services.

Psychological Problems

It is well recognised that a bond between patient and physiotherapist is created, possibly because of the nature of the treatment of the stroke patient which involves close physical contact, and physiotherapists should be aware of the possibility that 'transference' may occur at some stage of the treatment course.

Transference is a term used to describe the development of an emotional attitude in a patient towards a therapist. It is not unusual for a patient to experience powerful feelings of love, hate and so on with regard to the physiotherapist. The patient may also have certain fantasies about the physiotherapist and it is important that she is able to appreciate that such events are a normal consequence of many therapeutic relationships.

Apart from the psychological problems experienced by some stroke patients, there are also psychological problems for the physiotherapist when faced with a large contingent of such patients in the community. The work is usually heavy and demanding both in terms of time and effort, with the likelihood of emotional demands on the physiotherapist which are, on occasions, more exhausting than their physical counterparts.

The fact that the majority of the stroke patients are aged sixty-five and above (see Table 1) adds additional stress as many patients of this age are suffering from more than one pathological condition or present with a serious social problem unconnected with the stroke.

As the domiciliary physiotherapist is working in comparative isolation, it is probable that she is faced by more difficulties and the need to accept more responsibility for her patient than her hospital counterpart. It is not unusual for her to have to decide whether a patient should be admitted to hospital and then to make the appropriate arrangements.

Social Problems

In the hospital the patient is a part of a process which ensures that patients are fairly strongly regimented with regard to their treatment. If a physiotherapist shows the ward staff how to position the patient in a certain way this will usually be implemented whether the patient is able to agree or not. In the home the roles are reversed – the physiotherapist is a guest and if the patient does not wish to comply with her treatment procedures, he may refuse. It is vital that the domiciliary physiotherapist should gain the confidence and cooperation of the patient and his family as early as possible in the treatment course.

The physiotherapist will be teaching the family certain exercises and routines and she must rely on her own judgement as to the extent of family involvement for they are acting as unpaid helpers who will be providing care between visits. In such a situation it is not unusual for the physiotherapist to be seen as part of the family and she should retain her professional standing in order that role boundaries do not become unclear.

In dealing with any patient a friendly reserve should be adopted and it should be remembered that the dividing line between normal professional concern and friendship is easily misread. Making friends with a patient can lead to worry or even guilt; it is important to remember that some patients will misinterpret sympathy or similar attitudes which can lead him to develop unrealistic expectations about the clinical interaction. In this context 'friend' is taken to mean a person with whom a mutual need satisfaction can be realised. It is reasonable for the physiotherapist to express hopes, values and so on and to give support to the patient but she should not use the clinical interaction to support or satisfy her own needs or anxieties.

Problems with the Environment

The treatment of the stroke patient will normally require very little equipment. The main item of equipment missing in the home is a set of parallel bars and a high mat. It is often difficult, if not impossible, to get an elderly person with a stroke down on to the floor and the appropriate treatment will, therefore, be given while the patient is on his bed. Tables or chairs can sometimes be substituted for the parallel bars unless there is a family handyman who can easily construct such an item with suitable lengths of scaffolding. Full length mirrors are not always available in the home but lengths of mirror which can be screwed to the wall can be obtained quite cheaply and are well worth the investment.

With an efficient community store there should be few problems with aids such as chairs, commodes, bath seats, transfer boards and so on and time spent in developing a good relationship with the clerical staff in this store is well rewarded.

Communication Problems

As the physiotherapist is working single-handed within the community it is probable that she will experience problems arising from extended or non-existent lines of communication. To establish lines of communication is hard work and, initially, can be very time-consuming. These lines of communication are well established within the hospital but may be virtually unknown within the community. The general practitioner (GP), district nurse and health visitor may have an established communication procedure but often the physiotherapist can find herself having to contact these individuals separately which can prove both difficult and frustrating. Messages left with a third party are rarely delivered correctly and the domiciliary physiotherapist may have no option other than to spend several months establishing effective lines of communication with her colleagues in the community.

Diagnosis

Quite often the diagnosis which the domiciliary physiotherapist receives is superior to that provided for the hospital physiotherapist. There are always exceptions and sometimes it is difficult to contact the doctor on the day when he is needed. The establishment of group practices adds to this problem as some doctors may work only on certain days in the practice and cannot be contacted.

An additional task which, increasingly, is allotted to the domiciliary physiotherapist is the request from a consultant for her opinion as to whether the patient requires hospital admission for rehabilitation. She can also be asked whether she feels the patient requires surgery. This type of work is an example of the role extension possible within the community and adds greatly to the challenge presented by this type of work.

Supporting Services

Often the physiotherapist is the first person to recognise a particular need in a family and then she is faced with how to arrange for certain supporting services for the patient and his family. In areas where there is no community occupational therapist the physiotherapist may have to request for alterations to be made within the home. Invariably there will be a delay before a rehabilitation officer calls from the local social service department with an even longer delay before the alteration is made. This is an area of responsibility which ought to be extended to the domiciliary physiotherapist who is trained to recognise such a need and, more important, is probably one of the first experts to visit the patient.

SUGGESTED SOLUTIONS

All the above problems can be alleviated, if not prevented, provided a number of basic steps are taken at the commencement of treatment. If the preparation of the treatment plan, following the initial visit, is based on the problem oriented assessment approach this will allow the various problems to be listed in order of importance and enable the physiotherapist to define her role with regard to each separate problem. In this way the total problem presented by any patient can be broken down into separate tasks, some of which are the province of other specialties, and this will prevent the physiotherapist from attempting to do too much for any patient. The domiciliary physiotherapist will often be faced with a 'problem patient' who is excessively demanding or difficult. It is probable that the same patient is just as much a problem for the doctor or the district nurse as he is for the physiotherapist.

The sense of isolation which is sometimes experienced by the domiciliary physiotherapist can be helped by regular attendance at the weekly ward meetings and by regular visits to the GP practices. Many GPs meet at intervals to hold clinical discussions and these meetings are often supported by drug companies. Such meetings are worth attending and the combination of business with pleasure can be recommended; the social atmosphere encourages a good working relationship between the disciplines. Many GPs welcome the physiotherapist's call at the surgery and are willing to discuss the patient and compare notes.

It is recommended that the domiciliary physiotherapist participates in the hospital on-call and weekend rotas as this ensures frequent contact with her hospital colleagues as well as keeping her up-to-date with techniques. The domiciliary physiotherapist may be asked to visit luncheon and stroke clubs and such invitations should be accepted as they are a logical extension of her role in the community. She can enter a discussion about physical problems of patients and often performs a useful preventive role in this environment.

Frazer (1979) has suggested that the domiciliary treatment of the stroke patient is cost effective and it would therefore seem reasonable that the burden of car ownership and maintenance faced by the domiciliary physiotherapist might be eased by the provision of interest-free loans or alternatively by the provision of some form of sponsored transport within the community.

The social problems mentioned above require the physiotherapist to be adept at dealing with various social and ethnic groups. It is advisable that the domiciliary physiotherapist should have at least three years' experience since qualification, in order that she should have dealt with a wide range of people and conditions. Most university extra-mural departments organise courses on social behaviour or various aspects of sociology and it is recommended that intending domiciliary physiotherapists should attend such classes with the fees being refunded from the training budget.

The environmental problems are usually fairly easily solved. Many elderly people have their floors covered in rugs and carpets, laid one on top of the other, with a view to saving wear on the item underneath. Considerable tact is required to persuade them to remove these and it is often the case that they will be replaced as soon as the physiotherapist leaves! When the patient is beginning walking practice carpet can present a difficult surface; this can be overcome by laying a piece of plastic carpet protector over it. This can be bought in appropriate lengths from most carpet shops at a reasonable price.

The patient's bed may need to be transferred downstairs and if no relatives are available the department porter might be willing to help. A commode will be required in the early stages of recovery and a supply of disposable sheets and incontinence pads are useful, e.g. Kanga pants and Kylie sheets can be obtained from the community store.

The family who has a competent do-it-yourself member can avoid the long delays in having alterations to the home; provided the physiotherapist can give advice and instructions, many can do their own alterations.

The height of the bed can be adjusted either by using bed blocks or having the legs sawn off. The too soft mattress can be transformed by the use of a sheet of half-inch plywood of the appropriate size placed under it. If this should prove too expensive for the patient an old door, which often can be bought cheaply, is as effective.

If the family have insufficient pillows, paper pillow cases can be used to cover cushions or can be filled with foam off-cuts. While it is not suggested that the domiciliary physiotherapist should spend her time scrambling around junk yards, it is sometimes the case that she is the only person available and it is a measure of her resourcefulness that such tasks get completed.

The remaining problems mentioned above can be avoided by establishing effective communication and it is essential that this is carried out as a separate exercise before any domiciliary service is commenced. When the service is established it is important to remember that good communication demands constant effort.

PHYSIOTHERAPY

The routine which is adopted for the patient nursed at home is broadly similar to that used in hospital. The extension of physiotherapy into the community has enabled many stroke patients to remain at home and there is evidence to suggest that patients receiving their rehabilitation at home recover equally well as those treated in the hospital.

In hospitals which do not have a stroke unit, there can be differences of expertise within the different wards and it is sometimes difficult to engage the cooperation equally of all ward staff. In this respect the domiciliary stroke patient is at an advantage as the provision of care is directed and monitored by the domiciliary physiotherapist.

Early Stages

Treatment will begin as soon as possible following the stroke and will include positioning, passive movements and care of the chest. The domiciliary physiotherapist will have access to intermittent positive pressure breathing (IPPB) machines, ultrasonic nebulisers and chest suction equipment; if required she can also arrange the supply of a tipping frame. If there is a chest infection present it is possible for her to visit the patient frequently during the early stages of recovery.

A full range of passive movements should be given each day and the relatives will be shown these routines. Positioning of limbs should be taught and it is helpful to fix diagrams or pictures of the correct positioning above the patient's bed. Relatives are usually most anxious to be of assistance at this stage of rehabilitation and time spent in careful teaching is well rewarded.

POSITIONING

Cooperation between the physiotherapist and the district nurse is essential to ensure that the patient is placed in the correct position following routine nursing procedures. It is also important that the relatives receive consistent advice from both professions as there is nothing so detrimental as conflicting instructions.

It is usual for the district nursing officer to arrange study days when the domiciliary physiotherapist attends and demonstrates such techniques as positioning of limbs, bridging and handling the stroke patient. It is essential that the nurse and the relatives are shown how to lift the patient up and down and in and out of the bed. It must be repeatedly stressed that they should not support him underneath his affected arm as this can lead to the painful shoulder syndrome commonly found in the stroke patient. Provided the nurse, physiotherapist and family work closely together, it is possible to give a consistent service to the patient in the home.

BRIDGING

This simple procedure, which is taught to the patient and to his relatives from the earliest possible time following his stroke, makes it much easier to manage the patient in bed and facilitates such nursing procedures as sheet changing, care of pressure areas and use of the bedpan.

ROLLING

The ability to turn over in bed independently provides considerable stimulus to the patient and will contribute to an improvement in his morale. When it is appreciated that many stroke victims suffer depression which is often linked with the inability to move without help it can be seen that any independent movement will be important to the patient.

Bridging and rolling can be taught easily to the relatives and their use will make nursing considerably easier in the early stages of recovery.

Exercise Routine

The programme of exercise will closely follow those outlined in Chapters 10 and 11 although there may be occasional modifications depending upon the time available to the physiotherapist. Many of the procedures can be broken down into sections and then taught to the relative, for example re-education of balance can be taught in rotation starting with head control and progressing to the other elements described. It is possible for most relatives to cope with this 'sectionalised' approach and it ensures that the patient will be given a continuous and consistent treatment, even if it should be spread over a longer period with less professional input.

The programme of exercises assumes a bilateral approach to the restoration of function which constantly reinforces the awareness of the affected side. In the community where the patient is either too old or frail or his relative(s) is/are incapable of cooperating in the rehabilitation, the method adopted may have to concentrate on making the patient mobile by using the support of a walking aid, perhaps utilising some form of knee brace, such as the Swedish knee cage, or an ankle support.

The resulting pattern of walking is cumbersome and effectively prevents a return to independence as the patient can never carry anything or, while standing, manipulate any utensil. There may be occasions when the use of a below knee leg iron is justified, especially in cases where the patient is unaware that the ankle is inverted and suffering repeated minor trauma.

Walking

When the patient has achieved reasonable standing balance, walking can be attempted even before he has mastered the ability to swing his affected leg. The timing of this event will depend upon a number of factors including the morale of the patient and his family, his walking pattern and the space available within the home. The re-education of walking will be along the lines of that described in the preceding chapter.

ADVICE

It is recognised that the patient and his relatives will seek advice from the physiotherapist at all stages of his recovery. It is probable that the domiciliary physiotherapist is the person with whom the patient most readily relates and from whom advice most often will be sought. The advice which the physiotherapist is expected to provide is wide-ranging and she should beware of offering advice which is contra-dictory to that of the other professionals calling on the patient.

As far as advice on physical exercise is concerned it is probable that the physiotherapist is the person most suitable to provide it. In the cases where advice on medication, social or psychological matters is required, the doctor or the social worker can be approached by the physiotherapist and asked for their opinions. It has been found that the patient is more likely to talk with the physiotherapist than most other professionals, possibly because of the special bond which develops during the course of the treatment.

A delicate area is that of sexual activity. There have been a number of instances where a stroke patient has suffered a second one following such activity. Physiotherapists are often asked for their advice on whether such normal pursuits should be attempted. The fact that the patient should ask for advice of this nature suggests that he should be encouraged to follow his desires, as the object of treatment is the restoration of function where possible. It is helpful to be reminded that doctors, when faced with similar questions, are no more experienced than most physiotherapists!

FACTORS WHICH INFLUENCE RECOVERY

Patients who recover their muscle function within the first two or three weeks can be considered to have a good prognosis for rehabilitation. Neurological recovery is thought to begin at some point between the first and seventh week following the onset of the stroke, with little further neurological improvement following the fourteenth week. Functional recovery is closely linked with neurological recovery; Newman (1972) has suggested that much of the early recovery, including that of the upper limb, may be due to the restoration of circulation to ischaemic areas of the brain, with late recovery attributable to the transfer of function to undamaged neurones. One finding suggests that improvement can occur in performance two years after the stroke (Langton-Hewer, 1979). Factors which militate against recovery include severe spasticity, loss of sensation and mental confusion with inability to cooperate with the rehabilitation exercises.

The attitude of the relatives within the home is most important. Patients with many of the problems listed above can be maintained at home provided there is good family support. Such families will require long-term support from the domiciliary physiotherapist and it is common practice to keep such patients on the list of regular visits for periods of three or more years. There may not be any physical improvement in such cases but the weekly or fortnightly visit by the physiotherapist has been shown to be a significant factor in keeping the seriously impaired stroke patient at home. Any claim that the recovery of the stroke patient can be attributed mainly to circulatory and neurological factors can be questioned by examining a stroke patient who has been neglected for some reason. His limbs will be fixed in abnormal positions; contractures, pressure sores and incontinence will complete the picture and will all contribute to a severe nursing problem. The psychological state of the patient is an important factor in recovery and the sudden change in physical circumstances will, depending on his personality type, lead to depression or anxiety. The patient will worry about his future, especially with regard to his work and finances, and married patients may be concerned about a possible loss of attractiveness where their partner is concerned. All of these worries will depend upon the ability of the patient to be aware of his condition and are absent in a patient suffering from anosognosia. When these worries are superimposed upon either a speech defect or a perceptual difficulty, the physiotherapist needs constant patience and the ability to give continual reassurance.

Most physiotherapists will have had experience of a stroke patient who has been excessively agitated or who has struck out at them. These patients are depressed and it should be remembered that this depression is natural and, when the patient adjusts to his changed condition, should improve within a few months. The best therapy is improvement and any change for the better, no matter how minimal, must be highlighted by profuse praise and encouragement. There can also be a loss of self-esteem with a refusal to accept a changed body image, sometimes to the extent that the patient will deny that there is anything wrong with him. This state of mind is a serious impediment to progress and the use of portable video equipment may help the patient to adjust his self concept.

The economic, social and emotional effects experienced by the family as a result of stroke may be expressed in feelings of helplessness and frustration, often projected on to the physiotherapist in the form of criticism or by excessive demands for additional treatment. To counter this the family should be involved in all stages of the rehabilitation and should be encouraged to express their fears and anxieties. The family should also be prepared for the eventual termination of physiotherapy treatment and this process should commence from the first visit. The house-bound stroke patient is not able to mix with other stroke patients as is possible in hospital; such mixing in the ward encourages social skills and will facilitate interaction among the patients. In the case of the stroke patient at home, the physiotherapist will have to ensure that this element of rehabilitation is not overlooked and she may have to advise the family how best to achieve it. The tendency for the family to be protective and over-indulgent to the patient needs to be guarded against.

Although recovery is ultimately dependent upon the underlying pathology, it is evident that the sooner treatment begins, the better the outcome. The age of the patient is not significant although it has been claimed that the younger patient will have a stronger motivation to get better. Elderly patients are as likely to respond to treatment as well as younger ones.

Severe spasticity, if present, may be helped by drugs or by various surgical procedures, while muscle weakness is sometimes treated by electrical stimulators, such as the peroneal stimulator used in cases of drop foot. The painful shoulder, common to many stroke patients, is a constant problem for the domiciliary physiotherapist. She can treat it with positioning, ice, heat, interferential therapy or ultrasound. Connective tissue massage is useful in domiciliary treatment, while support from slings or the use of figure-of-eight bandages may provide some relief.

DISCHARGE

There are certain guidelines governing the discharge from treatment of the stroke patient, and these include:

1. Pressure of new referrals
2. The wishes of the patient and his family
3. Level of progress
4. Availability of follow-up services
5. Lack of further improvement

For physiotherapists, the lack of progress is likely to be the point at which discharge from treatment is considered. It should be remembered that the idea of 'discharge' is stressful for the patient and his family may respond by demanding further treatment, convinced that improvement will occur. Emotional language is often employed: 'left to rot', 'thrown out' commonly being used to express the fear felt at such a time. Because the domiciliary physiotherapist is often required to face this situation alone, she can experience acute discomfort and personal feelings of guilt. In order to avoid such problems, it is essential that the family is prepared for eventual discharge from the very first visit. This will require continual reinforcement on each subsequent visit and a possible routine is suggested:

1. Explain the nature of the illness and the possible plan of treatment.

2. Reassurance regarding the provision of other supporting services.

3. Praise and encouragement for the relatives.

4. Provide some indication regarding the probable number of weeks' duration of treatment. (The mean number of weeks of treatment in 160 cases within the South Birmingham Health District was twelve weeks.)

5. This routine should be repeated on each visit so that the family is conditioned to expect the eventual termination of treatment.

There will be cases where treatment will continue indefinitely on a restricted basis as described earlier.

The provision of adaptations within the home, the arrangement of visits to stroke clubs, day hospital, luncheon clubs and so on may all have to be organised by the domiciliary physiotherapist. Voluntary groups such as the Chest, Heart and Stroke Association (CHSA) volunteer stroke scheme provide valuable support in certain areas and the geriatric health visitor can help at this stage particularly with regard to holiday relief admissions to hospital. It may be necessary to provide certain patients with a wheelchair and to instruct them in its use prior to discharge, with possible adaptation of the home environment, such as the provision of wooden ramps or the removal of some internal doors.

In the case of the patient who will require long-term institutional care in either a young chronic sick unit or in a Cheshire Home, the contact with the domiciliary physiotherapist will assist the patient to endure the stress associated with such a transfer and will help him to adapt more readily to his new surroundings.

The domiciliary treatment of a stroke patient is undoubtedly cost effective although requiring considerable effort, ingenuity and dedication on the part of the physiotherapist concerned.

REFERENCES

Brocklehurst, J. C., Andrews, K., Morris, P., Richards, B. R. and Laycock, P. L. (1978). 'Why admit stroke patients to hospital?' *Age and Ageing*, 7, 2, 100.

Cochrane, A. L. (1970). 'Burden of cerebrovascular disease.' *British Medical Journal*, 3, 165.

Frazer, F. W. (1979). 'Evaluation of a domiciliary physiotherapy service to the elderly.' University of Aston.

Langton-Hewer, R. (1972). 'Stroke units.' *British Medical Journal*, 1, 52.

Langton-Hewer, R. (1979). 'How does arm movement recover?' *The Practitioner*, December issue (volume 223).

Mulley, G. and Arie, T. (1978). 'Treating a stroke: home or hospital?' *British Medical Journal*, 1, 30.

Newman, M. (1972). 'The process of recovery after hemiplegia.' *Stroke*, November/December issue (1972).

Opit, L. J. (1977). 'Domiciliary care for the elderly sick – economy or neglect.' *British Medical Journal*, 1, 30.

BIBLIOGRAPHY

Caillet, R. (1979). *Hemiplegia of the Shoulder*. F. A. Davis Co, Philadelphia.

Downie, P. A. and Kennedy, P. (1980). *Lifting, Handling and Helping Patients*. Faber and Faber, London and Boston.

Handling the Handicapped, 2nd edition. Woodhead-Faulkner Limited, Cambridge, in association with the Chartered Society of Physiotherapy.

Marshall, J. (1976). *The Management of Cerebrovascular Disease*, 3rd edition. Blackwell Scientific Publications Limited, Oxford.

See also Bibliography on pp.147 and 250.

Chapter 13

Multiple Sclerosis – Clinical

by J. M. SUTHERLAND, M.D., F.R.C.P.(Edin.), F.R.A.C.P.

Multiple sclerosis (MS), also known as disseminated sclerosis is primarily a disorder of myelin sheaths, nerve axons being affected in a secondary manner. Myelin derived from Schwann cells, envelops nerve axons in a winding process and has two functions: it controls the passage of ions on which transmission of nerve impulses depend; secondly, it has an insulating action. Thus, myelin sheaths are responsible for the normal propagation and conduction of nerve impulses. The process of myelination is completed in childhood and thereafter there is a slow metabolic turnover, replacement keeping pace with degradation.

Multiple sclerosis is characterised by the occurrence of patchy areas of demyelination (plaques) occurring in a widespread manner throughout the central nervous system (hence, 'multiple' or 'disseminated'). This active demyelination is usually followed by gliosis – 'scarring' (hence, 'sclerosis').

PATHOLOGY

The characteristic pathological feature of MS is the occurrence of plaques of demyelination, active and sclerotic, in the white matter of the brain, cerebellum, cranial nerves and spinal cord. Plaques, frequently giving rise to no symptoms, occur around the third and fourth ventricles. Elsewhere, plaques giving rise to focal neurological disturbances generally surround a small vein. It is therefore difficult to escape the conclusion that the agent responsible for demyelination may penetrate nervous tissue from the cerebrospinal fluid and from the blood.

In an area of active demyelination, myelin sheaths fragment and disintegrate. There is a cellular proliferation in the region and related axis cylinders show some evidence of degenerative change. Later, the plaque appears grey and shrunken; myelin has disappeared; axis cylinders are reduced in number; there is a lack of cellularity and a marked gliosis. It appears probable that in some plaques the active demyelinating stage may be followed by remyelination so that nerve conduction in the region is restored to normal or at least is not accompanied by obvious symptomatic effects. This concept of the pathogenesis of MS is summarised in Figure 13/1 (Lumsden, 1972; Adams, 1977).

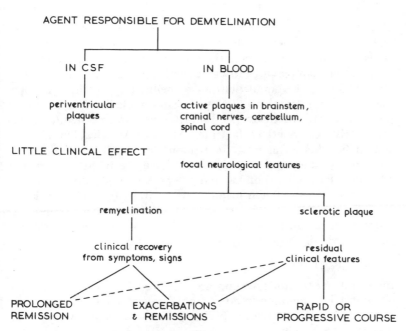

Fig. 13/1 Pathogenesis of multiple sclerosis

AETIOLOGY

Although some factors of aetiological significance in MS are well established the definitive aetiology remains hypothetical.

Established Facts

SEX INCIDENCE

In most series, female patients predominate slightly over males and this is particularly marked in low incidence areas. On the other hand, when the age onset is over 40 years male patients outnumber female.

AGE INCIDENCE

Multiple sclerosis is a disease of early adult life, the age of onset usually being between 20 and 40 years. Only a few cases occur in the second decade of life while an onset over 50 years of age, although not unknown, is unusual.

PREVALENCE AND GEOGRAPHIC DISTRIBUTION

One of the most remarkable features of MS is the increased incidence and prevalence in temperate as opposed to tropical and subtropical climates. This is true for both the Northern and the Southern hemispheres. For example, high risk areas with a prevalence in excess of 30 per 100,000 of the population can be defined in Northern Europe, Canada, North America and New Zealand while low risk areas with prevalence rates of 10–15 per 100,000 occur in the Mediterranean littoral, the deep South of the United States of America, South Africa and in Northern Australia. In Britain, the small communities of Shetland, Orkney and Aberdeenshire have the highest prevalence rates thus far reported of 150 and 125 per 100,000 respectively.

There is evidence that if an individual migrates from a high risk area (e.g. Shetland) to a low risk area (e.g. Northern Australia), the migrant retains the high risk of his country of origin unless migration occurs in childhood possibly before 15 years of age.

ETHNIC FACTORS

Independent of latitude MS appears to be prevalent in European stock while it is less common in other ethnic groups such as in Japanese, Indians, North American Indians, New Zealand Maoris and Australian Aborigines.

HEREDITY

Although MS is usually sporadic, the disease occurs some 20 times more often in the near relatives of MS patients than in the general population at risk.

OTHER FACTORS

It is difficult to determine the precise significance of factors such as trauma, emotional upset, intercurrent infections and pregnancy. Most neurologists have encountered instances when one or other of these factors appear to have triggered-off the onset of the disease or an exacerbation. While it is recognised that pregnancy is potentially harmful, it appears likely that physical fatigue and emotional tensions associated with the puerperium, rather than the pregnant state, are responsible.

The Aetiology – a Hypothesis

There is growing support for the concept that two factors are responsible for the development of MS, an environmental factor probably a virus or viruses, and an intrinsic factor – auto-immunity. Thus, it might be postulated that MS is due to a virus widespread in nature. Most individuals tolerate the virus and remain asymptomatic. Indeed, exposure in childhood as in low risk areas may result in the development of protective antibodies and immunity to demyelination. In high risk areas the infection is acquired in later life and demyelinating rather than protective antibodies develop.

It seems probable that whether the individual will tolerate the virus or not depends on his HLA antigen system. The human leucocyte antigen (HLA) system is the major histocompatibility complex of man. It consists of a series of closely linked genes some of which control the expression of antigen. There is evidence that HLA-A3 and HLA-B7 antigens occur commonly in individuals with MS and are infrequent in regions where MS is uncommon. This would account

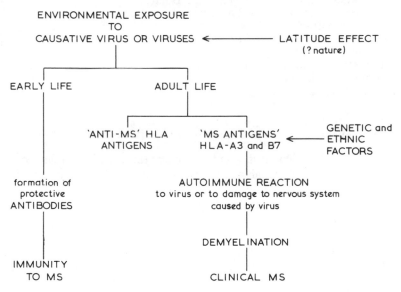

Fig. 13/2 Aetiology of multiple sclerosis – a hypothesis

for the genetic vulnerability to MS in near relatives of patients and to the resistance some ethnic groups show to the disease. This concept of the aetiology of MS is summarised in Figure 13/2 (Acheson, 1972 and 1977; Leibowitz and Alter, 1973; Fraser, 1977; Batchelor, 1977).

CLINICAL FEATURES

The Onset

The initial symptoms of MS may appear suddenly or insidiously. The first symptom is commonly referable to a single lesion in the central nervous system (e.g. impaired vision in one eye or diplopia), or symptoms may be multiple and referable to involvement of several areas of the nervous system.

Symptoms commonly encountered in the course of MS and the structures involved are indicated in Table 1.

Table 1. Symptoms of multiple sclerosis

SYMPTOMS	NEUROLOGICAL STRUCTURE INVOLVED
Blurred vision	Optic nerve(s)
Double vision	III or VI cranial nerves
Weakness of leg(s)	Pyramidal tract(s)
Paraesthesiae:ataxia	Posterior column(s)
Incoordination, ataxia intention tremor, slurred speech	Cerebellum
Incontinence of urine	Spinal cord
Emotional changes (euphoria:depression)	Hypothalamus

The Course

As discussed earlier, if the acute demyelinating lesion is followed by remyelination the initial symptom may, for practical purposes, disappear completely. Should, however, gliosis ensue there may be a residual neurological deficit. Typically, the course of MS is one of exacerbations and remissions so that after the initial symptom, or subsequent symptoms, intervals of months or years may ensue before another episode of demyelination occurs. With each exacerbation there is likely to be some degree of permanent neurological damage resulting in an overall course of step-like deterioration. In some cases, particularly when only the spinal cord is involved, the course may be slowly progressive with no significant remissions. In a number of cases a remission of 15 years or more may follow the initial symptom.

Paroxysmal Symptoms

Distinct from exacerbations of the disease process producing symptoms which may improve or clear over a number of weeks, paroxysmal symptoms lasting for moments to an hour or so may occur. These include an electric-shock like feeling in the back or legs on neck flexion, trigeminal neuralgia, tonic seizures and episodes of ataxia. A temporary worsening of symptoms may also follow exercise or exposure to heat.

Physical Signs

In an established case of MS the results of neurological examination reflect the scattered nature of the lesions. Thus, there may be evidence of atrophy of one optic nerve, impaired movements of the eyes or nystagmus, intention tremor in one hand, evidence of bilateral pyramidal tract dysfunction and impaired vibration sense or joint position sense in one leg. A change in emotional expression is common and although euphoria out of keeping with the patient's disabled condition may be striking, depression is more frequent.

At an early stage, MS is peculiar in that symptoms may outstrip physical signs of disease and give rise to an erroneous diagnosis of 'hysteria'. Conversely, in some patients, physical signs, for example active knee jerks and an extensor plantar response, may occur in the absence of related symptoms, such as weakness of a leg or legs.

LABORATORY DIAGNOSIS

There is as yet no specific laboratory test for MS. In an established case a history of the occurrence of symptoms scattered in time, and neurological findings indicative of lesions scattered in space throughout the central nervous system, generally indicate the diagnosis.

Lumbar puncture and examination of the cerebrospinal fluid (CSF) is the traditional means of excluding other conditions such as neurosyphilis and of yielding information which may support a diagnosis of MS. The typical CSF findings in MS are:

A slight increase in total protein content
IgG values in excess of 15 per cent of total protein
A positive colloidal gold reaction
Negative VDRL.

In patients presenting with clinical features which could be explained by a single lesion in the nervous system, two techniques are of value in disclosing subclinical or remyelinated lesions and by doing so indicate that lesions are indeed scattered and that the patient's condition is therefore consistent with MS. These investigations are:

1. *Visually evoked potentials*: When a stimulus such as light or black and white squares falls on the retina an impulse traverses the optic pathways to the occipital cortex where the electrical potential can be recorded by scalp electrodes. The time taken for the response to occur (the latency) can be measured. In normal optic pathways there is a fairly narrow range of latency. If demyelination has affected the visual pathways even in a subclinical degree there is delay in the conduction of the visually evoked potential (i.e. there is an increased latency).

2. *Computerised axial tomography* (CAT/CT): CT brain scans have been employed to detect subclinical plaques particularly around the ventricles of the brain.

DIFFERENTIAL DIAGNOSIS

Multiple sclerosis has been described as one of the great imitators and Table 2 indicates how early MS presenting with symptoms referable to a single plaque of demyelination may mimic many other conditions depending on the level of the nervous system involved.

PROGNOSIS

It seems probable that MS has been accorded an unjustifiably bad prognosis in that physiotherapists and doctors encounter for the most part deteriorating or advanced cases of the disease. In general, MS runs a protracted course of increasing disability over some 20–25 years. However, one in every four patients shows very little progress of the disease ('benign MS') while one in every twenty patients runs a rapid course terminating fatally within five years of the onset.

TREATMENT

In the sense of effecting a cure or preventing future exacerbations, there is at present no specific treatment for MS. This is not to be taken to mean that nothing can be done for patients with MS. In this section, current therapy, symptomatic measures and treatments being evaluated will be discussed.

Table 2. Multiple sclerosis – differential diagnosis

MS: SITE OF DEMYELINATION	PRESENTING FEATURES	EXAMPLES OF CONDITIONS ENTERING INTO DIFFERENTIAL DIAGNOSIS
Spinal cord	Paraplegia ± sensory ataxia	Spinal cord compression by tumour, spondylosis Friedreich's ataxia Motor neurone disease B_{12} neuropathy Syringomyelia Myelo-radiculitis
Optic nerve	Impaired vision	Other causes of optic neuritis Optic nerve glioma
III, VI cranial nerves	Diplopia	Aneurysm of Circle of Willis Intracranial tumour Myasthenia gravis
Cerebellum	Ataxic gait ± Intention tremor Slurred speech	Tumour, abscess involving cerebellum Alcohol Friedreich's ataxia
Combination of above		Neurosyphilis Encephalomyelitis Carcinomatous neuropathy Systemic lupus erythematosis

Current Therapy

On the basis that serum linoleate is reduced in MS patients, a low animal and dairy fat diet with linoleic acid and fat soluble vitamin (vitamins A, D and E) supplements has been employed. Linoleic acid is given in the form of sunflower seed oil (30ml twice daily) and there is some evidence that although exacerbations are not prevented, remissions last longer and exacerbations are less severe. A gluten-free diet has also been advocated.

Vitamin B_{12} is necessary for normal myelination and as an acute exacerbation subsides, vitamin B_{12} can be given intra-muscularly at weekly or twice weekly intervals for a period (cyanocobalamin, 1mg).

STEROID THERAPY

It appears probable that prednisone (100mg once daily on alternate days) or tetracosactrin (Synacthen Depot, 1mg intra-muscularly daily – weekly) are of value in lessening damage to the nervous system during an acute exacerbation of MS. These drugs given chronically over a prolonged period do not appear to influence the disease process and because of potential side-effects continuous treatment is not recommended.

Symptomatic Treatment

Measures employed to alleviate some of the symptoms of MS are indicated in Table 3. It should be noted that dosages given are 'average' for adult patients and because of side-effects dosage has to be individualised for each patient. This is particularly true of baclofen and dantrolene and it should be recalled also that these drugs may increase locomotor disability by reducing the 'splinting' effect of extensor muscle spasm in a weakened leg.

Treatments under Evaluation

Research into more effective forms of treatment in MS is based largely on the two factors most probably concerned in the aetiology of the disorder – antiviral therapy and immunosuppressive therapy.

Antiviral therapy with drugs such as amantadine, cytosine and arabinoside have been employed with, however, inconclusive results.

Immunosuppressive therapy with prednisone and tetracosactrin has already been mentioned. More intensive immunosuppression with azothioprine and cyclophosphamide appears to be of benefit in some patients while an even more intensive approach employing

Table 3. Symptomatic treatment in multiple sclerosis

SYMPTOM	TREATMENT	DOSE
Spasticity and muscle spasms	baclofen (Lioresal) dantrolene (Dantrium) diazepam (Valium) phenol in glycerine	15–30mg b.d. 100mg b.d. 5mg b.d.–t.i.d. 1ml 2% solution intrathecal
Precipitancy of micturition	belladonna alkaloids (Atrobel, Donnatab) propantheline (Probanthine) Percutaneous electrical stimulation over lower dorsal-sacral region	1–2 tablets b.d. or t.i.d. 15mg b.d.–t.i.d.
Incontinence of urine	Urinal or permanent catheterisation Percutaneous electrical stimulation over lower dorsal-sacral region	
Paroxysmal symptoms	carbamazepine (Tegretol) clonazepam (Rivotril)	200mg b.d.–t.i.d. 2mg b.d.

antilymphocytic globulin, prednisone and azothioprine is being evaluated. These and other research projects hold out hope than an effective treatment for MS may be forthcoming. However, it will be apparent that even when a curative treatment is available, patients will require assistance to overcome the results of the initial demyelinating lesions (McAlpine, 1972; Liversedge, 1977).

REFERENCES

Acheson, E. D. (1972). *Epidemiology* pp 3–80. Chapter included in *Multiple Sclerosis: A Reappraisal*, 2nd edition. McAlpine, D., Lumsden, C. E. and Acheson, E. D. Churchill Livingstone, Edinburgh.

Acheson, E. D. (1977). 'Epidemiology of multiple sclerosis.' *British Medical Bulletin*, **33**, 9–14.

Adams, C. W. M. (1977). 'Pathology of multiple sclerosis: progression of the lesion.' *British Medical Bulletin*, **33**, 15–20.

Batchelor, J. R. (1977). 'Histocompatibility antigens and their relevance to multiple sclerosis.' *British Medical Bulletin*, **33**, 72–77.

Fraser, K. B. (1977). 'Multiple sclerosis: A virus disease?' *British Medical Bulletin*, **33**, 34–39.

Leibowitz, U. and Alter, M. (1973). *Multiple Sclerosis: Clues to its Cause*. North Holland Publishing Company, Amsterdam, London. American Elsevier Publishing Company, New York.

Liversedge, L. A. (1977). 'Treatment and management of multiple sclerosis.'
   British Medical Bulletin, 33, 78–83.
Lumsden, C. E. (1973). *The Clinical Pathology of Multiple Sclerosis*
   pp.311–621. Chapter included in *Multiple Sclerosis: A Reappraisal*, 2nd
   edition. McAlpine, D., Lumsden, C. E. and Acheson, E. D. Churchill
   Livingstone, Edinburgh.
McAlpine, D. (1973). *Clinical Studies* pp.83–307. Chapter in *Multiple
   Sclerosis: A Reappraisal*, 2nd edition. McAlpine, D., Lumsden, C. E. and
   Acheson, D. E. Churchill Livingstone, Edinburgh.

BIBLIOGRAPHY

Acheson, D., Matthews, W. B., Batchelor, J. R., and Weller, R. (1980).
   McAlpine's Multiple Sclerosis. Churchill Livingstone, Edinburgh.
Forsythe, E. (1979). *Living with Multiple Sclerosis*. Faber and Faber, London
   and Boston.
Matthews, W. B. (1978). *Multiple Sclerosis: The Facts*. Oxford University
   Press, Oxford.

Chapter 14

Multiple Sclerosis – Physiotherapy

by J. M. TODD, M.C.S.P.

The previous chapter has described the clinical aspects of multiple sclerosis and this chapter will concentrate on the role of the physiotherapist in the care of multiple sclerosis (MS) patients. It is accepted that there are many MS sufferers who will never need physiotherapy because their disease process is either too mild or so slow that their activities are not restricted; nevertheless, advice for those with minimal signs is included.

Close inter-disciplinary teamwork is necessary to ensure the most effective management of the disability as well as sufficient support to allow the patient and his family to make the emotional and physical adjustments required to cope with a progressive handicap.

Hospital based therapists often encounter more people who are deteriorating or who already have established problems and consequently there is a tendency to think only of the progressive nature of the disease; a pessimistic attitude may, therefore, be adopted towards the efficacy of treatment and overall management when a more positive approach would be of greater benefit to the patient. It has been observed that MS patients respond well to an active programme and positive atmosphere provided by a rehabilitation unit or spinal injuries unit where staff and patients face the problems of handicap with an optimistic and enthusiastic attitude. In principle the symptoms presented by MS should be treated as they would be if they were the result of trauma or other disease. This approach will lead to a more active and positive treatment with the focus upon the strengths rather than upon the problems.

Where the disease leads to disability the patient should, from the earliest, be encouraged to take the responsibility for his own well-being particularly with regard to skin care generally, prevention of pressure sores, contractures, bowel and bladder function and the avoidance of infection.

The motor dysfunction seen in these patients arises from the disorganised neurological mechanisms of posture, balance and movement, and treatment should be aimed primarily at these central mechanisms. However, management of the disabled MS sufferer needs to be continuous and not confined to 'treatment' sessions. If certain postural mechanisms are stimulated during treatment and not reinforced between sessions, they will need to be retaught every time. If treatment is aimed at prevention of deformity and counteracted by bad positions and abnormal movement for the rest of the day then the effect will be wasted. It is therefore most important to consider the handling and equipment used throughout the 24 hours and not just during the treatment period.

The therapist must allow time to explain the rationale of treatment to the patient, his relatives and to any staff who may be involved, as well as teaching specific handling or positioning necessary to stimulate required responses. All those caring for MS sufferers must be shown which postures and movements to encourage, and which to avoid, i.e. which positions will make certain movements easier so that independence can be retained. Wherever possible, it is more effective if these activities can be incorporated into the daily routine so that a way of life is established which allows for continuous therapy.

Appropriate treatment will lessen the effect of any symptoms and, therefore, the earlier it is started the more opportunity is given for re-educating whatever potential abilities exist for decreasing deficit and avoiding secondary preventable complications. The therapist should encourage good relations with the neurologists and general practitioners who refer patients, to ensure they understand the role that the therapist can play in advising about ways of reducing to a minimum the effects of new symptoms or overcoming any functional difficulties, and the advantages of early contact with the therapist in the prevention of secondary handicap.

Periods of immobility for whatever reason should be stringently avoided. Special care is necessary at the following time: influenza, colds or infection; surgery; pregnancy; fracture or sprain of a joint and following the provision of a walking aid or wheelchair. At such times early activity and the need to be out of bed is normally stressed but MS sufferers tend to be kept immobile for longer. The need to stand, walk and balance in sitting on the side of the bed each day is vitally important. A refresher course of intensive physiotherapy after such an event will ensure the former level of function is regained.

CLINICAL PICTURE

According to the site of the lesions the clinical picture can present a broad spectrum of dysfunction. Damage can occur anywhere in the brain or spinal cord resulting in malfunction of any of the neurological mechanisms. As MS is usually a progressive disease with gradually increasing neurological deficit, the signs and symptoms are not static and may also vary from day to day.

It is a complex condition, not just a motor problem. As motor function cannot be isolated from other functions, it is important for the therapist to recognise that she is dealing with a multiple handicap. There will be handicaps arising from the original lesion and often secondary handicaps arising directly from these or resulting from inadequate management of basic defects. To illustrate this, paucity of movement leads to limited sensation and perception of everyday things. This lack of experience may also lead to apparent defects of perception such as agnosia or apraxia. If there is decreased movement in the legs and the patient is allowed to transfer like a paraplegic his ability to use the legs becomes further reduced. Lack of experience can also affect speech and lead to more rapid deterioration of language.

Behavioural and intellectual disturbance may be apparent, again as a direct result of pathology or due to inadequate emotional and social experience for which movement is necessary. Most people coping with a physical disability will experience increased anxiety, irritability or changes of mood from time to time.

Because of the variety of presenting symptoms, classification according to distribution is frequently used. To assist communication and discussion terms such as hemiplegia and paraplegia are used; they are often imprecise as other limbs may be slightly affected and, however minimally involved, one part will always affect movement throughout the body. Additionally, it is possible to use a broad classification according to predominant type, e.g. ataxic, spastic or mixed. As the lesion develops predominant features can vary either as a result of changing pathology or according to management.

SOME FEATURES COMMON TO ALL TYPES

Disturbance of Sensation

Disturbances such as paraesthesia or numbness and tingling are frequently early clinical signs. Sensory deficit may be due to the actual disease process or due to lack of experience or awareness. Abnormal afferent information will give rise to abnormal responses. Without correction, repetition of abnormal afferent sensation will eventually be learned and accepted as the normal.

Impaired Vision

Unfortunately, this is an added complication in a multiple handicap where eyes may have to substitute for proprioceptive loss.

Abnormal Tone

This may be of supraspinal or spinal origin and may present as hypotonia or hypertonia which is usually in the form of spasticity but occasionally rigidity is found.

Voluntary Movement

Once tone is normalised the active movement itself may vary in strength and coordination and it may not automatically occur during balance and maintenance of posture. Frequently, full use is not made of all available isolated movement for functional activities and disuse will often result in reduced ability, e.g. persistence in locking the knee in hyperextension when walking may contribute to loss of ability to take weight on a mobile knee. Using the better arm exclusively, because it is quicker, for feeding or dressing may lead to a more rapid deterioration of the other arm.

Involuntary Movement

This may be present and can be general or isolated to one joint or limb.

Disturbance of Posture and Balance Mechanisms

Postural reactions cannot be separated from voluntary movement but they deserve special consideration because training voluntary activity does not necessarily re-educate or stimulate the necessary postural reactions (see Chapter 2) which also do not seem to correlate with tone.

Prevailing Abnormal Postures

These may be as a direct result of abnormal tone, or may be because of excessive use of the influence of reflex patterns or attitudes, particularly the influence of the labyrinthine reflex, the symmetrical and asymmetrical tonic neck reflex either to aid movement or to achieve postural stability. It is important to watch that any unfixed deformities do not become fixed contractures as a result of adaptive shortening of soft tissues.

PRINCIPLES OF PHYSIOTHERAPY

The successful treatment of the neurological defects found in MS requires a combination of the skills developed in other specialised areas particularly from the treatment of stroke, head injury, spinal injury and cerebral palsy. The physiotherapist may be involved from the earliest signs to the terminal stages of the disease and she therefore needs to be acquainted with all the appropriate techniques required to treat any of the many possible signs and symptoms. At each stage specific techniques will be required to treat the neurological deficit and to allow any potential a chance to reveal itself. Every attempt must be made to facilitate normal movement or coordination which may have been lost during an exacerbation or period of immobility. Prompt intervention will reduce to a minimum the deficit and avoid the effects of forgetting due to lack of experience.

General principles of assessment and treatment are described in the early chapters of this book and readers are advised to refer to specialised sections for help with specific problems. Here, general advice for the planning of treatment will be given and, for convenience, special advice and points for emphasis will be indicated as though the course of the disease could be divided into four stages, although in practice one will merge with another.

AIMS OF PHYSIOTHERAPY

1. To re-educate and strengthen all available voluntary control.
2. To re-educate and maintain normal postural mechanisms.
3. To maintain full range of motion of all joints and soft tissues and to teach the patient and/or his relatives suitable stretching procedures to prevent contractures.
4. To incorporate treatment techniques into the way of life by relating them to suitable daily activities thus providing a means of maintaining any improvement.
5. To offer advice about sensible use of energy.
6. To prevent the use of abnormal movement which is inefficient and tiring in itself and may inhibit function.
7. To stimulate all sensory and perceptual experiences and

maintain the experience of normal movement throughout the course of the disease not only to exploit potential but to enable the patient to feel safer and move more freely when the assistance of relatives or helpers is required in the later stages.

General Preventive Measures

No two patients are alike in either their circumstances or their symptoms, thus no two treatments can be the same. However, whatever approach is adopted, there are certain problems seen in most patients with disability which must be anticipated and prevented.

PLANTAR FLEXED FEET

These can be prevented by avoiding the use of a total pattern of extension for weight-bearing; by attention to the posture of the feet when sitting; and by daily standing if walking is no longer functional.

A PREDOMINANT PATTERN OF EXTENSION AND ADDUCTION IN THE LOWER EXTREMITIES

This can be inhibited by training correct weight-bearing through a mobile knee; by attention to adequate flexion at the hip joint when sitting; and by the use of tailor-sitting to stretch the adductors.

KNEE FLEXION CONTRACTURE

This can be prevented if the hamstrings are stretched by touching the toes in long sitting while keeping both knees extended.

HIP FLEXION CONTRACTURES

These can be prevented by ensuring good hip extension when walking or standing. Daily prone lying should be encouraged.

FLEXED THORACIC SPINE

This can be avoided by active dorsal extension in sitting and when prone; stretching by supine lying over a pillow, or in sitting with hand support behind.

FLEXION AND INTERNAL ROTATION AT THE SHOULDERS

This can be counteracted by training balance reactions and by self-assisted full range shoulder elevation.

FIXED HEAD POSITIONS

These may be avoided by training adequate balance and postural reactions and preventing the use of abnormal movement patterns.

SPECIAL EMPHASIS NEEDED AT DIFFERENT STAGES

Early Advice

Initially the patient may complain of poor balance on the stairs, difficulty with fine finger movements or heaviness of one leg, and eye symptoms or some sensory disturbance may be present.

1. If the patient is referred to a physiotherapist at this stage, however minor the deficit appears to be, a thorough assessment of movement in all positions will enable suitable advice to be given about any potential lack of symmetry in posture, movement or balance which is observed.

2. If appropriate, emphasis can be given to certain activities in daily life which would stimulate postural and balance responses, e.g. going up and down stairs one foot after the other and standing from sitting without using the hands for balance; lifting one leg across the other when putting on shoes and socks; emphasis of dorsal extension during dressing or when reaching for objects. If suitable activities can be introduced as part of the daily routine it saves devoting time to special 'exercises'. However, if more specific emphasis is required additional work in standing or on a tilt board or large beach ball can easily be practised at home (see Chapter 11).

3. The benefit of resting in a position of side lying rather than supine can be explained, also that the patient must learn to lie in a prone position either over a pillow, foam wedge or suitable cushion, perhaps while reading or watching television, or even while sleeping.

4. The usual occupation and pastimes should be continued: during the assessment, work and leisure activities may be discussed with a view to conservation of energy; this is similar to the consideration which is given to joint preservation with arthritis sufferers. For the MS sufferer the danger of doing too much seems less than the danger of doing too little but slight adjustments made in the organisation of the daily routine may avoid undue fatigue and conserve energy for more enjoyable pursuits.

5. The patient should be advised to keep fit and healthy and encouraged to pursue some form of active exercise. Some neurologists prescribe the Rest Exercise Programme (REP) developed by Ritchie Russell. The programme is designed to influence the circulation around the spinal cord and brainstem and consists of two or three rest periods of 10 to 20 minutes each day preceded by a regime of stressful mat exercises such as press-ups, and weight lifting carried out until the patient is dyspnoeic and the heart rate increased. Other

neurologists prefer to encourage participation in sport such as tennis, badminton, and swimming or riding, which provides valuable recreation as well as keeping the patient active. Any abnormal patterns of movement observed during these activities should be corrected because if continued they will reinforce the abnormal at the expense of the normal.

6. After initial and intensive re-education and instruction during the early stage, patients may find it helpful to attend follow-up sessions every two or three months to evaluate the programme and to discuss any other problems. Regular out-patient physiotherapy should not be necessary nor encouraged if adequate adaption has been made to daily activities.

Slightly More Marked Signs but Walking Unaided

If the signs and symptoms increase, re-assessment is necessary and adjustments made to their management. It is helpful to involve relatives and, if necessary, visit both home and work to make further suggestions about sensible use of energy and ways of overcoming particular problems. The physiotherapist should be ready to ask the help of other members of the team, e.g. social worker, nurse, occupational and speech therapist and dietician. The same principles of management are continued but special attention may be needed in the following:

1. Diet: If necessary, advice should be sought as an increase of only 1kg (2.2lb) can affect mobility in a person with even minimal increased tone in the legs. Paradoxically, when ataxia is a feature, energy output is increased and this, in combination with tiredness and laboured feeding, could result in a gradual reduction in weight.

2. As the signs become more marked, concern about the future increases and social and psychological problems may arise. Frequently, some of the fear and depression can be relieved if the patient and family are given a fuller understanding of the symptoms, or practical guidance to overcome the physical or financial problems connected with employment, mobility or domestic arrangements. Occasionally, skilled counselling may be helpful to overcome specific marital, family or sexual difficulties. If some of the psychological stress can be alleviated, energy can be channelled more constructively towards enjoyment of life in spite of the handicap.

3. If the function of the bladder or bowel is affected the patient should understand that correct management of them could influence the amount of tone throughout the body. The bladder may be hypertonic or hypotonic and increased irritability or retention or any

infection will increase tone generally which, in its turn, could affect mobility. Bowel function should be managed to avoid constipation as this will cause increased tone and may also affect bladder function.

4. Particular attention will be required to overcome undesirable habits and to teach the specific stretching activities already mentioned to prevent any adaptive shortening.

5. Whatever type of abnormal tone is present there will usually be reduced rotation in the trunk in an attempt to maintain stability when walking; therefore, activities to encourage facilitation of this must be incorporated into treatment sessions and into home or work activities. For example, a suitable self-activity could be side sitting to inhibit extensor thrust, rolling both knees together from one side to the other – and if the arms are clasped above the head this will emphasise much needed dorsal extension. When ataxia is present the activity may be adapted during treatment so that approximation can be given through the arms in a 'lifting' pattern. In addition, always turning on to the side before sitting on the edge of the bed to get up, will facilitate rotation and head and trunk righting reactions.

6. Use of walking aids: Great care must be taken when an aid for walking becomes necessary and suitable activities which will counteract any detrimental effects should be encouraged. These effects may not be immediately apparent. Where possible, aids should be given during a refresher course so that proper instruction and evaluation may be carried out and arrangements made for a further follow-up. Typical points to watch would be:

(a) alteration in posture due to leaning on the stick or crutches;

(b) marked reduction in balance reactions of head and trunk through using the hands for balance resulting in increased difficulty with other functional activities in lying and sitting;

(c) possible alteration in distribution of tone throughout the body requiring extra care to maintain all the isolated movement available.

In a Wheelchair for Part of the Time

The chair should not be used full time until absolutely necessary and every effort must be made to keep ambulant if at all possible. However, it may be advisable to use a wheelchair for long distances in order to save time and to avoid unnecessary fatigue. This is a very dangerous period in management and many complications are directly related to insufficient guidance at this time. The inevitable reduction in amount of activity and increased use of the sitting posture usually lead to an alteration in patterns of spasticity and movement which will need specific treatment if potential problems are to be avoided.

1. The prescription of the wheelchair requires full consultation between the user, his relatives and all members of the team. There are many guides to assist the necessary decisions, but a few points will be mentioned as simple basic mistakes are frequently made with rather serious consequences. If the chair is not correctly measured it can cause or increase abnormal postures, especially if it is too wide. The height of the foot plates is particularly important; they should be able to be adjusted to achieve a right-angle at the hips and knees. Some elevating leg rests do not allow this and should be avoided. Heel straps which are fixed to the foot plate are frequently ordered; unless altered they hold the forefoot in an unsupported position and this leads to increased flexion of toes. The slightest tightness of toe or plantar flexors increases spasticity and could prevent walking or, later, the vital use of standing for transfers and maintenance. A strap behind the legs is more practical. Some reclining back rests will not raise sufficiently to allow a right-angle at the hips – a fact which may alter the management of tone and posture in the trunk and legs.

2. Wheelchair management should be very carefully taught. It is as important for the MS sufferer to receive the same detailed preparation and instruction in the use of the wheelchair which would be given to a person with traumatic paraplegia. This means meticulous attention to symmetry of posture with even weight distribution on both buttocks. The patient should be warned not to maintain asymmetrical positions for long periods, for example always leaning on the same arm could lead to a scoliosis and affect the tone in the trunk and legs. The degree of flexion at the hip will influence both the position of the head and trunk and the pattern of spasticity in the leg. Too much extension at the hip can increase extensor thrust in the leg. Hip retraction on one side can produce a pattern of flexion adduction and medial rotation with corresponding decrease in functional ability. The automatic use of the wheelchair arms should be avoided, unless necessary for safety; this will stimulate a more active sitting posture which will help to retain balance mechanisms. Sitting in a suitable ordinary chair makes a change from the wheelchair.

3. The period when there is increased use of the sitting position requires close supervision not only to ensure adequate management of the tendency of hypertonus to change from extension to flexion but also to prevent contractures. The patient must walk each day and if extra support is required in the way of gaiters, splints, bracing, a suitable walking aid or parallel bars, these should be readily available. Any interruption in the routine may mean not only losing the skill for ever but a risk of introducing a vicious circle of complications (p.176).

4. Extra care with stretching of muscle groups which tend to

shorten is vital. A pause to give an extra stretch each time a transfer is executed will help to maintain the length of the calf muscles and the hip flexors. The prone position and tailor-sitting will maintain range at the hip but specific stretching of hamstrings in long sitting is required. It is usually necessary to check full shoulder elevation, especially if ataxia is present, because this movement is performed so rarely in daily life (see pp.227–8).

5. There may be considerable changes during this period. Probably even part-time work will no longer be practical and alternative pursuits must be found to continue an interesting and stimulating life and to continue a responsible role within the family and social circle. Guidance may also be needed on various aspects to retain personal independence; this may include advice about suitable clothing and footwear as well as other aids which will enable the person to remain independent for as long as possible.

FULL TIME USE OF A WHEELCHAIR

1. Once walking is no longer feasible even for maintenance, additional provison must be made for standing. The physiological benefits of standing include reduction of spasticity, maintenance of length of hip and the knee flexors and calf muscles, more efficient drainage of the kidneys and possible benefits to counteract osteoporosis. Support for the knees in standing could include gaiters, plaster of Paris or polythene back slabs, or long-leg bracing. If needed, suitable apparatus must be supplied to assist standing at home (see Chapter 9).

In residential care or hospital a tilt table may be used with the patient prone or supine but care is required to obtain equal weight-bearing through both legs. It is of more benefit if standing can be an active and not just a passive experience. Correction of symmetry and posture, and activities to encourage balance can be practised while in the upright position.

2. Additional help may be needed to improve independence at home. Modifications to the bed or bathroom may retain independent turning and transfers or make it easier for helpers to assist. If the standing transfer has been maintained it is usually possible for relatives to manage a pivot transfer even when the disease is advanced (see p.221).

3. If necessary the patient may have to ask relatives to assist with positioning, stretching and pressure relief. If he is no longer able to correct the sitting posture himself extra care is needed to check that there is equal weight distribution and good alignment of the trunk and limbs. This is particularly important on some air filled cushions which

make balance more critical. Vigilant attention to such details will frequently overcome problems of balance and posture of the head and trunk which affect feeding and speech, or asymmetry in the lower limbs which could be the start of a vicious circle of complications.

MANAGEMENT OF SPASTICITY

Spasticity and its management has been fully discussed in Chapter 7 but it needs to be reiterated that managing spasticity in multiple sclerosis is of the utmost importance. The following points need to be continually remembered:

1. Diligent attention to educating the need for avoidance of positions and activities which increase tone or reinforce abnormal movement patterns.

2. Daily walking or standing for weight-bearing which has an inhibiting effect on hypertonus.

3. Constipation, bladder infections, pressure sores must be avoided.

4. Regular stretching of all potentially tight structures, especially at danger times, e.g. illness or the transition to a wheelchair. Contractures must be prevented at all costs; action must be taken as soon as there is any difficulty in obtaining full range by either increasing the amount of treatment or using some other adjunct.

5. Prolonged application of ice either locally or for total immersion can be used effectively for temporary reduction of hypertonus.

6. The inhibitory effect of drugs such as baclofen and diazepam is sometimes helpful but close monitoring is required as they may reduce arousal and active ability.

7. Use of splinting needs careful consideration as, without extra treatment, it may actually increase the problem. Removable splints are usually ineffective because the corrected position is not maintained and they are difficult to re-apply. However, at danger times splinting in the form of an all-round plaster of Paris cylinder for the leg or a below knee weight-bearing plaster can sometimes be considered to inhibit spasticity. If contractures do occur application of serial plasters can be used to correct the shortening.

8. Intrathecal injections of phenol may be useful but require knowledge of the neurological mechanisms involved as well as an understanding of the implication of any imbalance in a movement disorder. If ataxia is also present the possible reduction in stability should be considered.

9. Surgery may be required either to divide or to lengthen tendons, e.g. the hamstrings or tendo Achilles, or in the form of a partial or total

neurectomy, e.g. obturator. However, unless the original cause of the problem is eliminated or a different management is introduced the difficulty is likely to recur.

MANAGEMENT OF ATAXIA

Ataxia and its management has been discussed in Chapter 7 but, as with spasticity, ataxia requires understanding and continual treatment. The following points need to be remembered:

1. Attention to ensuring adequate experience of movement can easily be overlooked because of the voluntary control present which makes the lack of use less obvious to the therapist.

2. Many patients voluntarily restrict movement of the head and trunk to gain more stability and extra emphasis should be given to the stimulation of balance and righting reactions during treatment.

3. Instability and difficulty in performing activities against gravity often leads to the use of abnormal patterns of movement or reflex attitudes in an attempt to increase tone and achieve stability. This may appear to be an acceptable short-term answer but later on it may contribute to reduced functional ability, e.g. pressing the head into extension and rotation against the back of the chair can affect tone in the limbs and reduce the demand for already poor head control. Always folding the arms or pushing one arm into extension and medial rotation may assist sitting balance but will prevent use of the arms for more skilled functions and predispose to contracture.

4. A person with poor coordination tends to push against any available surface to achieve stability; therefore, any straps, aids or props used to assist certain functional activities, if permanently fixed, may actually increase abnormal movement and could eventually prevent the original function they were aiding.

5. Some approaches, e.g. those developed by Dr Frenkel and Professor Peto have emphasised use of cortical control in learning and training motor ability. The principle of using repetition of activities with variations in speed, rhythm and range, reinforced by speech, hearing and vision is valuable and can be superimposed on all functional activities.

ADDITIONAL MANAGEMENT

Respiration

Breathing exercises should be incorporated into the programme at all stages. If the muscles involved in respiration are affected, the patient and relatives can be shown suitable positions for postural drainage and how to assist coughing to clear secretions. In advanced cases, use of suction may remove secretions more effectively if coughing is tiring.

Feeding

It is particularly important to be aware of the effect of position and posture on a patient's ability to feed independently. Training balance reactions, head control, eye/hand coordination, could help to retain the basic motor skills required to bring the food to the mouth. Techniques to normalise tone, increase sensation and facilitate voluntary control within the mouth help to maintain patterns of chewing and swallowing necessary for efficient feeding.

Whenever possible the patient must be encouraged to feed himself and adaptations to cutlery, non-slip mats, and thermal plates can be helpful.

In many instances a liquid diet is given when what is really required is advice about suitable positions and instruction in facilitation of chewing and swallowing. With the right help it should be possible for a normal diet to be enjoyed. Solid food will help to retain the ability to chew, and stimulate lip closure and tongue and cheek movements. Maintaining good oral feeding patterns will also help to maintain speech patterns.

Communication and Mobility

A variety of systems to assist with the use of telephone, radio, typewriter and other communication aids can be supplied to allow more independence. Various forms of motorised transport are available for those who cannot manage a hand driven chair.

Bladder and Bowel Function

Incontinence can cause much embarrassment but problems arising from such distressing complications must not be accepted as an automatic outcome of MS. Adequate management is possible and dignity can be maintained. Much help can be gained by reference to the careful management accorded to bladder and bowel function in spinal injuries units. The initial responsibility for accurate diagnosis causing the incontinence belongs to the doctor but the therapist may be involved in establishing a suitable training regime. The therapist must be aware of the need to avoid infection of the bladder or retention of urine, as this can damage the kidneys and also have a marked effect on spasticity.

Constipation is a frequent problem with MS; it is aggravated by reduced mobility and has a marked effect on spasticity. It can be helped by allotting a regular time of day for bowel movement, a larger fluid intake and a high residue diet. If this is insufficient, regular aperients and suppositories every two or three days are used to train a convenient and regular routine.

The therapist can help the patient and his family to accept that effective management is possible in most instances and is of vital importance both medically and socially.

Prevention of Pressure Sores

Pressure sores can be prevented; if attention is given to stressing special positioning to inhibit spasticity and to the importance of relieving pressure in bed and in the wheelchair, the patient need no longer fear that pressure sores are inevitable. (See Chapter 9 for preventive measures.)

BIBLIOGRAPHY

Barton, A. and Barton, M. (1981). *The Management and Prevention of Pressure Sores*. Faber and Faber, London and Boston.

Davies, P. M. (1975). 'A physiotherapist's approach to multiple sclerosis.' *Physiotherapy*, **61**, 1, 5–6.

Gautier-Smith, P. G. (1976). 'Clinical management of spastic states.' *Physiotherapy*, **62**, 10, 326–8.

Lee, J. M. and Warren, M. P. (1978). *Cold Therapy in Rehabilitation*. Bell and Hyman, London.

Mandelstam, D. (1977). *Incontinence*. Heinemann Health Books Publication, London.

Nosworthy, S. J. (1976). 'Physiotherapy. A symposium on multiple sclerosis.' *Nursing Mirror*, **147**, 6 (5 August).

Ritchie Russell, W. and Palfrey, G. (1969). 'Disseminated sclerosis – rest and exercise therapy – a progress report.' *Physiotherapy*, **55**, 8, 306–10.

See also the Bibliography on pp.147, 250 and 276.

Chapter 15

Parkinsonism – Clinical

by R. B. GODWIN-AUSTEN, M.D., F.R.C.P.

Parkinson's disease and the parkinsonian syndrome comprise a group of disorders characterised by tremor and disturbance of voluntary movement, posture and balance. Parkinson's disease was first described by James Parkinson in 1817; its pathology was defined about one hundred years later and the treatment has been revolutionised since the 1960s by the introduction of levodopa.

The 'parkinsonian syndrome' is that group of disorders in which the characteristic symptoms and signs of parkinsonism develop but are secondary to another neurological disease (e.g. encephalitis lethargica, Alzheimer's disease, etc). Thus, whereas Parkinson's disease is a primary degenerative condition occurring in the latter half of life and following a progressive course, the parkinsonian syndrome has a natural history dependent on the cause. The word 'parkinsonism' is used to describe the symptoms and signs irrespective of the cause of the disease state. Where the parkinsonian syndrome is complicated by some generalised degenerative process (e.g. cerebral arteriosclerosis) treatment may be less satisfactory than in the uncomplicated case.

CLINICAL FEATURES

The patient with parkinsonism may present with the characteristic tremor. The diagnosis is then easily established although it is important not to label other forms of tremor 'parkinsonian'. More than 50 per cent of patients with Parkinson's disease do not have any tremor and the presenting symptoms are then much more diverse. The patient usually attributes the symptoms of the disease to 'old age' and is correspondingly grateful when treatment relieves them. Common presenting symptoms are slowness of walking and disturbance of balance with occasional falls or difficulty with fine manipulative movements such as dressing or shaving. Pain is a common presenting complaint and patients may attend a physiotherapy department for the treatment of cervical spondylosis, frozen shoulder, backache or osteoarthritis of the hip when their symptoms are in fact due to parkinsonism. The pain is rapidly relieved by appropriate treatment for their parkinsonism.

The general slowing up, associated as it often is by an apathy with depression, may lead friends and family to conclude that the patient is dementing. This is seldom the case. Patients with parkinsonism retain intellect and are the most cooperative patients to treat.

Early symptoms of the disease may include difficulty with specific movements such as writing; difficulty in turning over in bed or rising from a low chair; an excessive greasiness of the skin or an unusual tendency to constipation; and an inability to raise the voice or cough effectively. And all the symptoms tend to be disproportionately worse when the patient is under stress. Furthermore most patients discover that they have become much more subject to the effects of what would formerly have been regarded as trivial stresses. The patient therefore tends to avoid social engagements and to reduce the amount of work he does. The family may then conclude that it is all due to 'laziness' or psychological causes.

SIGNS

Posture

The patient with Parkinson's disease usually shows some disorder of posture. When standing there is a slight flexion at all joints leading to the 'simian posture' with the knees and hips slightly flexed, the shoulders rounded and the head held forward with the arms bent across the trunk (Fig. 15/1). More rarely the abnormality of posture will be a tendency to lean backwards with a rather erect stance.

When sitting the patient tends to slump in the chair often sliding sideways until supported by the arm of the chair. The head again may fall forwards on the chest.

The abnormal posture can be voluntarily corrected but only temporarily and with considerable effort and concentration.

Balance

When standing, these patients characteristically have a tendency to topple forwards. They are unable to make the quick compensatory movements to regain balance and so are easily knocked over. When

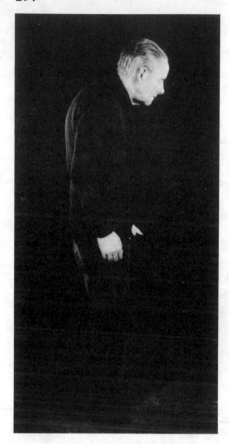

Fig. 15/1 The typical posture of a man with Parkinson's disease

they start to walk there is difficulty in shifting the centre of gravity from one foot to the other so their paces become short and shuffling – and the patient may lean too far forward in walking so that he has to 'chase' his centre of gravity if he is to avoid falling forwards.

There are specific difficulties in turning round or initiating the movements of walking. The patient describes the feeling 'as if the feet are glued to the floor'. If he is pulled, he will fall over and an important part of physiotherapy is to teach the patient and his family how to overcome these problems (see Chapter 16).

Getting out of a chair may be difficult because the patient can no longer automatically judge how to place his centre of gravity over his feet. Thus he falls back into the chair each time he attempts to rise.

Learnt and Voluntary Movements

All movements are reduced in range and speed (akinesia). In walking the patient tends to take small paces and to walk more slowly. Speech becomes slower and softer. Handwriting tends to get smaller and after writing a few words slows down and becomes increasingly untidy. Cutting up food may become impossible and buttons and shoelaces likewise. Repetitive movements such as stirring and polishing are often particularly affected.

By contrast some complex coordinated movements such as driving a car may be relatively little affected. And similarly the preparation of meals and tasks such as cleaning a house or using a typewriter may pose few problems, although slower than normal.

Automatic Movements

These are specifically reduced or lost in Parkinson's disease. The patient blinks infrequently and has an expressionless 'mask-like' face giving the spurious appearance of stupidity. There are none of the restless associated movements of the hands seen in the normal. When walking the patient does not swing his arms but instead walks with them hanging slightly flexed at the elbow.

Automatic swallowing of saliva is also impaired so that these patients tend to dribble involuntarily particularly when they sit with the head flexed on the chest.

Coughing as an automatic reflex response to clear the airway may be defective and there is therefore a risk of respiratory infection.

Unfortunately treatment does not restore any of these defects of automatic movement to any significant degree.

Rigidity

Muscle tone is increased in parkinsonism but the resistance to passive movement at a joint is uniform throughout the range of the movement (in contrast to spastic hypertonia). Two types of parkinsonian rigidity are described – 'lead pipe' where the resistance is smooth or plastic; and 'cogwheel' where the resistance is intermittent.

Although rigidity does not account for the poverty of movement which characterises parkinsonism it undoubtedly contributes to it. Similarly it is the rigidity which plays a part in the causation of the muscle pain already described. Relief of the rigid hypertonia is an important part therefore of the treatment.

Rigidity may be very asymmetrical or even unilateral. It may occasionally only affect one group of muscles to any significant degree – such as the neck muscles, forearm or thigh muscles. And it increases with nervous tension or in a cold environment.

Tremor

Like rigidity tremor is usually asymmetrical or unilateral. It consists of an alternating contraction of opposing muscle groups causing a rhythmical movement at about four to six cycles per second. Tremor is usually maximal at the periphery and affects the arm more frequently than the leg.

Tremor is more of an embarrassment to the patient than a handicap because it is maximally present at rest but reduces or disappears on voluntary movement. Thus the patient is able to lift a glass to his mouth steadily without spilling the contents but the hand when relaxed on the lap is constantly shaking. Furthermore any anxiety or self-consciousness increases the tremor so that the embarrassment of any social occasion may become intolerable.

AETIOLOGY

The symptoms and signs of parkinsonism stem from a disturbance of function in two regions of the basal ganglia – the substantia nigra and the corpus striatum (caudate nucleus and putamen). These central nuclear masses of grey matter contain practically all the dopamine in the human brain. Dopamine is a chemical substance and one of the neurotransmitter amines (like adrenaline and noradrenaline) which carry the electrical message from one neurone to the next across the synapse. In parkinsonism there is a specific reduction of dopamine concentration at the synapse. This lack of dopamine results from a degeneration of neurones in Parkinson's disease or in the degenerative parkinsonian syndromes (such as Alzheimer's disease) or from focal damage in the parkinsonian syndromes following encephalitis lethargica, head injury or manganese poisoning. There is a chemical block to the action of dopamine in parkinsonism due to phenothiazine drugs.

Parkinson's disease accounts for the great majority of cases of parkinsonism. The cause of the degeneration in the substantia nigra and corpus striatum is unknown but it is a progressive process with a time course from onset to death between 10 and 15 years. Some cases progress more rapidly. Others so slowly that deterioration may be undetectable. And modern treatment has so improved the prognosis that there is now no overall excess mortality from Parkinson's disease when comparison is made with individuals of the same age.

In the worst cases increasing immobility leads eventually to weight loss, pressure sores and respiratory complications which are the usual cause of death.

In parkinsonism secondary to phenothiazine drugs or following encephalitis lethargica (now very rare) involuntary spasms of the eyes (oculo-gyric crises) may occur. Post-encephalitic parkinsonism is often non-progressive and may be associated with widespread brain damage causing behavioural disorder, spastic weakness and visual disturbance.

Features of the parkinsonian syndrome may occur in patients following a single severe head injury or following multiple head injuries (e.g. in boxers). Such cases are generally resistant to drug treatment, and like those cases in whom parkinsonism is part of a generalised degenerative process there is commonly intellectual impairment further reducing therapeutic responsiveness.

TREATMENT

The treatment of the patient with parkinsonism must be multidisciplinary and above all designed to be appropriate to the individual case. Thus the patient with only tremor is going to require very little treatment, whereas disturbance of locomotion or severe slowness of movement of the hands (bradykinesia) may require treatment involving drugs, physiotherapy and occupational therapy. The more disabled patients usually require the advice and assistance of medical social workers, welfare officers and disablement resettlement officers.

Drug treatment and physiotherapy are the most important forms of treatment in this condition with surgical treatment being only occasionally appropriate.

Drug Treatment

The depletion of brain dopamine characteristic of this condition causes a reactive increased production of acetyl choline in the basal ganglia. Treatment is designed therefore to replenish the dopamine by administering the dopamine precursor levodopa – and reduce the acetyl choline with anticholinergic drugs such as benzhexol (Artane) or orphenadrine (Disipal). Levodopa is usually given in combination with a chemical which prevents its metabolism outside the brain and these combined tablets are marketed as Sinemet (levodopa plus carbidopa) and Madopar (levodopa plus benserazide).

Levodopa-containing drugs are the most effective treatment for the severe case and provide relief from most of the symptoms and signs especially the slowness and poverty of voluntary movement which is the main cause of disability. They also relieve the rigidity and substantially reduce the tremor. While on treatment with these drugs many patients lose all the manifestations of the disease and appear 'cured' although as soon as the treatment is stopped symptoms recur. On this treatment improvement may increase over many months.

Side-effects may be troublesome at the start of treatment (nausea and vomiting, postural hypotension, confusional states) or become manifest only after months or years of treatment (choreiform involuntary movements of the face or limbs, and 'on-off' attacks in which for periods of 30 minutes to two hours the patient becomes profoundly akinetic and unable to move).

Anticholinergic drugs, while less effective than levodopa have an additive therapeutic effect with particular benefit to rigidity. They produce dryness of the mouth, slight blurring of near vision and occasionally hesitancy of micturition and confusional states.

The side-effects of both types of drug are dose dependent, disappearing when the dose is reduced.

Amantadine is sometimes used in the mild case. It acts by releasing dopamine in the brain but it is less potent and effective than levodopa.

Bromocriptine is a synthetic compound which mimics levodopa in all its actions and side-effects but has a slightly longer period of action.

The value of destructive surgical procedures on the thalamus in cases of parkinsonism was discovered in 1958 by a happy accident. During an operation on the brain of a patient with Parkinson's disease a small blood vessel had to be tied because of a haemorrhage. The resulting 'stroke' far from increasing the patient's disability led to the abolition of tremor and reduction of rigidity on the other side of the body. Tremor continued to be treated by surgical means until the advent of levodopa which is a more effective and safer method of treatment in most cases.

General Care

None of the drug therapy is effective unless the patient takes advantage of his improvement and returns to more normal activity. The slowness of movement and difficulties with walking make the patient disinclined to be active and tend to make him over-ready to accept help and become dependent on others. This leads to a dependent state of mind and chronic invalidism. Furthermore relatives tend to be over-anxious to help, and must be advised to allow, and indeed encourage, the patient to remain independent however long it takes him, for example, to dress or wash. Regular exercise should be encouraged, and the patient should remain at work if possible and continue to maintain an interest in hobbies, sport and social activities.

It is rarely necessary, even for the most severely afflicted cases, to require hospital care – even on a day basis. Home nursing is normally satisfactory following occupational therapist advice on aids and appliances – such as a high chair (and raised lavatory seat), zips and Velcro fastenings to clothes, electric razor and toothbrush.

The occasional patient is bed or wheelchair-bound but here the nursing care required is no different from that of any other patient unable to stand or walk. In such cases particular attention has to be paid to respiratory infection and pressure sores since intercurrent illness greatly exacerbates the parkinsonian disability, and reduces the benefits of drug treatment.

Physiotherapy

See Chapter 16.

BIBLIOGRAPHY

Marsden, T. D. and Parkes, J. D. (1977). 'Success and problems of long-term therapy in Parkinson's disease.' *Lancet*, i, 345.

Matthews, W. B. and Miller, Henry (1979). *Diseases of the Nervous System*, 3rd edition. Blackwell Scientific Publications Limited, Oxford.

Parkinson's Disease: A Booklet for Patients and Their Families, by R. B. Godwin-Austen and published by the Parkinson's Disease Society.

Chapter 16

Parkinsonism – Physiotherapy

by M. A. HARRISON, m.c.s.p.

Physiotherapy may be required for the patient who is also receiving drug therapy or who has undergone surgical intervention or, in fact, for the patient who is having no other form of therapy.

It is important to appreciate that the patient should be given help and advice by the physiotherapist as early as possible. Many patients are given a diagnosis of parkinsonism while in its very early stages, and may be given no help at all because they are considered 'not bad enough' to warrant drug therapy, physiotherapy or surgery. This may be true of drug therapy and surgery but it is not true of physiotherapy. The sooner the patient can be seen by the physiotherapist the better, because it is easier to prevent loss of normal movement patterns than it is to regain them after they have apparently disappeared and abnormalities have become a habit. Less time is required for the initial treatments and a few more months or years of relative independence may be gained by the patient.

If the patient has had surgery or is receiving drug therapy, he may still benefit from the help of the physiotherapist. By this time he may well have had the disease for several years. The onset tends to be gradual and the patient adapts to his symptoms, so that the various movement problems become a habit to such an extent that he is unaware of the true degree of his abnormality. Drugs and surgery may dramatically change the situation and make more normal reactions fairly readily available. However, the patient may have 'forgotten' the patterns and then will never realise his full potential without some help.

It is important to appreciate that physiotherapy cannot bring about a reversal of the changes which have occurred in the central nervous system as a result of the disease process. It is only possible to help the patient to minimise the effect of these changes by encouraging activities to remain as normal as possible. The patient's nervous system can only do its best in the circumstances, and the physiotherapist can only help it to exploit its full potential.

Assessment

All patients should be assessed carefully, since symptoms will vary according to the stage of the disease and the effect of other therapy being used. Assessment procedures should follow the lines indicated in Chapter 5 and a functional assessment for daily living activities should preferably be conducted in the patient's home surroundings.

Treatment Programme

When the assessment has been carried out, an individual programme, appropriate to the patient's needs, can be planned with emphasis being placed on improving speed, mobility and coordinated movement. As the patient will never recover from his illness, it is important that an initial intensive treatment programme should be succeeded by reassessment and 'booster' programmes at intervals as necessity dictates.

Rigidity and Balance Reactions

Treatment will almost certainly need to include activities to minimise rigidity and to improve the quality of balance reactions. The reader is referred to Chapter 7 which emphasises these activities. Application of ice packs prior to activity sometimes helps to promote relaxation of rigidity.

The patterns used in proprioceptive neuromuscular facilitation techniques (PNF) may be used to facilitate both limb and trunk activities. Isotonic techniques rather than static posturing and stabilisations should be used as these patients tend to be static anyway as a result of the disease process; one of their greatest difficulties being to initiate movement. Therefore, a rhythmical technique is used to reinforce initiation of movement. The physiotherapist moves the part to be exercised passively through a small range of pattern several times, thereby setting up a pace or rhythm for the patient to follow. After several passive movements the patient is asked to assist the physiotherapist in the same pattern, still utilising the rhythm set up with the passive movement. These small range reversals can gradually be increased in range and speed.

This 'pumping-up' into an activity can be used as a preparation for all activities, and the patient may ultimately learn to prepare himself for movement by carrying out repeated simple swaying movements until he is sufficiently loosened to be functioning effectively. The patient needs practice in carrying out movement rapidly and smoothly.

Patients who have difficulty in initiating walking may be helped by marking time on the spot first, and once the smooth rhythm is established can then proceed forward. It is sometimes useful to include rhythmical activities to music to assist gait. Arm swinging needs to be encouraged, a lengthening of the stride and also practice in stopping as well as starting, walking backwards, sideways and turning without overbalancing.

Control of Head and Neck Activities

In the parkinsonian patient there is a tendency for the head to drop forwards and for the thoracic spine to show an exaggerated primary curve of flexion (see Fig. 15/1, p.294). This is not good for the respiratory movements, makes equilibrium reactions even slower and inhibits speech, mastication and deglutition. Such patients may also complain of pain and discomfort in the neck and shoulder regions which is due to irritation of the cervical nerve roots. Conservative physiotherapy may help to relieve this pain, and the general activities already mentioned may well have the effect of automatically improving the functional posturing of the head and thorax. Far-reaching effects are often achieved by using trunk and balance activities without the need for specific head and neck activities. However, if automatic improvement of the head and neck posturing does not occur, some emphasis may be put on the cervical spine by giving assisted active head movements, suitably coordinated with the movements of the body as a whole. The patient should be encouraged to lead the upper trunk by using head and neck movements, and if upper limb reversals are used the patient should follow his hands with head and eye movements. Specific proprioceptive neuromuscular facilitation techniques may be used for the redevelopment of head and neck patterns, and the methods used are similar to those advocated for the limbs. Guided reversals through increasing ranges should be encouraged and stabilisations avoided. In addition, respiratory exercises should be encouraged so that the danger of chest complications is minimised.

Many people advocate the use of cervical collars for advanced cases and they may, indeed, be necessary if there is a danger of peripheral nerve root compression or cord damage. However, collars will inhibit movement and should only be used if absolutely necessary.

Problems of Mastication, Deglutition and Speech

These are present in many patients demonstrating parkinsonism, and are particularly obvious in the more severely affected patients and those who have difficulty in controlling the position of the head.

Inactivity of the facial muscles and, in particular, of buccinator allows food and saliva to escape from the mouth and collect in the area between the cheeks and the teeth. This results eventually in distressing and unsightly dribbling at mealtimes and even at other times during the day. The patient becomes very embarrassed by this and feels socially unacceptable, which in fact he is, particularly to people who do not fully understand his condition. The tongue and supra- and infrahyoid muscles will also present problems, and difficulty with deglutition will be experienced. Speech is affected by the inactivity of all of these muscles and also by difficulty in vocalisation due to respiratory impairment.

Stimulation of the tongue, facial muscles and hyoid muscles may be brought about by icing inside the mouth, the surface of the tongue, face and anterior aspect of the neck. Light stimulating massage may help to activate the facial muscles while respiratory exercise and chest percussion may help vocalisation. Great attention must be paid to head posture, since deglutition and tongue movements can be severely impaired if the neck is in a non-functional position. For this reason it is important to see that the patient with poor head control is upright and well supported at mealtimes, with the head and neck in a good position for performing the functional movements associated with eating. Icing the tongue, cheeks, face and neck prior to attempting to eat may help the patient to cope with the problem and make mealtimes more enjoyable. Inexperienced nurses and relatives often need help on these matters if undue distress to the patient is to be avoided.

Advice and Assistance for the Patient at Home

Relatives and the patient should understand that prolonged periods of inactivity are detrimental to the patient. There are many ways in which help can be given. One of the worst times for the patient is on waking in the morning, because he has probably retained one sleeping posture all night and become genuinely stiff and immobile by the morning. If the problem is severe the relative may be required to loosen the patient passively by helping him to rotate his trunk. The less severe patient can help himself by turning over a few times before trying to get out of bed and by sitting on the edge of the bed.

Clothing can be made easy to fasten and of materials which are not too resistant to stretch. Clothes can be placed on both sides of the patient so that he has to turn and therefore rotate his trunk to pick up each article.

The patient can learn to help to loosen himself by swaying his bodyweight in different directions before he stands up and attempts to walk. Any job he does about the house should be as active as possible, and sedentary work should not be carried out over long periods. Such patients are often unable to detect fatigue in themselves, and while encouraging movement it is important to avoid overdoing any one activity. Frequent changes of activity are helpful.

A few weeks of intensive physiotherapy and advice to both the patient and those with whom he lives will help him to realise his full potential. Thereafter the management should be restricted to check-ups and occasional 'booster' periods of treatment. It is useful to visit the patient occasionally at home to see him in his own surroundings and relatives will, in this way, be kept fully in the picture regarding his capabilities.

Occupational therapists and physiotherapists need to collaborate closely, since many patients can retain their functional independence with the help of some simple gadgets and instruction from the occupational therapist. The help of the social worker may be needed in certain circumstances, and the local authority can be approached if alterations to the home are required.

BIBLIOGRAPHY

Brain R. (rev. Bannister, R.) (1978). *Clinical Neurology*, 5th edition. Oxford University Press, Oxford.

ACKNOWLEDGEMENT

This chapter is based largely upon that which has appeared in the previous editions and the author is indebted both to Miss Joan Cash and Mrs H. W. Atkinson for allowing her to use their material.

Chapter 17

Peripheral Nerve Injuries

by M. I. SALTER, M.B.E., M.C.S.P.

STRUCTURE

A peripheral nerve is composed of sensory, motor and autonomic fibres collectively known as the nerve trunk. These trunks contain afferent fibres carrying impulses towards the spinal cord, and efferent fibres carrying the impulses outwards to effector organs and muscles. This trunk of nerves is surrounded on the outside by a loose construction of connective tissue making up the epineurium. Contained within are the bundles of individual nerves further encased in a strong sheath, the perineurium. Each of the individual nerves is again enclosed by a layer known as the endoneurium. Individual nerve cells of the trunk are called neurones (Fig. 17/1). Each consists of a cell body and its projections, the dendrites, and the axon or nerve fibre. The nerve fibre is the long process of the neurone with the properties of excitability and conductivity. The sensory and motor fibres, which are myelinated, consist of the following structures from within outwards: a central semi-fluid core, the axoplasm, which flows from the cell body to the periphery and vice versa; separating the axoplasm from the surrounding structures is a cell membrane, the axolemma; wrapped around this are rings of insulating myelin sheath consisting of Schwann cells (Fig. 17/2). In the axoplasmic flow material such as neurotransmitters, enzymes, proteins and glycoproteins are transported and it is thought that these substances may be involved with the passage of information from the nerve cell to its terminations and across nerve and muscles fibres thus acting as a monitoring system.

The myelin sheath is interrupted at intervals by the nodes of Ranvier. These nodes are important in conduction. As the impulse travels down a fibre it 'leaps' from node to node, a process known as saltatory conduction (*saltare*, Latin, to leap).

The speed of conduction varies with the diameter of the nerve and

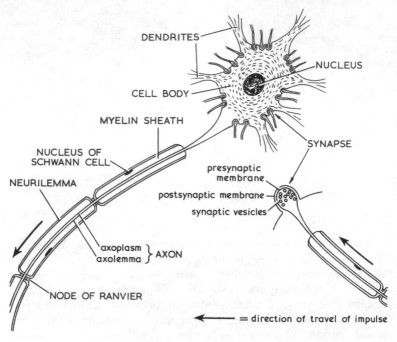

Fig. 17/1 Structure of a neurone

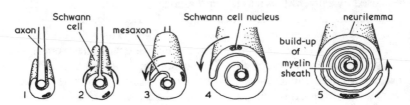

Fig. 17/2 Myelinogenesis

distance between nodes (less resistance is offered with larger diameters and therefore the impulses travel faster). The speeds range from 2 to 120 metres per sec, i.e. 270 miles per hour. If this mechanism was not present the impulses would travel directly along the nerve, i.e. by 'cable conduction', at a speed approaching 5 metres per second instead of the normal 50 metres per second. Very slow velocities are in fact found in diseases which attack the myelin sheath causing segmental demyelination (e.g. infective polyneuritis and diabetes).

The motor unit consists of one anterior horn cell, its peripheral axon and many muscle fibres, the number varying with the precision of the muscle concerned. The sensory fibres convey impulses from the skin, muscles, joints and other deep structures to the posterior root ganglia and then to the spinal cord. The sympathetic fibres of the autonomic nervous system are post-ganglionic from the sympathetic ganglia. These fibres innervate involuntary structures such as blood vessels and sweat and sebaceous glands.

CAUSES OF INJURY

Peripheral nerves are frequently injured by laceration, particularly the median and ulnar nerves which are susceptible to damage at the wrist where they may be divided by glass or by knives. They may also be damaged by pressure following a fracture of the humerus which can cause a radial nerve lesion, or the nerve may be trapped in the callus formation as the fracture heals. In rheumatoid arthritis, inflammation of the synovial sheaths of the flexor tendons as they pass under the flexor retinaculum may lead to compression of the median nerve in the carpal tunnel. Pressure from tourniquets and badly applied plasters may also lead to interference in nerve conduction. Industrial and traffic accidents and gunshot wounds may cause both the division of a peripheral nerve and widespread soft tissue damage.

Stretching of a nerve can occur with an increasing cubitus valgus deformity following an elbow injury and may produce a delayed paralysis of muscles supplied by the ulnar nerve. Traction injuries can cause brachial plexus lesions, these commonly occurring in motor cycle accidents, because the head is forcibly side flexed and the shoulder depressed when the victim hits the ground, while still holding on to the handlebars of the machine.

TYPES OF INJURY

The main classifications are neurapraxia, axonotmesis and neurotmesis, but there can also be a combination of the first two types of lesions.

Neurapraxia is defined as a non-degenerative lesion. Electromyographic studies may show slight evidence of degeneration suggesting a mixed lesion. It is possible to stimulate the nerve electrically below the site of the lesion but not above it. There is a total motor paralysis, but sensation may sometimes remain normal depending on the cause and severity of the lesion. Recovery usually occurs within six weeks, but a severe neurapraxia can take longer.

Axonotmesis. The term axonotmesis is used when the axon

degenerates but the nerve sheath remains intact. The nerve fibres mostly regenerate to their original end organs. Recovery should be good if muscles, joints and skin have been maintained in good condition.

Neurotmesis. The term neurotmesis is used when the lesion affects both the axon and the sheath. Nerve suture must be carried out to allow the regenerating axons to grow down the sheaths to their peripheral end organs. Motor and sensory fibres rarely re-grow to all their correct end-plates, so that there will be incomplete restoration of power and faulty localisation of sensory stimuli. Re-education is therefore essential if a good functional result is to be obtained.

Degeneration

Following an axonotmesis or neurotmesis retrograde degeneration occurs proximally for 2–3cm, and changes also occur distally. The process whereby the axis cylinder breaks up and the myelin sheath gradually turns to oily droplets is known as Wallerian degeneration. The debris is cleared away by macrophage activity, and Schwann cells fill the endoneurial tubes within three months.

In the muscle fibres changes also occur, and the coarse striation becomes less apparent. Muscles are gradually replaced by fibrous tissue, this fibrosis being complete within two years if nerve regeneration does not occur.

Regeneration

If the nerve ends are in apposition, sprouting axons will regenerate down the endoneurial tubes. Several fibres may grow down each tube, but after two to three weeks all degenerate except one which continues to grow to the periphery. The myelin sheaths begin to develop after fifteen days, and these take a long time to mature. When the axon reaches the nerve ending it may establish a connection, but the end-plate formed depends on the function of the parent cell, so may not be appropriate to the structure re-innervated.

The rate of recovery depends on the age of the patient and the distance between the lesion and destination of the regenerating nerve fibres. The average rate of peripheral nerve recovery is 1.5mm per day in the early stages, but the rate decreases later, and is also lower in elderly people.

If accurate alignment of the nerve ends is not achieved by the surgeon, or if much fibrous tissue forms, many of the sprouting axons will be unable to regrow down their endoneurial tubes, and a neuroma will form.

EFFECTS OF PERIPHERAL NERVE INJURIES

There are motor, sensory and autonomic effects.

Motor

Interruption of a motor nerve produces a lower motor neurone lesion with loss of reflexes, of tone, and of any active contraction of the muscles which it supplies. There is atrophy of muscle and soft tissue. Patients should be made aware that even with intensive treatment wasting will occur. Deformities are caused by the unopposed action of the unaffected muscles, e.g. the claw hand of the ulnar nerve lesion. The strong pull of the long finger flexors and extensors is unopposed when the intrinsic muscles are paralysed and therefore clawing occurs.

Due to lack of movement, adhesions may occur between tendons and sheaths and fibrous tissue may form in muscles and joints. These complications can be prevented by maintaining full range of movement and good circulation.

Sensory

The sensory effects are loss of cutaneous and proprioceptive sensations. The initial size of the anaesthetic area will decrease around its periphery, due to adjacent sensory nerves taking over. Loss of temperature sensation means that patients are liable to become burned and repeated warning should be given of the dangers of cigarettes, kettles, radiators and hot plates. Even hot soup has been known to cause a burn. Similarly, intense cold, as from refrigerators and ice boxes, can cause blistering of the skin.

Autonomic

Damage to sympathetic nerves causes a loss of sweating and the skin tends to become scaly, and later thin and shiny. The nails become brittle and the skin is more liable to pressure sores. If trophic lesions occur they will be slow to heal. The limb will take on the temperature of its surroundings and so, to maintain an adequate circulation, it is essential to keep the hand or foot in a warm glove or sock during cold weather.

OPERATIVE TREATMENT

A divided nerve must be sutured if it is to regenerate. If the patient is seen within six hours and the wound is clean and the patient fit, an experienced surgeon will perform a primary suture immediately. Otherwise the nerve ends should be approximated and secured to prevent retraction, and the suture delayed for two or three weeks. Scarred ends of the nerve may need resection, then an epineural or fascicular repair is carried out with the aid of the microscope to ensure accurate alignment. Releasing and transposition of the nerve may be necessary to prevent tension on the sutured ends, e.g. the ulnar nerve may be transposed to the anterior aspect of the elbow and temporarily immobilised in a plaster of Paris splint.

Other Surgical Procedures

Provided that the ends are not too far apart there are a variety of techniques available for bridging the gap with a graft. The sural or medial cutaneous nerve of the arm may be used for a free graft; a pedicle graft may be selected as it maintains its blood supply in its transposed position. If a nerve is compressed by scar tissue a neurolysis is performed to free it.

If nerve repair is not feasible, or regeneration does not occur, then reconstructive surgery of joints and muscles should be considered. For example, in non re-innervation of opponens pollicis, the tendon of flexor digitorum superficialis to the ring finger is transferred into the extensor pollicis longus expansion at the base of the proximal phalanx of the thumb to restore opposition. In non-recovering radial nerve lesions the tendons of pronator teres and flexor carpi ulnaris can be transferred to provide some wrist, finger and thumb extension.

Useful motor function is regained only if there is sufficient return of sensation. In special circumstances, where there is permanent loss of cutaneous sensation of median nerve distribution, neurovascular skin island transfers may be carried from the ulnar side of the hand. An area of skin from the ring finger plus its neurovascular bundle is transferred to the thumb and index finger to provide the sensation necessary for precision grip. Sensory re-education is then essential to gain sensibility of the recipient area.

POSTOPERATIVE CARE

To prevent undue stretch of the nerve ends, a plaster of Paris dorsal slab is applied for two to three weeks with the adjacent joints positioned to reduce tension, and the limb is initially supported in elevation to prevent oedema. Care must be taken not to put any passive stretch on the nerve for at least eight weeks. In the upper limb shoulder exercises are given to maintain joint mobility.

PHYSIOTHERAPY

The treatment of peripheral nerve injuries involves a team led by the surgeon or rehabilitation specialist and backed by the skill of physiotherapists and occupational therapists. In a peripheral nerve injury the loss of movement and sensation, particularly in the upper limb, may have a profound effect on the patient's personality and outlook and this should be considered when planning treatment. Frequently it is complicated by tendons and other structures having been divided, and it has been found that a programme of physiotherapy and occupational therapy for all or half a day for a short period is more effective and economical than less intensive treatment over a long period. The doctor and therapists should see the patient together to plan and to integrate treatment. The patient should be given a full explanation of the reasons for treatment so that he will cooperate and work hard both in the department and at home. The social worker may need to be involved at an early stage so that support may be provided for the patient and his family. Prospects of future employment should be considered and discussed. Unless the patient is cooperative and well motivated the most skilled therapy is unlikely to be successful.

Stage of Paralysis

The principles of treatment whether surgery has been performed or not are as follows:
1. To maintain and improve the circulation and reduce any oedema
2. To maintain or obtain full movement
3. To correct deformity
4. To encourage function
5. To increase the power of unaffected muscles
6. To control pain.

A thorough assessment should be made prior to treatment. It is easy to be confused by trick movements and variations of nerve supply in the upper limb. If the muscles of the thenar eminence are contracting in a median nerve lesion, it may be a partial lesion, or the muscles may be supplied by the ulnar nerve. One person in five has an anomalous nerve supply in the hand, and this can be confirmed by electrical stimulation. Range of movement should be measured and recorded. Both extension and flexion of each joint is measured with a goniometer to indicate deformity; the distance of finger tips towards and away from the palm is measured with a ruler. These measurements are repeated weekly. They can also be used to show the patient that progress is being made, and to encourage him to continue working at home. Muscle power is recorded by using the 0-5 Medical Research Council Scale, and sensory charts showing the areas of diminished or absent sensations are made periodically.

First priority of treatment must be given to reducing oedema. If the limb is allowed to remain oedematous, fibrin is deposited, and the tissues become bound down, causing permanent stiffness.

The upper limb should be supported during the day in a sling, with the level of the hand above that of the elbow, and the fingers free to move. At night the arm should be supported in a roller towel slung from a drip stand or other suitable means, until the oedema is controlled. In the lower limb, oedema should be controlled during the day by the use of an elastic bandage, and a well-fitting shoe is essential. The bed should be elevated at night.

Ultrasound should be given around the scar, and pulsed diathermy is also considered an effective treatment in promoting healing and reducing formation of fibrous tissue and adhesions. Massage in elevation using oil will improve a dry scaly skin and, combined with the use of oedema controlling apparatus, will help to reduce swelling. When well healed, deep lanolin massage should be given to the scar if adherent to the underlying structures. A warm water or saline soak may precede this, the patient being encouraged to move the limb in the water. This is found preferable to wax baths. If wax is used great care must be taken to lower the temperature to 45°C (115°F) maximum or burns will occur.

The use of cold is contra-indicated for peripheral nerve lesions, as the limb remains cold for a long time after this form of treatment. It is essential to maintain a good circulation by keeping it warm, and a glove or warm footwear should be worn out of doors in cold weather.

Active movements are encouraged where possible, otherwise joints must be moved passively. It is important that the accessory movements of roll, spin and slide (*Gray's Anatomy*, 1980) are used to maintain or increase the range, but the movement of the sound side should be compared so that the joints are not over-mobilised. Facilitation techniques are used to maintain or increase available muscle power, to increase range of movement by use of the relaxation techniques and as a means of maintaining the pattern of movement in the patient's mind. Compensatory or trick movements are taught, as they are useful for maintaining function, particularly when lively splints are provided. Lively splints may be used to correct or prevent deformity and to increase function. Details are given under the individual nerve lesion.

If pain becomes a problem, this must be controlled as the patient will probably be unwilling to use the limb (see p.314).

Stage of Recovery

Motor and sensory re-education begins at this stage. As re-innervation occurs a muscle will be found to contract first as a synergist and later as a prime mover. Each muscle should be re-educated individually in middle to outer range at first, and later into inner range as the power improves. Facilitation techniques, springs, games and specific activities in the occupational therapy department are programmed to improve function. For the larger joints and muscles hydrotherapy and swimming are of great value. Sensory re-education details are given under the treatment of a median nerve lesion (p.323).

Tinel's sign is a useful means of testing regeneration of the nerve (Henderson, 1948). Tapping from distally to proximally over the nerve trunk sets up a sensory discharge and the point of regeneration can be located and measured.

As the patient's ability to work increases, a functional assessment should be carried out by the occupational therapist. Results of this are valuable in giving guidance about future employment prospects, and the patient is encouraged to return to work as soon as is suitable.

Throughout treatment the physiotherapist must check that the patient is carrying out his own treatment at home, particularly if he is unable to attend the physiotherapy department regularly.

PERIPHERAL NERVE INJURY IN THE UPPER LIMB

The methods already outlined apply to the following injuries, but some specific points will be discussed.

BRACHIAL PLEXUS LESIONS

Injuries to the plexus may be partial or complete, and may combine the three types of lesions, neurapraxia, axonotmesis and neurotmesis. Upper trunk lesions are more common than lower.

The plexus may be damaged by traction as in motor cycle accidents, by gunshot or stab wounds, by fractures of the clavicle, dislocation of the shoulder and by carcinoma of the lung. The motor and sensory changes will vary according to the site of the lesion.

Complete Lesions

All the muscles of the upper limb are involved except trapezius and there is complete anaesthesia apart from a small area on the medial side of the arm which has T2 root supply. The limb hangs limply in medial rotation, the head of the humerus may subluxate due to the lack of tone in the deltoid, the elbow is extended and the forearm pronated. The hand loses its normal contour and becomes blue and swollen when dependent.

Partial Lesions

Upper trunk lesions affect the muscles around the shoulder and the elbow flexors. Causalgia is a feature of partial lesions. It is an intense burning pain which radiates down the arm and may be precipitated by sudden noise and shock. The transcutaneous nerve stimulator will reduce this pain in a proportion of cases if used for several hours a day. The only drug which might relieve causalgia is chlorpromazine (Largactil). If these treatments are not effective then a stellate block or sympathectomy should be carried out, but a cordotomy has sometimes to be performed as a last resort.

Site of Lesion

It is important in complete lesions to determine whether the damage is pre- or post-ganglionic, as recovery cannot occur if the injury is proximal to the ganglion. The following methods are used to indicate the position of the lesion.

A sensory conduction test is carried out using electromyographic equipment. If a sensory action potential is obtained from a ditigal nerve, then the peripheral axons are in continuity with the posterior root ganglion, so that the lesion for that root is pre-ganglionic. It is usual to wait ten days after injury before performing these tests to allow Wallerian degeneration to occur, otherwise inaccurate results may be obtained.

If no sensory action potential is found, the lesion will be distal to the posterior root ganglion, and recovery might occur. However, there may be a pre-ganglionic lesion also, and a myelogram should therefore be carried out in these cases. Meningoceles will indicate that the dura has been torn and therefore the prognosis for that root is hopeless.

SURGICAL TREATMENT

A plexus lesion from a direct injury may be suitable for surgery if the patient is referred to a specialist hospital within a day or two of his accident. It takes many hours by a specialised team of surgeons to expose the plexus and possibly repair or graft the nerves. If damage is extensive then an attempt is made to provide for re-innervation of the proximal muscles, and elbow flexors.

In complete pre-ganglionic lesions it used to be recommended that the arm should be amputated above the elbow, the shoulder arthrodesed and a prosthesis fitted as soon as possible. However, it was discovered on reviewing these patients some years later that very few used their prostheses. Now an external modular splint can be provided instantly with a variety of attachments (Fig. 17/3). The patient learns to use the splint quickly before he has time to adapt to life with only one arm.

In partial lesions time should be allowed to see how much recovery is going to occur before embarking on reconstructive surgery, and the same modular splints should be worn during this waiting period. If regeneration does not occur, a variety of muscle and tendon transfers are available which can restore function, e.g. strong wrist flexors may be transferred to the wrist and finger extensors, if these are paralysed, to restore wrist and finger extension.

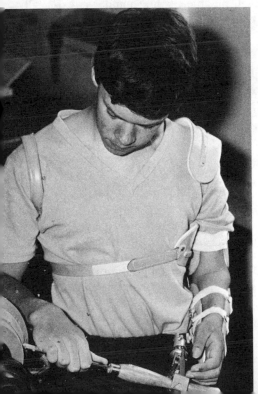

Fig. 17/3 Patient with a brachial plexus lesion wearing a flail arm splint while working with tools at a lathe

PHYSIOTHERAPY

Motor and sensory charting should be carried out and a regular reappraisal made in the case of post-ganglionic lesions. Passive movements to the affected joints should begin as soon as possible, but delay may be unavoidable if there are un-united fractures. A full range of movement should be given twice a day, and the patient taught to carry this out for himself. Lateral rotation of the shoulder and abduction and supination of the forearm quickly become limited and the thumb web becomes tight and the metacarpophalangeal joints very stiff if not regularly mobilised. If stiffness occurs it takes weeks of intensive treatment to rectify. Hydrotherapy techniques will help to increase the range of stiff joints, and progressive resisted exercises in water are introduced when recovery occurs. Compensatory movements should be encouraged as they assist in maintaining function.

AXILLARY NERVE INJURY

This nerve supplies deltoid and teres minor and may be injured with fractures of the surgical neck of the humerus and in dislocations of the shoulder. There is marked flattening of the contour of the shoulder and an area of sensory loss on the lateral side of the upper part of the arm. Powerful elevation can be restored if the shoulder joint is mobile by teaching compensatory movements. When lying supine with the elbow flexed, the patient will be able, if the shoulder is externally rotated, to elevate the arm using the long head of biceps. The clavicular head of pectoralis major and serratus anterior help to complete the movement. As the patient's ability improves, the back of the plinth is gradually raised until it is vertical, and he is able to perform the movement without support. Some patients learn this movement by themselves while with others it may take a few weeks of intensive rehabilitation. When re-innervation occurs and deltoid regains strength, the trick movement will disappear.

ULNAR AND MEDIAN NERVE INJURY

The ulnar and median nerves are frequently divided at the wrist as the result of putting the hand through a window. Tendons and arteries are usually damaged at the same time. The tendons of flexor pollicis longus and flexor digitorum superficialis are often divided at the same time as the median nerve, and flexor carpi ulnaris with the ulnar artery and ulnar nerve. It is usual for primary tendon suture to be performed. Both nerves may be involved in elbow injuries, more com-

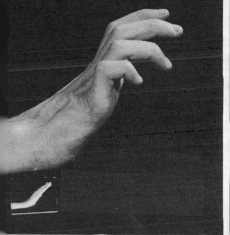
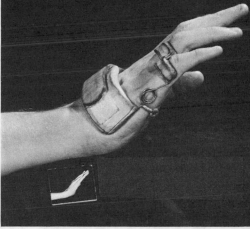
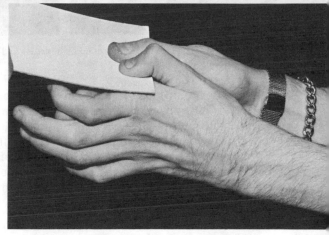

Fig. 17/4 (a) (above left)
The claw hand deformity of
an ulnar nerve lesion. (b)
(above right) Deformity
corrected by a lively splint.
(c) (right) Showing trick
adduction of the thumb
using flexor pollicis longus

monly the ulnar nerve with the medial epicondyle. The median nerve
may be compressed in the carpal tunnel, but this can be relieved by
surgical division of the flexor retinaculum.

The deformity of an ulnar nerve lesion is the claw hand (Figs. 17/4a.
b. c.). There is hyperextension of the metacarpophalangeal joints of
the ring and little fingers, due to action of extensor digitorum being
unopposed by the paralysed medial two lumbricals, and the interossei. There is flexion of the interphalangeal joints of these two fingers,
due to the strong pull of the long flexors unopposed by the paralysed
intrinsic muscles. If the lesion is at the elbow there will also be
paralysis of flexor digitorum profundus to these two fingers. The
sensory loss does not impair the patient's function severely, though
burns may result on the affected fingers and ulnar border of the hand.

The deformity of the median nerve lesion is the monkey hand (Figs.
17/5a. b.). The thumb is held alongside the index finger by action of

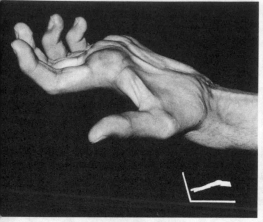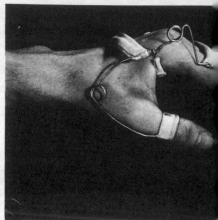

Fig. 17/5 (a) (*left*) Deformity of combined median and ulnar nerve lesions. (b) (*right*) Deformity corrected by a lively splint

extensor pollicis longus, unopposed by the paralysed abductor pollicis brevis and opponens pollicis. The thenar eminence becomes flattened due to atrophy of the underlying muscles. The sensory loss is a severe disability, as sensation is lacking over the thumb, index and middle fingers and a large area of the palm. The patient is therefore unable to recognise objects, and the lack of cutaneous sensation and proprioception greatly impairs motor function, especially precision grip.

Progression of Treatment Following Suture of Median and Ulnar Nerves

If the suture is at the wrist, this joint is usually immobilised in flexion by a plaster splint for three weeks. If at the elbow, and an extensive resection has been necessary, a turnbuckle plaster may be applied to maintain the elbow in flexion. After three weeks the elbow is gradually extended by use of the turnbuckle, which allows flexion, but controls extension. Full movement is regained within three to five weeks.

ONE TO THREE WEEKS

Active movements of the unaffected joints of the upper limb are encouraged.

THREE TO FIVE WEEKS

The daily treatment follows the routine described for a peripheral nerve lesion, avoiding tension on the sutured nerve ends. Patients must be warned, for instance, not to allow the hand to hang palm uppermost over the edge of the table thereby applying tension on the sutured ends. The nails should be cut by the physiotherapist to prevent the patient damaging his anaesthetic skin. If there are unhealed areas, or if trophic lesions have occurred, saline soaks are used and the wounds cleaned with half-strength Eusol.

Treatment should be repeated three to four times daily and alternated with periods of occupational therapy. If this is not possible the patient must be made aware of how important it is to carry on his own treatment.

SIX TO EIGHT WEEKS

Deeper massage with lanolin is given to help free adherent scars, and soften indurated areas.

It is essential to differentiate between deformities caused by over-action of the antagonists, those caused by joint stiffness and those caused by tendon adherence. In the contracture following laceration of the flexor aspect of the wrist, flexor digitorum superficialis may become adherent to the scar and the proximal interphalangeal joints will be held at 90° flexion. This deformity will disappear if the wrist and metacarpophalangeal joints are flexed and the tension on flexor digitorum superficialis is released. It reappears as the wrist and metacarpophalangeal joints are extended. Graduated resistance is introduced and facilitation techniques are used. The flexion ab-duction pattern encourages wrist and finger extension. If these movements are limited, strengthening and relaxation techniques may be employed in bilateral and unilateral patterns. Games, such as table tennis and darts progressing to badminton, are useful and encourage the patient to use his whole arm, but volley ball, where the hand may be forcibly extended, is not suitable. Precision movements may be encouraged, by playing with such things as cards, matches and Pik-a-Stik.

When full passive mobility has been restored, lively splints are needed to prevent stretch of ligaments and capsules of joints, and to improve function.

The aim of the ulnar lively splint is to correct the hyperextension of the metacarpophalangeal joints when the patient extends his fingers, and to give support to the proximal phalanges so that the long exten-sors may extend the interphalangeal joints. The splint should also maintain the palmar arch and allow full flexion and extension of the fingers. Shaped bars are fitted over the dorsum of the hand and over the proximal phalanges of the two medial fingers, with a pad under the palm. A coil of wire, in line with the metacarpophalangeal joints, acts

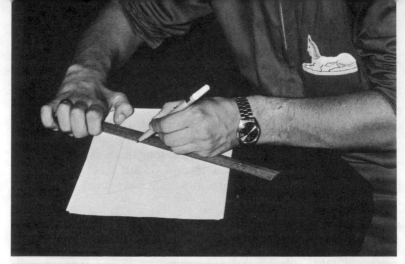

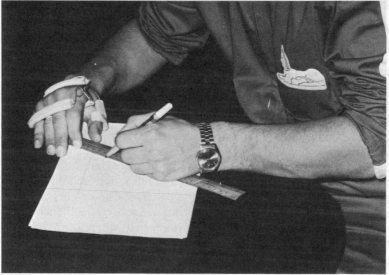

Fig. 17/6 Patient with median and ulnar nerve lesions attempting to hold a ruler. (a) (*top*) Without a splint. (b) (*above*) Wearing a lively splint

as a spring and maintains these joints in slight flexion while the hand is at rest (Fig. 17/4b).

The aim of the median lively splint is to place the thumb in a functional position of palmar abduction, rotation and opposition, and to prevent permanent flattening of the thumb. A pinch grip to the index and middle fingers can then be made by using flexor pollicis longus. A strip of rubber is looped round the metacarpophalangeal joint of the thumb and taken across to the ulnar side of the wrist where it is fixed by a leather cuff, and so maintains the thumb in the functional position.

The splint for the combined median and ulnar lesion works on the same principle as that of the ulnar. The proximal bar extends over the dorsum of the whole hand and the distal bar over the proximal phalanges of all four fingers. There is a spring wire attached from the lateral side which supports the thumb in a functional position (Figs. 17/5b and 17/6a. b.).

EIGHT WEEKS ONWARDS

More vigorous resisted exercises are now introduced. Passive stretching is required if full mobility has not been regained. The stretch should be slow and steady and combined with relaxation techniques. Serial stretch plasters are necessary in stubborn cases, and this is a skilled technique which must be applied with care and with medical agreement. Plaster of Paris and Polyform are both found to be suitable materials as they conform well to the contours of the hand, therefore maintaining it in the desired position. The splint is applied by the physiotherapist who treats the patient so that no more than the correct amount of stretch is given. If plaster of Paris is selected, twelve layers 10cm wide are used with a crescent cut out to allow free movement for the thumb. Vaseline petroleum jelly is applied to the skin if it is hairy, to prevent adherence. The layers are soaked in warm water, squeezed out and smoothed well so that no wrinkles remain. They are placed directly on to the skin of the palm and forearm, and held so that the maximum extension of the wrist and fingers is obtained. Care is taken to prevent both hyperextension of the metacarpophalangeal joints, and ulnar deviation of wrist and fingers. The position is held until the plaster has set. When dry the plaster is lined with cotton wool and the forearm placed on the plaster. The fingers are then extended into position and a thin layer of cotton wool placed between each to prevent friction. The splint is held in position by a crêpe bandage, keeping the fingertips free so that the circulation may be checked (Fig. 17/7a. b.). The splint should be worn free for about one hour only during the day, and a check made by the physiotherapist on its removal. As soon as the patient has increased his range of movement and is able to lift his fingers from the splint, a new one should be made. The splint should only be worn at the allotted times so that function is maintained. Plasters must be used with extreme care where there is complete anaesthesia especially in combined median and ulnar nerve lesions, as trophic lesions can easily be caused by a badly applied splint. In-patients should, at night time, wear the splint made the previous day, so that any correction obtained during the day is not lost. This,

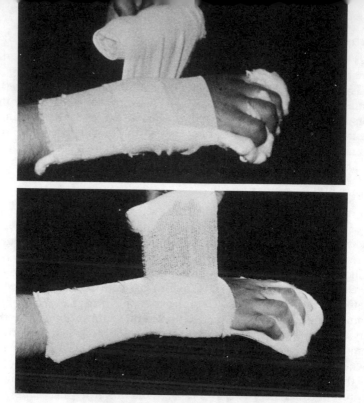

Fig. 17/7 (a) and (b) Patient with median and ulnar nerve lesions with adherence of the flexor tendons at the wrist having a serial stretch splint applied

however, may need to be modified for out-patients who have sensory loss.

Special care must be taken to assess the patient's suitability to wear these splints. He must be sufficiently intelligent to understand the significance of the instructions concerning the circulation and to observe that the limb remains warm and the colour normal. If he is an out-patient he must be able to attend the hospital for the splint to be checked regularly. Contra-indications to the use of stretch plasters include oedema, circulatory impairment, infections and unhealed areas. Their use, when there is intracapsular joint damage is limited in value and they should be used with great care. If the nerve is unlikely to regenerate, the use of passive stretches and serial plasters must be limited to prevent the joints from becoming hypermobile. When the optimum degree of mobility and function has been achieved the patient should be able to care for his hand at home and may be able to return to work.

The doctor checks his progress at intervals and treatment is resumed when re-innervation takes place.

In an ulnar nerve lesion, the first muscle to recover is abductor digit minimi, on average 90 days after a suture at the wrist, and it will contract first as a synergist in opposition of little finger and thumb. It is easy to be misled by the tightening produced by the pull of flexor carpi ulnaris on to the pisiform bone or on to an adherent wrist scar.

In a median nerve lesion, flexor pollicis brevis is the first muscle to recover followed shortly by abductor pollicis brevis, the average of the former being 80 days and the latter 90 days. Before a contraction can be felt, there is an improvement in the position of the thumb due to increasing tone.

Intensive rehabilitation is essential and should include individual and group re-education of muscles and functional activities. Facilitation techniques should be used as the threshold of the anterior horn cells is high following a nerve lesion and maximum excitation is necessary to produce a contraction.

SENSORY RE-EDUCATION

Sensibility is the interpretation by the brain of the sensory stimuli that it receives and the hand is one of the main sensory organs of the body. It is thought that the differences in sensation are produced by the coding of varying combinations and speeds of impulses transmitted along the axons from the peripheral receptors. Good motor function is dependent on feedback of cutaneous and proprioceptive sensations. Wall (1961) points out that a passive stimulus is very rare in normal life and that sensory stimuli usually need motor participation. The function of both is therefore very closely interlinked and sensation combined with active movement needs re-education (Wynn Parry and Salter, 1976).

When there is some return of sensation to the median distribution of the fingers, sensory re-education is started so that the patient may use any altered sensation for stereognosis, i.e. recognition of objects.

Large blocks of wood of differing shapes, weights and sizes are used at first. The patient, with eyes shut, is asked to describe the blocks, and also coins, materials and everyday objects (Fig. 17/8). An assessment is made, with a re-appraisal every month on the same objects. Training on similar items, looking if necessary and feeling before closing the eyes again, helps to build a visual-tactile image.

Any incorrect localisation caused by crossed re-innervation, can be improved by localisation training. The patient is asked to point, while his eyes are closed, to the place where he is being touched. If incorrect he is told to look so that he may learn to interpret his

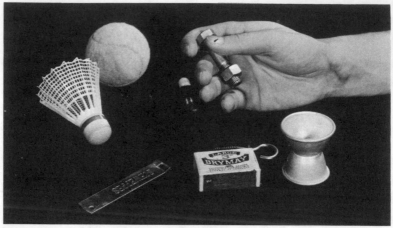

Fig. 17/8 Sensory re-education for a recovering median nerve lesion

altered localisation correctly. Gradually he will say that it feels in one position but that he knows it is elsewhere, until he eventually points directly to the correct spot.

RADIAL NERVE INJURY

The radial nerve is most frequently damaged at the point where it winds round the humerus as a result of fractures or by pressure from callus formation. It may also be damaged in the axilla by pressure from an axillary crutch.

Complete interruption of the nerve in or above the axilla causes paralysis of the extensors of elbow, wrist and fingers. If the injury is below the axilla the triceps will not be affected. Although there is inability to extend the wrist or metacarpophalangeal joints, the inter-phalangeal joints can be extended by the interossei, and the thumb by abductor pollicis brevis, as it has an insertion into the extensor expansion of the thumb.

Damage to the posterior interosseus branch will spare the brachioradialis and extensor carpi radialis longus muscle.

A simple lively splint of wire should be worn with a pad under the palm and a coil acting as a spring on either side of the wrist which will allow the fingers and wrist to be flexed and then return the hand to a functional position. It also prevents the weight of the hand from producing a stretch of the ligaments of the wrist joint. Leather loops suspended from wires should not be used as these tend to hyperextend the metacarpophalangeal joints. The patient sometimes finds, however, that the addition of a spider splint is useful for finger release in precision movements and large grasp. This consists of four plastic-coated wires, fixed by a cuff round the base of the proximal phalanx of the thumb, spread out and looped under the proximal phalanges of the fingers (Fig. 17/9). This allows full flexion of the fingers and holds the metacarpophalangeal joints in slight flexion when relaxed.

Reconstructive surgery may be carried out if regeneration of the nerve does not occur, by transferring one or more flexor tendons into the extensors, to restore active extension of wrist and fingers.

PERIPHERAL NERVE INJURY IN THE LOWER LIMB

The sciatic nerve may be severed by wounds of the pelvis or thigh, and quite commonly is damaged either completely or partially by dislocation of the hip. In a complete lesion there is paralysis of the hamstrings and all muscles distal to the knee, and sensory loss also which is extremely disabling. The common peroneal branch may be damaged by fractures of the neck of the fibula or by pressure from a badly applied plaster cast. A foot drop occurs as there is paralysis of the anterior tibial and peroneal muscles. The sensory loss is over the dorsum of the foot and lateral side of the leg. The patient walks with a high-stepping gait to clear the floor when gravity and the unopposed calf muscles cause the foot to drop into equinovarus. This can be corrected by the use of a toe-raising spring, or a foot-drop device fitted into the heel of the shoe.

Passive movements should be given daily to prevent contracture of

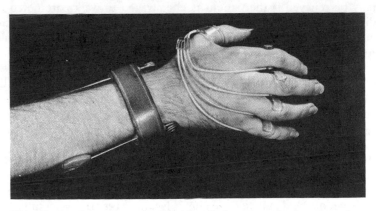

Fig. 17/9 A radial nerve palsy splinted in a lively cock-up for the wrist and a spider splint for the fingers allowing the interossei to extend the · interphalangeal joints

the calf muscles and clawing of the toes. The patient can carry this out for himself by standing with the affected foot on a low step and pushing his bodyweight forward over his foot. A night splint should be made to support the foot at 90° dorsiflexion and in the mid-position between inversion and eversion. The splint should extend for 2.5cm distal to the toes to keep the weight of the bedclothes off the foot, and should be lined carefully to avoid causing pressure sores. If contractures have developed, correction is necessary by passive stretching and the use of serial stretch plasters. Particular care must be taken however when using these plasters if there is total anaesthesia of the skin. During the recovery stage, facilitation techniques are used for re-education. Balance reactions are effective for stimulating the peronei and anterior tibials and a balance board is also useful. The board may have a rocker underneath or a rounded shape which allows it to roll in all directions. Balance boards are also valuable forms of equipment for re-educating proprioception in the lower limb.

As the power of the dorsiflexors increases, the strength of the toe-raising spring is reduced. Postural re-education and correction of gait is important throughout treatment.

Lesions of the tibial branch of the sciatic nerve may occur in supracondylar fractures of the femur. There is paralysis of the calf, posterior tibial and plantar muscles. Contracture of the plantar fascia may follow paralysis of the short muscles of the foot.

Trophic lesions are liable to occur on the sole of the foot, due to lack of sensation and vasomotor changes. It is therefore essential that shoes fit well. A well-fitting Plastazote insole will help to prevent these lesions. During sensory recovery, hyperaesthesia may be severe. This may be relieved if the patient is encouraged to walk barefooted on different surfaces such as lineoleum, carpet and tiles and in summer out of doors on the grass. Use of the cutaneous stimulator will usually reduce the discomfort.

Lesions of the femoral and obturator nerves are rare. With paralysis of the quadriceps the knee gives way and the patient cannot lift himself up on the affected leg to climb stairs. However, he quickly learns to compensate by hyperextending the knee and achieves a surprisingly good walk. Paralysis of the hamstrings proves a greater disability than paralysis of the quadriceps. There is inability to extend the hip and a loss of stability of the thigh on the lower leg, and the patient has difficulty in walking.

Surgical procedures may be indicated if there is irreparable nerve damage, or the distance from site of lesion to the paralysed muscle is too great. With lack of dorsiflexion or plantar flexion the ankle joint is arthrodesed. With lack of eversion a triple arthrodesis is performed.

Electrical Stimulation

Electrical stimulation is believed to maintain protein metabolism and to preserve the bulk of muscle fibres if carried out regularly. To be effective, though, it must be maintained daily for a considerable period of time. Results from intensive rehabilitation, which maintains the circulation and function, have been so good that routine stimulation has been stopped. Patients with brachial plexus lesions who have received no electrical stimulation have been seen with worthwhile recovery in the hand two or three years after injury.

Stimulation is useful for detecting anomalies of nerve supply and for re-education in the stage of recovery if the patient is having difficulty in relearning the feel of a muscle contraction.

REFERENCES

Gray's Anatomy, 36th edition (ed. Warwick, R. and Williams, P. L.) (1980). Chapter on *Arthrology*. Longman Group Limited, Edinburgh.

Henderson, W. R. (1948). 'Clinical assessment of peripheral nerve injuries: Tinel's test.' *Lancet*, 2, 801.

Wall, P. D. (1961). *Two transmission systems for skin sensations*. In *Sensory Communication*, pp. 475–96 (ed. Rosenblith, W. A.). MIT Press, Cambridge, Mass.

Wynn Parry, C. B. and Salter, M. (1976). 'Sensory re-education after median nerve lesions.' *Hand*, 8, 250.

BIBLIOGRAPHY

Caillet, R. (1975). *Hand Pain and Impairment*, 2nd edition. F. A. Davis Co Philadelphia.

Maitland, G. (1977). *Peripheral Manipulation*, 2nd edition. Butterworths, London.

Rob, C. and Smith, Sir R. (eds.) (1977). *Operative Surgery*, 3rd edition. Volume *The Hand* (ed. Pulvertaft, R. G.). Butterworths, London.

Wynn Parry, C. B. (1981). *Rehabilitation of the Hand*, 4th edition. Butterworths, London.

ACKNOWLEDGEMENTS

The author wishes to acknowledge the very large contribution which Barbara Sutcliffe, M.C.S.P., made to the first edition of this chapter. She also acknowledges the help and encouragement received from Dr C. B. Wynn Parry, M.B.E., D.M., F.R.C.P., F.R.C.S. She also thanks Mr Norman Chandler for his valuable assistance with the photography, and she is grateful to the Director General, Medical Services Royal Air Force, for permission to publish this chapter on peripheral nerve injuries.

Chapter 18

Polyneuropathy

by J. M. LEE, B.A., M.C.S.P., DIP. T.P.

Polyneuropathy is a collective term for a syndrome which includes all inflammatory and degenerative diseases involving the peripheral nervous system. The main presenting features include widespread sensory and motor disturbances of the peripheral nerves and it often appears as a symmetrical involvement of the nerves but this is not always so. The syndrome is usually seen in the young or middle-aged adult, men being affected more frequently than women.

Polyneuropathy and polyneuritis are interchangeable terms: strictly speaking polyneuropathy refers to the primary degenerative diseases which begin in the nerve parenchyma and are initiated by toxic, metabolic or vascular causes; whereas polyneuritis covers all primary inflammatory diseases of the connective tissue in peripheral nerves which are due to toxic or allergic substances and infections.

Before looking at the various polyneuropathies an understanding of the organisation and functioning of the peripheral nervous system is essential. The anatomical and physiological descriptions which follow are at a superficial level and serve only to refresh the memory.

Formation of a Peripheral Nerve

The peripheral nervous system is composed of fibres from both somatic and visceral nervous systems, together with their associated ganglia containing nerve cell bodies, and supportive connective tissue. All the above elements are situated distal to the pia-arachnoid membranes of the spinal cord.

A mixed spinal nerve is made up of parallel bundles of nerve fibres – these fibres are divided into two functional systems: somatic and visceral.

The somatic system consists of afferent and efferent nerve fibres.

The afferent fibres conduct impulses from sensory receptors in the skin, joints, muscles and subcutaneous tissues to the central nervous system. These fibres are the long dendritic processes of the sensory nerve cell body which is situated in the dorsal root ganglion. The efferent fibres are axonal processes of nerve somata in the ventral horn of the spinal cord; they are classified as α, β and γ neurones and convey impulses to the skeletal muscles.

The visceral nervous system includes the parasympathetic and sympathetic divisions which innervate glands, viscera and unstriated muscle. The afferent side of this system is in many ways similar to that of the somatic nervous system. The cell body of the afferent fibre being situated in the dorsal root ganglion of the spinal cord and the nuclei of the facial (VII), glossopharyngeal (IX), and vagus (X) cranial nerves.

The efferent pathway is very different from the somatic system. The cell body of the (preganglionic) efferent fibre is found in the lateral grey column of the thoracic and upper lumbar spinal segments. The parasympathetic efferent cell is found in the nuclei of the occulomotor (III), facial, glossopharyngeal, vagus and accessory (XI) cranial nerves and in the lateral grey column of the sacral segments of the cord.

The two divisions of the visceral nervous system normally operate at a subconscious level and are broadly antagonistic in action. The sympathetic nervous system has a more general effect in preparing the body for activity, whereas the parasympathetic has a more localised action on individual viscera, in general producing a more tranquil state of affairs in the body. The afferent pathways of the visceral nervous system are responsible for sensations of nausea, visceral pain, hunger etc, all of which are perceived as conscious sensations.

Gross Structure of a Mixed Peripheral Nerve (see Fig. 17/1, p.306)

The larger diameter somatic afferent and efferent nerve fibres are wrapped in a layer of lipid material, the myelin sheath. This is formed from the membrane of the Schwann cell. At regular intervals along the nerve a gap occurs between adjacent Schwann cells and the axolemma is exposed. This gap, the node of Ranvier, is essential for saltatory conduction along the nerve fibres. The small diameter somatic sensory and visceral nerve fibres are non-myelinated, that is to say that one or several fibres are loosely enclosed by Schwann cells and because of this their conduction velocity is considerably reduced.

The outer layer of the Schwann cell was at one time known as the neurilemma sheath but this term is now not in common usage.

Individual nerve fibres are surrounded by a delicate tissue, the endoneurium, which serves as support for not only the nerve fibres but also for the rich vascular system supplying a peripheral nerve; these nerve fibres are gathered together into small fasiculi and supported by perineurium, and the fasiculi in turn are surrounded by a dense connective tissue sheath, the epineurium, which serves as the outer layer of the peripheral nerve trunk.

Transport Systems in the Nerve Fibre

Running the length of the nerve fibre are intracellular microtubules which are more prominent in the axoplasm than in dendrite processes. These microtubules are not surrounded by a membrane as are other cell organelles, e.g. lysosomes, but the walls are composed of repeating sub-units of glyco-proteins, resembling those found in cilia and spermatozoa and are thought to have similar contractile properties. The peristaltic-like movement occurring in microtubules from the cell body to the distal end of a nerve process would allow them a role in intracellular transport.

Experiments have already shown that the axon has two transport systems in the distal parts. One is relatively slow and has been estimated at 1–2mm per day, the other is much faster moving at a rate of 200–400mm per day. Different substances are thought to be transported by each system and current thinking is that the fast flow component transports cell organelles, e.g. lysosomes and large molecules, whereas the slower system carries structural proteins.

From this brief revision of nerve cell organisation it can be seen that metabolic disorders which affect the cell body will rapidly result in dysfunction in the ability of the neurones to conduct a nerve impulse and transport molecules which are essential for synaptic transmission and the continued integrity of the distal parts of the nerve process. It may also explain why the first symptoms and signs of a peripheral neuropathy appear in those neurones with the longest line of communication, that is, the feet and lower limbs, closely followed by the hands.

AETIOLOGY OF POLYNEUROPATHIES

There is still argument as to the precise metabolic dysfunction which results in some polyneuropathies but the following classification of causal agents is commonly accepted.

1. Infective condition
   (a) local infections of peripheral nerves:
   e.g. virus – herpes zoster
   bacteria – leprosy, brucellosis
   (b) polyneuritis complicating a current infection:
   e.g. dysentery, influenza, mumps
   (c) infections with organisms whose toxins have an affinity for the peripheral nervous system:
   e.g. diphtheria, tetanus, botulism.
2. Post-infective polyneuropathy
   e.g. Guillain-Barré-Landry syndrome.
3. Toxic substances
   e.g. heavy metals – mercury, lead, arsenic, gold and copper organic chemicals – aniline, cyanide, triortho-cresyl-phosphate
   drugs – isoniazid, thalidomide and nitrofurantoin, vincristine.
4. Deficiency, metabolic and blood disorders
   e.g. alcoholism, porphyria, leukaemia, diabetes mellitus, chronic uraemia, liver failure and various vitamin deficiencies.
5. Trauma
   e.g. physical (compression/stretching), electrical (earth shock) or radiation injury to nerves.
6. Connective tissue disease and allied disorders in which abnormalities in metabolism of serum proteins occur
   e.g. polyarteritis nodosa, systemic lupus erythematosus, amyloid disease, sarcoidosis and carcinoma.
7. Genetic disorders
   e.g. hereditary sensory radicular neuropathy (Denny-Brown), hypertrophic interstitial neuritis (Déjèrine-Sottas), peroneal muscular atrophy (Charcot-Marie-Tooth), Refsum's disease.
8. Pure vascular disorders
   e.g. atheroma, collagen disorders, diabetes mellitus, Buerger's disease.
9. Polyneuropathy of unknown origin

PATHOLOGICAL CHANGES IN PERIPHERAL NEUROPATHY

The pathological changes produced by the causal agent can be divided into two groups – parenchymal and interstitial.

Parenchymal

In parenchymal neuropathies it is the neurone and/or Schwann cell which undergo degeneration. There are three types of lesion:

1. *Axonal degeneration* (sometimes called Gombault's degeneration). The nerve processes and soma atrophy, with associated breakdown in the myelin sheath. Recovery from these changes is slow and incomplete.

2. *Segmental degeneration*. This involves the loss of myelin from sections of the nerve fibre usually in the more proximal parts. The recovery of nerve function is rapid and complete.

3. *Wallerian degeneration*. This occurs when both axon and myelin sheath undergo disorganisation; the demyelination process occurring some time after the destruction of the axon, the nerve soma undergoes chromatolysis. Recovery from Wallerian degeneration is slow and often incomplete.

In all three types of parenchymal pathology nerve conduction is outside normal limits, and due to the loss of conduction capability the muscles supplied will atrophy.

Interstitial

In the polyneuropathies of interstitial origin it is primarily collagen changes in the vascular structures which produce the neural changes. The connective tissues supporting the nerve processes can also be involved in producing pathological changes in nerve trunks, e.g. amyloid and tumour tissue.

CLINICAL FEATURES

The clinical picture of peripheral neuropathy comprises a lower motor neurone paralysis, especially in the limbs, the lower one being more involved than the upper limb.

The patient exhibits atrophy, muscle flaccid paralysis, weakness and ataxia, usually complaining of the inability to walk over rough ground – stumbling, even falling, he may present with a chronic ankle sprain due to the balance problems. In the upper limb the patient indicates problems in manipulating small coins, matches, knives etc, and may drop objects unintentionally.

Foot drop and wrist drop are present and joint contractures and deformity may be seen in hands, feet and spine.

Tendon reflexes are sometimes absent and often sluggish, the latter being due to a reduced nerve conduction velocity and impulse volley dispersal. The ankle jerk disappears before the knee jerk and the plantar response is flexor. Impairment of both cutaneous and proprioceptive sensory modalities are seen initially in the extremities but later progressing proximally. Paraesthesia is a common complaint and if muscle groups or nerve trunks are palpated with a deep pressure pain is often produced.

The loss of proprioception will also contribute to the 'drunken' (ataxic) gait described above. Severe joint disorganisation (Charcot joints) is seen as a result of persistent injury which is not felt due to loss of pain sensibility, resulting in damage and eventually destruction of the joint.

Trophic changes in the skin of the extremities are shown by the red, glossy skin which on palpation seems to have 'double thickness'; later, thickening of the nails is seen. Trophic and sensory changes in their most extreme form are seen in leprosy where loss of digits may occur.

In more serious neuropathies there may be associated myocardial damage, resulting in cardiac arrhythmia and labile blood pressure.

In addition to the above clinical features a history of exposure to toxic chemicals may produce their own symptoms, e.g. the pigmentation in arsenic poisoning.

CLINICAL DIAGNOSIS

First, the existence of a neuropathy needs to be established, then its cause must be determined and treatment prescribed.

The first stage is fairly easy as the clinical history and presenting signs and symptoms may be those associated with a particular neuropathy. The symmetrical and distal distribution of muscle atrophy and weakness together with sensory impairment is characteristic of peripheral neuropathy. But it is more usual for other clinical diagnostic tests to be needed to determine the existence and cause of the disease.

Biochemical tests may be used which will establish the presence of certain metabolic or toxic substances or the absence of nutrients. An electromyelograph (EMG) will differentiate between a neuropathy and a myopathy, or a disorder of the neuromuscular junction.

The measurement of nerve conduction velocity can be a help in determining the type of pathological changes occurring in the neurone. It is usual to find in Wallerian degeneration that conduction velocity is reduced by up to 30 per cent. In segmental demyelination conduction velocity is often slowed by more than 40 per cent (Gilliatt, 1966).

The nature of the neuropathy can sometimes be determined by the biopsy of the sural nerve (the resultant sensory loss is minimal).

MEDICAL MANAGEMENT

The medical management will depend on the speed of onset and the patient's clinical presentation.

In the more severe cases, e.g. Guillain-Barré-Landry the full services of an intensive care unit may be required whereas in others, e.g. diabetic neuropathy, the patient may receive treatment on an outpatient basis.

The indicator for ventilatory assistance is when the vital capacity is reduced to 800ml and a PaO_2 below 60mm Hg. Patients who are thought to be entering respiratory problems should have hourly assessment of vital capacity. As ventilatory help is required for several weeks it is usual for a tracheostomy to be performed and a cuffed tracheal tube inserted. Tracheal toilet and suction is needed to prevent lung infection but antibiotics are not as a rule prescribed unless there is evidence of an infection. Respiratory support is given by an intermittent positive pressure ventilator.

Normal nursing care to the bladder, pressure areas, skin care, and mouth toilet is required. In some cases hypotension occurs, usually in the elderly patient, and pressor drugs are required to support blood pressure. The fluid balance of the patient is important so that dehydration does not occur, a nasogastric tube is usually present in patients with bulbar palsy, and depending on the patient's condition may be used to feed them, though intravenous feeding can be used.

Analgesia may be required if pain is a problem and, as pressure can produce pain, a bed cradle is used to relieve the weight of blankets. Careful positioning of the patient's joints is needed to prevent discomfort as well as contractures occurring. In most cases of severe infective neuropathy improvement occurs, the mortality of such patients is approximately 5 per cent if care is given in an intensive unit, compared with about 25 per cent mortality for admission to a general ward. It is important to remember that the patient is conscious and can feel pain, though he may need assistance with breathing and cannot move. Hospital personnel and relatives who have contact with the patient must remember this and not discuss the more depressing aspects of the patient's condition within earshot or treat the patient as an imbecile.

The patient who is not so severely affected and who can maintain his own airway and is somewhat more independent is in a better position. For these patients rest in bed is often required and is essential if there are signs of cardiac involvement. Analgesia may be required to mini-mise spontaneous pain and a bed cradle to support the bedclothes. Some medical regimes include a high caloric diet and vitamin therapy especially of the B complex; careful positioning is again necessary to preserve joint integrity.

If toxic substances have been absorbed, removal from the cause will lead to improvement; in some cases, e.g. lead or arsenic poisoning, chelating agents are given to provide an alternative chemical 'acceptor' for the causal metal agent; the drug used for lead or arsenic neuropathy is dimercaprol.

In polyneuropathy due to vitamin deficiency, e.g. beri-beri, a good diet plus vitamin replacement therapy will facilitate recovery which though slow is usually complete as malnutrition must be prolonged for Wallerian degeneration to have occurred.

Most cases of polyneuropathy, once the cause has been removed, show signs of improvement; in other cases, the disorder persists for some time before improvement begins and yet again in other neuropathies no change is seen.

PRINCIPAL POLYNEUROPATHIC SYNDROMES

The list of polyneuropathic syndromes is very extensive and it is not possible to cover all of them in this text. The more commonly met polyneuropathies are listed below.

A. Acute Ascending Polyneuropathy
   Guillain-Barré-Landry
   porphyria
   diphtheria
   mononucleosis
B. Sub-acute Sensorimotor Polyneuropathy
   (1) symmetrical
       arsenical
       lead
       thalidomide
       alcoholic
   (2) asymmetrical
       polyarteritis nodosa
       diabetic
C. Chronic Sensorimotor Polyneuropathy
   (1) acquired
       carcinoma
       amyloid
       rheumatoid arthritis

(2) genetic
peroneal muscular atrophy (Charcot-Marie-Tooth)
hypertrophic interstitial neuritis (Déjèrine-Sottas)
hereditary atactica polyneuriformis (Refsum's)

ACUTE ASCENDING POLYNEUROPATHY

Guillain-Barré-Landry Syndrome

This syndrome which affects both sexes at any age, peaking at 20–50, is found world-wide and in all seasons. Its cause is unknown, though current authorities consider it to be due to hypersensitivity or allergy to unknown viruses or allergens. In around 50 per cent of cases the onset of symptoms is preceded by a mild gastro-intestinal or respiratory infection.

Clinically, the syndrome presents as a symmetrical weakness of muscle; there is some wasting, hypotonia and a partial or complete loss of the associated deep tendon reflexes. The motor symptoms start distally and move proximally, with lower limb involvement preceding that of the upper limb, the disease may progress to involve the trunk and cranial muscles. Pain is a variable symptom, though there is usually tenderness on deep pressure, especially to motor points in muscle and nerve trunks. Paraesthesia is often described in the limbs.

Both sensory and motor nerve conduction velocities are reduced. Autonomic functions are sometimes affected, usually cardiac muscle, which may lead to sinus arrhythmias and variable blood pressure.

Visual impairment is rare, though papilloedema is occasionally seen. The hearing is not usually affected and cerebral symptoms rare.

The symptoms may progress for one or several weeks until the disease 'peaks and plateaus out' gradually regressing symptoms in reverse order of onset.

PATHOLOGY

The disease process affects the spinal roots and nerve processes, primarily involving the Schwann cell and this results in segmental demyelination of the nerve process initially, later there is a proliferation of Schwann cells. The axon remains intact though demyelinated and can conduct an impulse with a much reduced velocity.

There is an associated perivascular lymphocytic inflammatory exudate of the peripheral nervous system, and other organs such as the heart, lungs or kidney may show this. Recovery takes place by remyelination of peripheral axons, though the myelin sheath is thinner and the internodal distances less, but eventually the conduction velocity returns to within normal limits.

PROGNOSIS

In epidemics the mortality is high but usually in a single incidence of this syndrome most patients recover completely. The more favourable ones in three to six months although more often the time scale is one to two years.

COMPLICATIONS

In severe cases who need respiratory assistance, infections of the lower respiratory tract can be a hazard. Deep vein thrombosis due to paralysis affecting the limbs and thereby removing the muscle pump effect, and the temporary loss of an effective respiratory system, can also occur.

The retention of urine is an uncommon complication.

Cardiac arrhythmias and labile blood pressure have already been mentioned as a possible complication.

TREATMENT

If respiratory assistance is required for the Guillain-Barré-Landry patient ideally it should be managed in an intensive care unit as the chance of life expectancy is enhanced under these conditions.

The normal nursing care for fluid intake, skin and pressure area care is needed. Sometimes ACTH is prescribed for these patients to reduce the inflammatory response but clinical results vary.

PHYSIOTHERAPY MANAGEMENT

A. UNDER INTENSIVE CARE IN THE ACUTE PROGRESSIVE STAGE

During this period of treatment when the patient is to all intents and purposes a tetraplegic with respiratory distress the aims of treatment are to:

(a) maintain a clear airway
(b) prevent lung infection
(c) maintain anatomical joint range
(d) support joints in a functional position to minimise damage or deformity
(e) assist in the prevention of pressure sores
(f) maintain peripheral circulation
(g) provide psychological support for the patient and relatives.

Methods

1. MAINTENANCE OF A CLEAR AIRWAY

2. PREVENTION OF LUNG INFECTION

The patient's breathing will be assisted by intermittent positive pressure ventilation (IPPV) via a cuffed tracheostomy tube. This leads to some limitation of the positions in which the patient may be placed to posturally drain areas of lung tissue. Some compromise is necessary and, in the absence of lung infection, two-hourly turning into supine or side lying positions will aid the removal of secretions from all parts of the lung.

A suction catheter is used to remove secretions from the respiratory passages, until the cough reflex reappears.

Manual techniques used to assist in maintaining and clearing the airway include vibration with/without over pressure. To enhance expansion a two to four litre anaesthetic bag can be used for patients with tracheostomy tubes, although care is needed as a reduction in cardiac output can occur as a result of 'bagging'. Two people are necessary for this technique, one to squeeze the bag, and another to apply chest manipulations.

To simulate a cough, rib-springing techniques are useful, although a faulty technique may produce fractures of the ribs! As chest care is relatively long term for these patients, a 2.5cm thick piece of foam rubber placed under the physiotherapist's hands makes rib-springing more tolerable for the patient.

Once the patient is weaned off the ventilator, respiratory care is a shared responsibility between patient and physiotherapist and adequate expansion in all areas of the lung and effective coughing must be taught to the patient. As neurones recover their function and muscle once again responds to a nerve impulse active assisted/active exercises to those muscles may commence. Patients at this stage tire fairly quickly and there are still some 'aches and pains' in the limbs.

3. TO MAINTAIN NORMAL JOINT MOVEMENT

Gentle passive movements should be given through full range at least three times a day. Multi-joint muscle groups should also be placed on full (normal) stretch. Patients appreciate these simple procedures as they comment (later) on a feeling of tension 'cramp' building up in the limbs, and this sensation is relieved by passive movements.

The hip joint must be fully extended at least daily when the patient is in the lateral position. The shoulder joint range also should be maintained, care being taken that movements occur at the gleno-humeral joint and not just the shoulder girdle. The tempero-mandibular joint should not be forgotten. Ankles, wrists, hands and feet also need accurate passive movement applied; as these areas will be the last to recover, serious loss of joint and muscle extensibility with functional loss and unacceptable cosmetic appearance could be due to sloppy passive movements.

4. SUPPORT OF JOINTS

Light splintage using Plastazote is required to support the peripheral joints in a comfortable and functional position during the time of flaccid paralysis. Splintage will prevent abnormal movements and untoward damage occurring to the joints. Bed cradles should be used to avoid pressure on the joints from bedclothes.

The general position of the patient in bed will alternate between supine and side-lying positions; sandbags and pillows must be used to stabilise these positions and if splints are used a careful check should be made to avoid damage to other parts of the body from pressure or rubbing by the splint.

5. PREVENTION OF PRESSURE SORES

The physiotherapist joins the nurse in having a responsibility towards frequent checking of the patient's pressure areas. The patient is normally on a two-hourly turning regime to prevent chest complications and pressure sores.

As the physiotherapist usually times her visit to coincide with these turns she can check the new and old pressure areas. Should a pressure sore develop the physiotherapist may be required to give ultra-violet radiation or ice-cube massage to the sore to enhance the healing process.

6. MAINTENANCE OF CIRCULATION

The passive movements described in (3) will assist in increasing venous return. Additionally, gently but firm effleurage massage may be given to the lower limbs, although by some method of communication the patient should indicate if this produces extreme discomfort.

7. PSYCHOLOGICAL SUPPORT

The patient with this syndrome has *unimpaired* cerebral functions, therefore his perception is unclouded. As treatment is commenced, the patient should be involved in his treatment; he must be told what is to be done to him, very simply and undramatically. Include the patient in conversation if another member of staff is present. Never discuss his prognosis or condition with a colleague within earshot.

The patient's relatives should be briefed on the points above and must be reassured that the prognosis, though slow, is excellent so that visiting time is a supportive experience rather than a frustrating and upsetting time for the patient.

B. RECOVERY STAGE

When the patient can maintain his own airway and ventilation and some motor recovery is occurring an assessment of the patient's problems is required to define treatment priorities.

The assessment should be detailed under the following headings:
  (a) respiratory system; rate, depth and pattern of breathing should be noted. Vital capacity and chest expansion recorded.
  (b) joint range on active and passive movement; also noted should be joints which still require splint support.
  (c) motor power of the recovered and recovering muscles.
  (d) sensation; all cutaneous modalities including vibration and two-point discrimination. Proprioception.
  (e) balance in various functional positions together with details of methods of support needed to stabilise a position.
  (f) independence of self-care.
  (g) motivation and general psychological approach to life in general.

Physiotherapy

As patients recover at different rates it is impossible to outline a course of treatment to suit them all. However, certain basic principles should be common to all treatment programmes and these are defined below. Some or all of the principles listed are applicable in an on-going scheme of treatment.

In general during recovery of nerve function, motor improvement occurs more rapidly than sensory and treatment plans should take this into account.

Principles of Physiotherapy

1. MAINTENANCE OF THE AIRWAY AND VENTILATORY CAPACITY

Care of respiratory function is an aim for some time during the recovery phase. Patients can be taught breathing techniques and adequate coughing together with instruction on frequency of practice, i.e. three to four times a day, say, prior to each meal.

2. MAINTAIN AND IMPROVE JOINT RANGE

The more peripheral joints will require splintage and passive movements for some considerable time. The patient's relatives can be taught care and application of splints and effective and safe passive techniques of movement.

The patient will now be allowed out of bed and in sitting should sit squarely on the buttocks with shoulders level.

3. STRENGTHEN AND RE-EDUCATE NORMAL MUSCLE FUNCTION

The proximal muscles recover first and to facilitate voluntary contraction of muscle some of the following techniques may be useful:

  (a) neuromuscular facilitation techniques
  (b) afferent stimulation of skin
  (c) free active exercises
  (d) equilibrium and righting reactions
  (e) progressive resistance exercises
  (f) hydrotherapy
  (g) suspension
  (h) springs/pulleys
  (i) simple, progressing to more difficult, circuits for power and endurance.

The patient should have a short programme of 'core' exercises which he must practice for a certain number of repetitions (which are increased daily) and frequency throughout the day.

4. RE-EDUCATION OF SENSORY AWARENESS

(1) cutaneous stimulation: the use of different materials, textures, shapes and weights will assist in perceptual re-education.
(2) proprioceptive: the use of equilibrium and balance responses.
(3) use of alternative systems, i.e. vision.

To protect the integrity of the skin the patient or his relatives must be made aware of the importance of skin care both of hygiene and protection (especially the hands) against thermal or mechanical damage.

5. RESTORATION OF NORMAL FUNCTION

1. Lower limbs
Various gait aids and orthoses may be required initially to restore a safe walking pattern appropriate to the weakness, incoordination and proprioceptive loss.

2. Upper limbs
Some splintage is often necessary and certain aids to daily living are

required to enable the patient to be independent in his personal care, e.g. hygiene, toilet, feeding and dressing.

6. RESTORATION OF MAXIMAL INDEPENDENCE

In some cases recovery may not be complete and the patient's environment must be restructured to accommodate his disability and his needs.

7. MOTIVATION

Most patients in the acute stage will not believe that they will recover. It is sometimes, but not always, useful for the patient to see a person who has recovered well from the same illness. The physiotherapist must help the patient and often the relatives to gain the will to join in the treatment and so regain a productive and happy life again.

PORPHYRIC POLYNEUROPATHY

This polyneuropathy is inherited as an autosomal dominant trait which produces a liver defect which results in an excess of porphobilingogen and d-ammalaevulinic acid (precursor to porphyrin) being found in the urine. The onset of the neuropathy is rare before puberty and affects men more than women. The onset can be precipitated by drugs affecting porphyrin metabolism, e.g. barbiturates, oral contraceptives and methyldopa. The clinical presentation is a severe, rapid onset, showing symmetrical motor symptoms beginning in the feet and ascending, and later involving the upper limb and moving centrally. Sensory symptoms are less well marked. Associated with these symptoms are abdominal pains and tenderness with vomiting and constipation. The classical symptom is of urine which becomes port-wine coloured if left to stand.

Cerebral symptoms of confusion, delirium and occasionally convulsions are usually present.

Other symptoms include, tachycardia, leucocytosis and fever.

The prognosis of this neuropathy is variable, a disturbance in cerebral function precedes the more severe rather than milder forms. The milder form often regressing and, at the other extreme, a severe form which may progress rapidly to be fatal within days.

Pathology

In most peripheral nerves, typical Wallerian degeneration of nervous tissue is found, along with some segmental demyelination of the remaining nerve fibres.

SUB-ACUTE SENSORIMOTOR POLYNEUROPATHY

Symmetrical Polyneuropathies

The use of heavy metals in industrial processes has for many years been subject to legislative controls in their use, to minimise the health risk to persons who need to handle these substances.

However, occasionally a polyneuropathy is seen which is the result of poisoning by a heavy metal.

One of the most common is lead poisoning; this is increasing in incidence, and is found more often in children whose home or school is close to a motorway or industrial process using lead. The radial nerve is most commonly affected, also the proximal muscles of the arm and shoulder girdle in the upper limb, and the common peroneal nerve in the leg. Arsenical poisoning is more rare and the symmetrical neuropathy is slow to develop. Associated symptoms are intestinal problems, anaemia, a typical brown skin jaundice and excess of the metal in hair and urine samples.

In all poisoning by heavy metals the symptoms are slow to develop, taking many weeks to reach their peak, and last a variable time. The typical clinical presentation of polyneuropathy is present, i.e. pain, paraesthesia, muscle weakness, atrophy and tenderness.

PATHOLOGY

Initially, myelin changes are present but later Wallerian degeneration occurs especially of the larger fibres.

MEDICAL AND PHYSIOTHERAPY MANAGEMENT

Chelating agents are given to remove the heavy metal from the body.

Physiotherapy care depends upon the severity of the disease, and is symptomatic (see p.337 et seq).

ASYMMETRICAL POLYNEUROPATHIES

The two most commonly encountered in this group are due to polyarteritis nodosa and diabetes mellitus.

POLYARTERITIS NODOSA

In this condition 75 per cent of cases show nutritional changes in nerve tissue due to thrombosis of the vasa nervorum. The clinical finding is either of a diffuse, more or less symmetrical polyneuropathy or more often a mononeuropathy multiplex.

The onset is usually abrupt, pain and numbness being present, together with motor weakness, and sensory loss of cutaneous and proprioceptive modalities.

The medical care may include corticosteroid therapy and symptomatic physiotherapy, but the prognosis is poor in most cases.

DIABETIC POLYNEUROPATHY

This is a common finding in diabetics over 50 years of age. It appears clinically in two forms, distal symmetrical polyneuropathy and mononeuropathy multiplex.

Distal Symmetrical Polyneuropathy

This is the most common type exhibited by patients and its clinical features include sphincter weakness, numbness and tingling in the lower limbs, which is worse at night; trophic changes are seen in the distal areas of skin (ulcers may be multiple) and joints. There is usually areflexia of the tendo Achilles reflex and mild muscle weakness. The resultant weakness and sensory loss leads to an ataxic gait. The symptoms mimic tabes dorsalis, but evidence of raised blood sugar provides the differential diagnosis.

Mononeuropathy Multiplex

This form affects older patients who have a mild or undiagnosed diabetic condition; it usually involves nerve trunks supplying the pelvic and upper leg muscles.

The presenting symptoms are frequently a complaint of pain in the lumbar or hip region which is more severe at night, the quality of the pain is described as sharp and lancinating. There is also muscle weakness and atrophy in the affected groups. The deep and superficial sensation is variable in involvement and may only be mildly affected. There are, however, usually sphincter disturbances and urinary incontinence may become a problem.

PATHOLOGY

Changes in the motor-end plate in the form of expansion of the terminal ending are thought to precede the segmental demyelination of peripheral nerves. It is thought that the metabolic activity of the Schwann cell is altered by the disease process, although a causal agent may be ischaemic changes secondary to the disease which occurs in the vasa nervorum.

MEDICAL MANAGEMENT

The treatment of both forms of diabetic neuropathy includes:
1. The stabilisation of the diabetic condition
2. The inclusion of vitamin supplements to the diet
3. The management of pain.

PHYSIOTHERAPY

The patient with diabetic neuropathy often presents with other problems, such as osteoarthritis of hip or knee, not associated with the diabetic condition.

The aims of treatment are to:
1. Restore the normal range of joint movement
2. Increase muscle strength and/or endurance
3. Improve balance in sitting and standing
4. Teach the patient a safe walking pattern with aids if necessary
5. Teach skin and joint care if there is sensory loss
6. Advise on the fitting and use of orthoses
7. Advise on alterations or best use of the patient's home environment
8. Help the patient achieve a satisfactory life-style.

CHRONIC SENSORIMOTOR POLYNEUROPATHY

ACQUIRED

A polyneuropathy associated with carcinoma is slow to develop, and may occur prior to the malignancy being found, usually in lung and/or stomach.

The symptoms are typical of a neuropathy and a mixed sensori-motor type is more common.

Rheumatoid polyneuropathy develops in some patients, and is usually a painful neuropathy with minimal sensori-motor loss or reflexive changes. Little is known of the link with rheumatoid disease, but it may be due to arterial lesions.

In amyloid polyneuropathy it is usual for both sensory and motor systems to be affected. Amyloid tissue is found in many older individuals and can be considered as part of the ageing process. The symptoms are initially confined to the autonomic nervous system, and the symptoms affecting the somatic nervous system often mimic syringomyelia, though ECG abnormalities in amyloidosis differentiate between the two conditions.

GENETICALLY DETERMINED

The main polyneuropathies in this are peroneal muscular atrophy (Charcot-Marie-Tooth disease) and hypertrophic interstitial neuritis.

Peroneal Muscular Atrophy (PMA)

This is due to an autosomal dominant or recessive gene, the onset occurring in late childhood/early adolescence. It is a neuropathy rather than a myopathy despite its name.

The initial manifestations are a symmetrical weakness and wasting of the peroneal muscles, and later the anterior tibial and intrinsic foot muscles are affected. The muscle weakness spreads to involve the proximal parts of the leg but halts its progress at the distal third of the thigh and the typical picture of 'inverted champagne bottles' is produced.

Involvement of the hands and forearm comes later. There is usually a stocking and glove distribution of sensory loss, and areflexia of the tendon reflexes of affected muscles. The course of the disease is slow and it is not severely disabling.

PATHOLOGY

Changes occur mainly in the cells of the ventral horn and its peripheral processes. The dorsal horn is involved to a lesser degree. Chronic demyelination occurs in nerve trunks, leading to degeneration of the large diameter motor and sensory nerve fibres, leaving connective tissue only. There is degeneration of the posterior columns of the spinal cord.

MEDICAL AND PHYSIOTHERAPY MANAGEMENT

There is no specific medical treatment. Physiotherapy is aimed at relieving symptoms and advice on splinting may also be required. If foot deformities occur, i.e. pes cavus or talipes equinovarus, orthopaedic surgery may be needed.

Hypertrophic Interstitial Neuritis

Also known as Déjèrine-Sottas syndrome and is due to an autosomal dominant gene. Symptoms appear in childhood or infancy and slowly progress. The first symptoms are seen distally in the legs, in a symmetrical weakness and wasting of muscle. Pain and paraesthesia are early features of the disease. The symptoms progress to the hands and move centrally to the trunk. There is areflexia of the involved muscles.

It is a slowly progressive disease which is more disabling than PMA and patients frequently deteriorate and have to lead a wheelchair life. Deformities of the feet and hands occur, e.g. talipes equinovarus, claw foot/hand and, in more severe forms of the disease, a kyphoscoliosis may be found.

PATHOLOGY

There is a proliferation of perineurium tissue in the nerve trunk and this leads to a palpable painless thickening of peripheral nerves. The Schwann cells undergo changes leading to a thinning of the myelin sheath and axonal degeneration.

MEDICAL AND PHYSIOTHERAPY MANAGEMENT

No specific medical treatment. Physiotherapy is symptomatic with advice on wheelchair life, home adaptation and aids to daily living.

REFERENCE

Gilliatt, R. W. (1966). 'Nerve conduction in human and experimental neuropathies.' *Proceedings of the Royal Society of Medicine*, **59**, 989–93.

BIBLIOGRAPHY

Chusid, J. G. (1976). *Correlative Neuroanatomy and Functional Neurology*. Lange Medical Publications, California.
Gray's Anatomy, 36th edition (ed. Warwick, R. and Williams, P. L.) (1980). Longman Group Limited, Edinburgh.
Lenman, J. A. R. and Ritchie, A. E. (1977). *Clinical Electromyography*, 2nd edition. Pitman Medical Publishing Company Limited, Tunbridge Wells.
Passmore, R. and Robson, J. S. (jt. eds.) (1974). *A Companion to Medical Studies*, volume 3. Blackwell Scientific Publications Limited, Oxford.

See also Bibliography on p.327.

ACKNOWLEDGEMENT

The author thanks Mrs M. Loughran for kindly typing the original manuscript.

Chapter 19

Spina Bifida and Hydrocephalus

by O. R. NETTLES, M.C.S.P., O.N.C.

The three major and most common neurological conditions found in the newborn are anencephaly, hydrocephalus and spina bifida cystica. The last is the most common crippling congenital condition in this country.

ANENCEPHALY

Literally this means absence of the brain and the condition is not compatible with life. It is said to be the commonest of the three conditions and it is known that it is more common in the Eastern hemisphere than in the West.

HYDROCEPHALUS

Hydrocephalus occurs when there is an increase in the cerebrospinal fluid circulating in and around the brain. Normally the fluid is formed by the choroid plexuses, circulates through the ventricular system (under increased pressure) and central canal of the spinal cord and reaches the subarachnoid space through the median and lateral foramina in the fourth ventricle. It bathes the surface of the brain and cord and is reabsorbed into the cerebral venous sinuses via the veins on the surface of the hemispheres and the granulations.

Should any blockage occur in any part of this system pressure of fluid will build up in the ventricles causing enlargement and in the neonatal stage a consequent enlargement of the skull. Occasionally hydrocephalus occurs in utero and is easily detected if the size of the head interferes with the normal delivery of the baby. Much more often the head is normal at birth and only grows abnormally during the early months.

In 80 per cent of all cases hydrocephalus is associated with spina bifida cystica and when this condition is present the doctors will be prepared for hydrocephalus. In the remaining 20 per cent it may only be detected when the head grows abnormally and the anterior part bulges. Often the health visitor or infant welfare doctor may spot this during routine visits because they have the detailed knowledge of child development which is required to ascertain whether the circumference of the head is outside the normal limits.

Aetiology

In the 80 per cent of cases of hydrocephalus associated with spina bifida, the excess of fluid is due to malformations associated with the spina bifida. Known as the Arnold-Chiari malformation, it is a displacement of the medulla and part of the cerebellum into the foramen

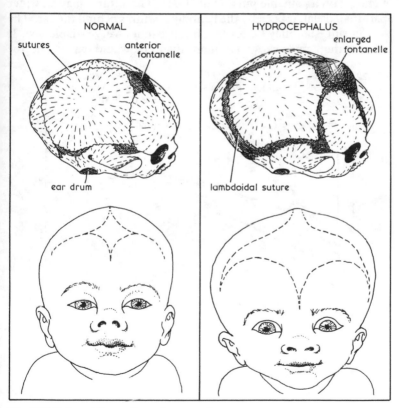

Fig. 19/1 Enlarged fontanelles and separated sutures

magnum, causing a damming up of the cerebrospinal fluid. In a few cases this blockage may be complete but in the great majority of cases it is only partial.

Hydrocephalus may occur as a result of prematurity, a precipitate birth, or toxaemia in the mother. During birth the baby's head may be damaged due to haemorrhage and this may result in an interruption in the flow of the cerebrospinal fluid. The blockage may be by a blood clot, in which case the damage may only be temporary.

Again, hydrocephalus may occur after birth if a newborn baby develops an infection causing meningitis. The inflammation of the meninges may narrow the channels through which the cerebrospinal fluid has to flow and this will produce symptoms of hydrocephalus.

When the baby is born it may be possible to recognise the hydrocephalus at once. The head may be larger than average or deformed. The brow may be bulging, the fontanelles larger than usual and bulging with a palpable pulse (Fig. 19/1). The sutures may be wider apart than usual, especially the lambdoid sutures behind the ear. The 'setting sun' sign may be present but it is not a very reliable one. If present, the baby's eyes stare more than one would expect and the

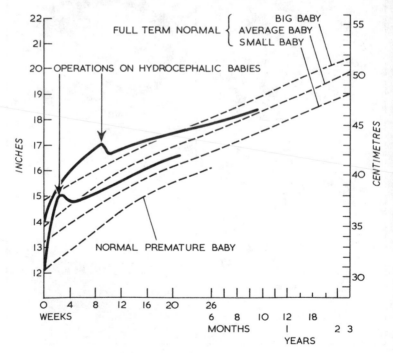

Fig. 19/2 Head circumference chart

cornea is large with the sclerotic visible above but not always visible below. If there is any doubt the circumference of the head is watched closely, and a chart of this is kept. This usually gives a very accurate estimate of abnormal growth (Fig. 19/2).

Treatment

Until 1956 no effective treatment for hydrocephalus was available, but some time before this a child, whose father John Holter was an engineer, was born in America with this complaint. This father together with a neurosurgeon, Mr Eugene Spitz, perfected the Spitz-Holter shunt (Fig. 19/3A) which is designed to drain the excess cerebrospinal fluid from the ventricles into the circulatory system (to be disposed of in the usual way).

This shunt comprises a right-angled catheter, the 'proximal' catheter, one end of which is inserted through the skull into the ventricle of the brain while the other end is attached to a piece of clear plastic compressible tube about 4cm long. This has at either end a non-return valve encased in metal and at the lower end is the 'distal' catheter

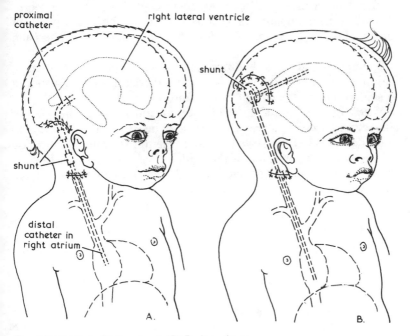

Fig. 19/3 (A) Spitz-Holter shunt. (B) Pudenz shunt

which in turn is usually inserted into the jugular vein and thence into the right atrium of the heart. The whole shunt runs beneath the skin with the valve just behind the right ear. To a trained eye the catheter in the neck is just visible looking very much like a prominent vein, while the shunt is soon covered by the growing hair.

To insert the shunt, a half-moon incision is made behind the right ear and another one over the jugular vein. As the child grows it may become necessary to lengthen the distal catheter to ensure that drainage into the heart is maintained.

Once the shunt is in position it begins to drain away the excess cerebrospinal fluid, the bulge in the fontanelles disappears and the space between the sutures returns to normal. The valves in the shunt only work when the pressure in the ventricles is excessive, and it has been found that in many children the shunt may only be operational for short spells during the day. At the present time the shunts are not removed but remain in situ indefinitely. Other types of shunts have been used, notably the Pudenz (Fig. 19/3B).

This method of control of hydrocephalus was first used in this country by the late Mr G. H. Macnab at the Hospital for Sick Children, Great Ormond St, London, and for some time was the standard procedure in all cases of hydrocephalus in the newborn. Nowadays the treatment is more conservative and the future quality of the life of the child is assessed before the surgeons come to a decision on surgery.

Spontaneous arrest of hydrocephalus does happen in a few cases. This has always been the position and it is these cases which managed to survive before the advent of the shunt.

When hydrocephalus appears without spina bifida, there is, of course, no flaccid paralysis but there may be spastic paralysis due to brain damage. Left untreated, the damage to the brain will increase especially once ossification of the skull bones has occurred. In such cases the degree of spastic paralysis will increase and mental retardation will result. Hydrocephalus often causes a squint even when treated, but if untreated blindness may result.

PHYSIOTHERAPY

Such children are treated exactly as other children with cerebral palsy (see Chapter 20).

Before a baby with a shunt is allowed home the parents are given instructions in its care. Blocking of the shunt is an ever-present danger and the ward sister makes sure that the parents know the signs to look for. The valve in the shunt can be tested by compressing the soft tube which normally empties and fills quickly. If the proximal catheter in the brain blocks the valve will stay flat as no cerebrospinal fluid can pass into it when pressure is released. The onset of the symptoms may be sudden or gradual depending on the extent of the blockage.

FALSE FONTANELLES

One operation which is sometimes performed is to create 'false fontanelles'. Before the child's fontanelles close naturally, it is very easy to keep a check on the functioning of the shunt. If this is pumping satisfactorily the fontanelles are soft and look normal, but when there is any malfunction in the shunt the fontanelles very soon begin to bulge and this acts as a warning sign. Once they have closed naturally this method of checking is denied to the parents and medical personnel. In order to maintain this accurate indication surgeons may now remove a small circle of bone, usually from behind the right ear, so that there is a more permanent aperture in the skull through which any increase in the intracranial pressure may be watched.

TYPES OF SPINA BIFIDA

There are two main types of spina bifida:
1. Spina bifida occulta
2. Spina bifida cystica (or aperta or manifesta)
    (a) with meningocele
    (b) with myelomeningocele.

SPINA BIFIDA OCCULTA

This is a bifid or split spinal column but a perfectly normal and unaffected spinal cord (Fig. 19/4A).

In its mildest form an occult spina bifida may go undetected throughout that person's life, or may only be diagnosed if there has to be a spinal x-ray for some completely different reason, but other cases may have slight muscle imbalance, often in the muscles of the feet. This may not become apparent until the child is in his early teens when he puts on a spurt of growth during which his cord, already 'tethered', causes the nerve roots to be stretched and consequently damaged. The defect in spina bifida occurs in the first month of development, so the cord is 'tethered' at a much lower level in relation to the bones than the normal level in the upper lumbar vertebrae. This in turn interferes with nerve conductivity and so causes the imbalance. This usually results in a pes cavus deformity but in any

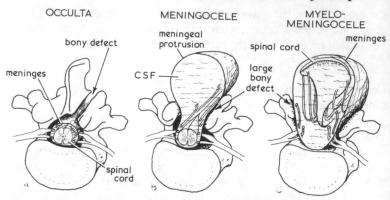

Fig. 19/4 Classification of spina bifida. (A) Normal vertebra (spina bifida occulta). (B) Incomplete vertebral development (meningocele). (C) Incomplete vertebral development with flat protruding spinal cord plate (myelomeningocele)

unusual abnormal pattern of foot growth an occult spina bifida cannot be ruled out without an x-ray. Such cases are frequently seen in children's orthopaedic clinics.

An occult spina bifida is sometimes detected at birth by a number of outward signs. These are: a hairy patch over the vertebrae; naevi; unusual dimples; and/or a small fatty lump over part of the spina. Provided the baby exhibits all the normal reflexes and is normal in other respects, he does not require urgent surgical treatment but a careful watch is kept on his progress.

Cases of spina bifida occulta are not the ones usually associated with the condition as they may never be diagnosed as such. Recognised cases of spina bifida cystica are those associated with either a meningocele or a myelomeningocele. In each type the baby is born with either an open wound over the area or a sac covered with skin.

SPINA BIFIDA CYSTICA

Spina bifida cystica is a neural tube defect – a defect in the structure of the bones of the spine with an incomplete closure of the vertebral canal and often associated abnormalities in the spinal cord itself, and other abnormalities in the body. It is one of the conditions that comes under the general heading of rachischisis (Greek: a cleft spine) an alternative name being rachischisis posterior. It is also known as dysraphism. A raphe is the ridge or furrow marking the line of the union of the two halves of symmetrical parts. Dysraphism is a failure of these two parts to join to form the raphe.

Incidence

Spina bifida occurs in about two per thousand live births in this country but its incidence varies from area to area. The Welsh and Irish have a higher incidence than the English and over the world the incidence is higher in Europe than in Asia, and, unlike anencephaly, it is more common in the Western hemisphere than in the Eastern. It is estimated that between 2,500 and 3,000 babies with spina bifida are born annually.

Before the design of the shunt to control hydrocephalus 90 per cent of all known cases died, leaving only about three hundred surviving annually. Some of these were only mildly affected but many were so disabled that they spent their lives in institutions and were not integrated into the community. Between 1960 and the early 1970s all children born with spina bifida were so treated. If a myelomeningocele was present this was operated on as soon as possible after birth and subsequently the shunt inserted into the head to overcome the hydrocephalus. About 60 per cent of such children lived beyond the age of five years and, although the subsequent death rate was higher than expected, many attained adulthood. Apart from the difficulties for the child himself and his family, this presented the medical, paramedical, education and employment authorities with very big problems as quite a number were too disabled to live a normal life and had to have sheltered employment and/or accommodation. With this in mind, much consideration is now given to the quality of life any baby can reasonably expect before embarking on neonatal surgery.

Aetiology

The cause is unknown. After years of research the present conclusion is that the cause is multifactorial and that genetics, environment, diet and/or drugs all play a part in the development of these defects.

The defect occurs in the early weeks of pregnancy, usually the fourth week, before the mother is really sure she is pregnant. At this stage of the zygote a primitive streak develops which is later to become the brain and spinal cord. This normally becomes covered with cells which later develop into the bony casing, the skull and vertebrae, but occasionally these cells fail to fuse completely and spina bifida results. This may appear anywhere from the occipital bone in the back of the head (encephalocele) to the sacrum, but about 70 per cent are in the lower thoracic and lumbosacral region. Figure 19/5 shows the distribution of lesions and the incidence of hydrocephalus in a series of 262 cases studied by two surgeons. Spina bifida in each area has its own characteristics.

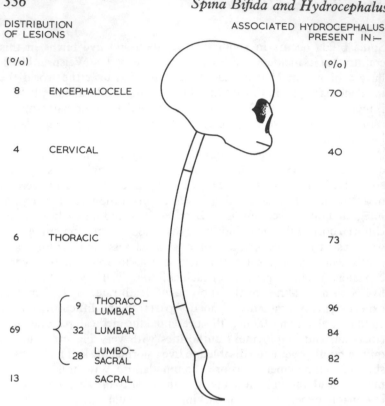

DISTRIBUTION OF LESIONS (%)			ASSOCIATED HYDROCEPHALUS PRESENT IN:— (%)
8	ENCEPHALOCELE		70
4	CERVICAL		40
6	THORACIC		73
69	9	THORACO-LUMBAR	96
	32	LUMBAR	84
	28	LUMBO-SACRAL	82
13		SACRAL	56

Fig. 19/5 Incidence of spina bifida

Once a child with spina bifida has been born into a family, although apparently random in the case of the first child, the chances of having a similarly affected second child is greatly increased. Whereas the initial risk of any family having a child with spina bifida is about one in five hundred, once one baby is born the risk increases to about one in twenty-five for the second and one in eight for the third.

Recently it has become possible to diagnose some cases of anencephaly and spina bifida before the child is born, by examination of the amniotic fluid surrounding the fetus. In early intra-uterine life the substance alphafetoprotein (AFP) is the main circulating protein in the fetus, and some of this substance is present in the amniotic fluid. In a procedure known as amniocentesis a sample of this fluid is taken from the uterus, and if the fetus has a neural tube defect the amount of AFP in the sample is raised. Other tests on the same sample may show the presence of other congenital defects, notably Down's syndrome and other conditions associated with chromosome abnormalities. This test is a complicated one and is carried out during the second trimester of pregnancy, between the sixteenth and eighteenth week. If the test is positive the parents are informed and are offered an abortion. The test can only be offered to parents who are known to be at risk, e.g. those who have already had one abnormal child, or where there is a history of abnormal births in the immediate family, or where the mother is over 35 years of age (when the risk of an abnormal birth, especially Down's syndrome, is considerably greater). AFP is also present in the blood plasma of the mother, and the viability of screening every pregnant mother by a blood test is now under discussion. If the AFP level is raised in the plasma, the parents are offered an amniocentesis to confirm the suspicions, and if the result of this is positive an abortion will be offered, but the final decision always rests with the parents.

As has been stated, hydrocephalus occurs in 80 per cent of all cases of spina bifida and 20 per cent of affected children have hydrocephalus alone. Conversely, there are 20 per cent of spina bifida cases where

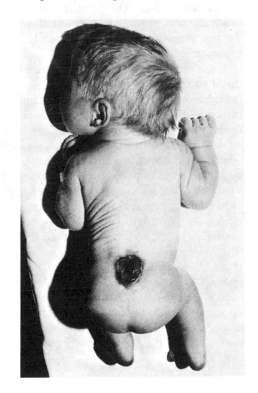

Fig. 19/6 Spina bifida in the lumbo-sacral region

hydrocephalus does not occur. These cases are usually the milder ones in any region but the majority are the ones affecting the sacral bones (Fig. 19/6).

SPINA BIFIDA WITH MENINGOCELE

This may occur at any spinal level or in the occipital bone in the back of the head. The sac or lump has a meningeal lining but no tissue of the spinal cord itself so that paralysis does not result from a meningocele. Meningoceles may be covered with a thin skin, or with an abnormally thick skin and a pad of fat, but not all lumps covered with a skin are simple meningoceles. This condition may be associated with hydrocephalus.

SPINA BIFIDA WITH MYELOMENINGOCELE

This unfortunately is much more common and in these cases the spinal cord or cauda equina protrudes into the sac or lies on the surface of an open wound. The nerve roots are malformed or damaged and this leads to a partial or complete flaccid paralysis below the site of the malformation. There may also be loss of sensation and loss of sphincter control.

Some spastic paralysis may be present in some muscles. The cord distal to the lesion may not be damaged in which case the muscle innervation is normal but the path of messages to and from the brain is interrupted (either partially or completely) by the lesion. Uncontrolled or spastic movements may occur in the limbs and in the newborn it is very difficult to decide, when movement is present, whether it is uncontrolled or volitional. This type of spina bifida may be accompanied by a bony deformity of the spine causing scoliosis, kyphosis or lordosis – either over the site or in the length of the spine. Other deformities are often present, especially foot deformities – often talipes equinovarus. The hips may be dislocated or 'at risk' with a limitation in abduction, or the child may lie with his hips fully flexed (this is usually associated with a lesion in the L 3 area) and the knees may be deformed, stiff or abducted. These deformities may be caused either by an associated skeletal defective development or by the muscle imbalance. This imbalance is due to difference in tone in opposing groups of muscles, either hypertonicity if there is uncontrolled action or hypotonicity where some muscles are flaccid. This unequal pull of the muscles will cause an abnormal bone growth and consequent deformities.

DIASTOMETAMYELIA

Diastometamyelia is spina bifida in which there is a bony spur in the spinal canal. The spinal cord splits into two, one side of which may be normal and the other damaged. This does not occur often but when it does it is recognised because one leg is virtually normal while the other is paralysed to some extent – one half of the spinal cord being affected while messages can travel normally up and down the cord in the other half. There is usually some nerve supply to the sphincters and such children are trainable. In its mild form, as in spina bifida occulta, this may only become apparent during growth.

If a mild diastometamyelia or spina bifida occulta is suspected, a myelogram may be done and this will show that the conus or tip of the spinal cord is at a lower level than normal. In spina bifida occulta the tethering is by the filium terminale (a fibrous band) whereas in diastometamyelia it may be a peg of bone or soft tissue separating the two cords.

MYELODYSPLASIA

This is a disordered development of the spinal cord associated with the bifid spine.

HEMIVERTEBRAE

This is another condition associated with spina bifida in which one or more of the vertebrae are wedge-shaped or malformed in such a way that part of the vertebra is missing, causing a scoliosis.

SYRINGOCELE

This is a form of spina bifida in which herniation of the spinal cord contains a cavity.

SYRINGOMYELOCELE

A form of spina bifida in which a cavity in the protruding sac is connected with the central canal of the spinal cord and that central canal is distended.

CRANIUM BIFIDUM

A cranium bifidum is present when there is a malformation mostly of the occipital bone, but may be frontal, vertical or basal and this may produce a meningocele, but if the brain protrudes it is called an encephalocele. If the former, the prognosis may be good, although hydrocephalus is usually present. If it is accompanied by an encephalocele the outlook is poorer and the child is often mentally retarded and hydrocephalus is a complication. Expectation of life is not good.

Lesions here do not produce a flaccid paralysis as, being a brain lesion, the descending and ascending tracts may be involved with a consequent spastic paralysis. There is not usually any sensory loss or consequent circulatory sluggishness and whether or not the child can be toilet trained depends on his mental ability rather than on his muscular control. This condition may be associated with micro-cephaly, i.e. a very small brain, which also causes retardation.

From the physiotherapist's point of view, a case of encephalocele is treated as a child with cerebral palsy (see Chapter 20) and not as a child with spina bifida with the resulting paralysis.

SPINAL AREAS AFFECTED

Where a myelomeningocele has occurred the resulting damage depends on the extent of the malformation and the area in which it has occurred. Although the typical spina bifida patient is one in whom the disease is in the lumbo-sacral area, the condition is seen in all parts of the spine (Fig. 19/5).

Cervical Spine

Spina bifida occurs less frequently here (about four per cent of all cases) than in any other area. There is often a cervical scoliosis causing a torticollis and there may be deformities of the shoulder girdle. There may also be an inability to raise the arms above the head and the fine movements in the hands are impaired, this being due to paresis and underdeveloped muscles of both arms.

Only in rare cases is the paralysis complete and lower limb para-lysis, if any, is usually of a spastic nature but ataxia is occasionally present. Control of the sphincters is unaffected and as a result there is no incontinence.

Thoracic Spine

With a thoracic spina bifida there is often considerable deformity of the rib cage. This is because the ribs are attached to the thoracic vertebrae and any malformation of these will cause a scoliosis and a consequent rotation of the ribs. It is in this area that hemivertebrae are most likely to appear. Occasionally a child is completely paralysed from a thoracic lesion and needs a considerable amount of splintage for walking. More often there is a paresis of the legs and sometimes a spastic paralysis; poor chest expansion and chest ailments are common and incontinence may be complete in severe cases, but some children with a thoracic lesion are trainable in this respect.

As well as the treatment given to all children with spina bifida (pp.366–374), physiotherapists may be called on to teach breathing exercises and to train the patient to use what chest muscles are present to the full and so help to prevent frequent and debilitating chest illnesses.

Lumbar Spine

This, together with the last two thoracic vertebrae, is the area which produces the typical spina bifida patient and 70 per cent of all myelomeningoceles occur in this region. The flaccid paralysis may be complete or only partial and the legs may be quite flail or some groups of muscles may have slight innervation. There is also, at best, a weakness of the hip muscles, especially the extensors, resulting in unstable hip joints with hips that may be dislocated at birth or 'at risk'. The hip is a shallow joint as normally the acetabulum is not a deep socket at birth, and the joint is largely kept stable by the tone of the muscles and fascia surrounding it, so that when this tone is missing as in a flaccid paralysis, instability of the joint results.

Incontinence is common, sometimes only of urine but it may be of faeces as well. Circulation in the legs is poor due to an impairment of the sympathetic nervous system. Due to the poor circulation and lack of use, the condition of the bones is not good and they are thinner than normal. This results in frequent fractures which may go undetected as the patient cannot feel pain. The first indication that there has been a fracture may be the lump of callus formation during the healing process, but usually the swelling is noticed shortly after injury. The leg may become reddened with the associated warmth of the skin. These fractures may not be as serious as in an unaffected child as displacement does not often occur. Healing is usually fairly quick but can be delayed due to the poor general condition of the paralysed limb, and unless care is taken the injury can recur once ambulation is resumed.

Lack of sensation is one of the more serious symptoms. The patient cannot feel hot or cold, pressure or pinpricks, and great care must be taken in the handling of such children. Parents must be taught to make the examination of the child's legs and feet an automatic part of the general hygiene of the child. Physiotherapists must be continually aware of this and avoid anything that is likely to cause continual rubbing which, in turn, causes friction burns. Hot water bottles, radiators, or anything hot are other hazards to be avoided.

Hydrocephalus is present in most cases of lesions in the lumbar regions.

Sacral Spine

Spina bifida in this area causes a mild paralysis usually below the knee joint with paresis of the glutei and hip extensors. Hydrocephalus is rarely a complication and the highest survival rate is in these lesions. Conversely, incontinence is a major problem in this group, both of bladder and bowel, as innervation of the genito-urinary muscles comes largely from the sacral plexus and there is an associated sluggishness in the sympathetic nervous system. Lack of sensation is again a problem as in cases of lumbar lesions.

In all cases of spina bifida where there is some flaccid paralysis there may also be symptoms of spasticity. This is due to the fact that there may be some part of the spinal cord intact below the area of the lesion but impulses cannot travel to the brain because of the blockage caused by that lesion. Reflex action may then take place in the muscles controlled by the isolated cord and physiotherapists should be aware of this in order that they are not too optimistic when slight movement occurs. Occasionally even in fairly severe spina bifida cases some slight communication is left, although only a few fibres of the cord are intact and this (according to the nerves involved) may result in some bladder or bowel control or in some action in a few muscles.

THE COCKTAIL PARTY SYNDROME

The character of the typical child with spina bifida has been described thus – most of the children are happy, lovable extroverts with a quick wit, full of uninhibited questions and ready answers. This tends to convince their parents, and others, that they are exceptionally bright. Unfortunately only a few live up to this early prognosis and on expert assessment it is found that their retention of knowledge may not be as good as expected. In fact the intelligence of any group of children with spina bifida seems to be much the same as that found in any other group of children, i.e. 25 per cent are below the range of normal intelligence, 50 per cent within the average range and the remaining 25 per cent above normal. Physiotherapists should be aware of this and not be over-optimistic about their future scholastic prowess.

INCONTINENCE

One of the most distressing complications of spina bifida cystica is incontinence. This may be of the bladder only or of both bladder and bowel.

Incontinence of Urine

This is a major problem facing the parents of a child with spina bifida. It is caused partly by lack of sensation and partly by the lack of a motor nerve supply. Those whose motor nerve supply to the sphincters may be intact may have no sensation so that they may not realise the feeling of fullness of the bladder that indicates to most of us the need to urinate. This incontinence may take three forms.

1. There may be neither control nor sensation; the bladder does not store the urine as the sphincters are always open. There is a continual trickle of urine, the patient is always wet and there is no residual urine in the bladder. These cases rarely get an infected bladder as no stasis occurs and equally they will never be trainable.

2. There is no sensation at all, but there is slight involuntary control of the sphincters. The patient has no conscious control so the bladder keeps filling but as sensation is absent he cannot tell when he needs to urinate and cannot control the sphincters. The bladder continues to fill until there is an overflow or 'stress' incontinence which is followed by a dribble until pressure is eased. The bladder is never really empty, and the residue becomes stale and infected. Left untreated this infection may travel via the ureters to the kidneys and this will soon cause kidney infection with serious consequences.

3. There is no sensation, but there is some muscle control. In these cases the bladder fills normally and automatically empties, but with no sensation, and the patient has no idea when the need arises. This group may be dry for long spells and are often trainable by finding out how long they can stay dry and giving them attention regularly and gradually increasing the time between this attention.

In the second type, manual expression is possible and may be advised to keep the bladder as empty as possible and perhaps keep the child dry for up to three hours. In the other two types expression has no place.

TREATMENT

The problem of urinary incontinence especially in girls is the social one. Changing one's own nappy when chairbound is almost impossible, there is always the danger of pressure sores (the more so when there is anaesthesia) and the risk of a smell; in fact, one is not socially acceptable when incontinent.

Appliances are available for boys and men and there are a number of different ones to choose from, depending on the requirements of the individual. No such appliances are available for girls but indwelling catheters are used for some cases of either sex and in a few cases intermittent catheterisation may be the answer. The method chosen must depend on the consultant concerned and in some cases a urinary diversion operation may be performed if the surgeon feels there is a risk of infection and that there is no hope of getting control.

In this operation (sometimes called a uretero-ileostomy or ileal loop) a short section of the small intestine is isolated from the rest and sealed at one end – the small intestine itself being sutured together again. The ureters are then passed from the kidneys into this segment, the open end of which is passed through the body wall usually on the right hand side just below the waist. This provides a stoma (or spout) through which the urine may pass into a bag which is attached to the skin by a variety of methods (Figs. 19/7 and 19/8).

By this means the girl becomes completely independent and is socially acceptable. This operation has proved so successful for girls that it is now being performed more and more on boys in preference to the penile appliance. It is irreversible and once done is there for life but this is preferred to the only alternative of nappies or pads. Modern diagnosis enables surgeons to decide at a very early age whether control will eventually be possible and this diversion operation may be

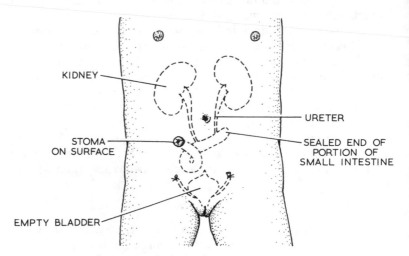

Fig. 19/7 Uretero-ileostomy or ileal loop with stoma

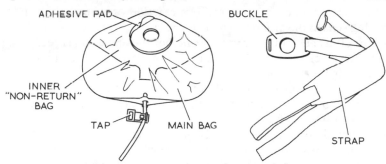

Fig. 19/8 One type of bag and belt for ileal loop stoma

performed while the child is still a baby so that no damage is caused to the ureters and kidneys by infection.

Incontinence of Faeces

Lack of bowel control occurs very occasionally in cases of thoracic spina bifida but much more often when the lesion is in the lumbar and sacral regions.

It is from the same sacral roots that the pudendal and other pelvic nerves arise that are responsible for the urinary incontinence. In some cases the lumbar lesion may be complete and the sacral nerves may not be damaged so that the sphincters function but are uncontrolled by the brain as no messages can pass the lesion. There is then no idea of the need for defaecation and again the lack of sensation means that there is no feeling of fullness.

It is ironical that it is in children with the milder motor paralysis that the faecal incontinence is most marked, and this is the group which is sufficiently mobile to attend normal school. It is difficult for the child to do so if his bowel action is unreliable and he is not socially acceptable because of an offensive odour.

In some cases there is a continual looseness and in others a severe constipation with a large faecal mass in the rectum. This may result in an apparent diarrhoea as the spastic contraction of the sphincters does not allow the child to excrete this mass and liquid faeces are all that can pass it.

Occasionally it is necessary for a colostomy to be performed as well as a urinary diversion operation but by far the greater majority of children manage to get some control. Since the popularity of the urinary diversion operation it has been found that once such a child is dry the bowel action seems to become more controllable. Whether this is due to some sympathetic nervous reaction or whether the child, having sensed the difference in no longer being wet, makes an unconscious effort at control, or indeed whether the operation is performed at a time when the years of routine and regular training are producing results, is not known.

The use of suppositories and/or medicines may be necessary to gain regularity but this is such a highly individual problem that the answer may be different in every case.

Although physiotherapists are not directly concerned with the questions arising from incontinence, the whole subject is one of such concern to the parents that physiotherapists will inevitably be asked about it. Physiotherapists working in hospitals will be able to refer the family to the appropriate department but this knowledge is necessary for those who work in the field where specialist information may only be obtainable when the parents travel to the hospital.

TREATMENT OF SPINA BIFIDA

The active treatment of spina bifida has only become a realistic possibility since the introduction of the shunt to control the hydrocephalus. Before this the repair of the back lesion was not considered for some months as most of the babies died in the neonatal stage (i.e. within the first few weeks of life) and only when it was found that the baby survived and hydrocephalus did not develop was an operation undertaken to repair the lesion. Even then hydrocephalus sometimes developed and with no treatment to control it, the result was a grossly enlarged head with consequent brain damage and mental subnormality.

With the advent of the shunt it became the usual practice to repair the back lesion as soon after birth as possible, preferably within the first 24 hours. The theory underlying this was to prevent further damage to the exposed nerves, as nerve fibres cannot live uncovered and soon deteriorate.

Modern thinking now takes a line somewhere between these two courses of action, and before selecting any neonate for surgery many aspects of the condition are discussed. The prognosis, the probable quality of life that can be expected, the possible mental and physical abilities of the child, as well as the number of major operations likely to be needed before the child can walk, all have to be taken into account, and often surgery may be delayed for some weeks for a full assessment.

The following pages refer to the treatment of surviving babies with neural tube defects, whether they have been treated conservatively or by surgery.

Neonatal Physiotherapy

As well as the paediatrician, paediatric or neurosurgeon, orthopaedic surgeon and experienced nursing staff, the spina bifida team also includes a physiotherapist who has a very important role to play from the day the baby is born until he becomes independent.

As soon as the baby is admitted the physiotherapist is called upon to make a physical assessment of the child and this early assessment, if correctly done, can give a fairly accurate indication of the future physical ability of the child. The movement of the legs in some babies appears to improve after the back is repaired but when an assessment is made after about one year it nearly always relates very closely to the neonatal one.

This assessment – both of movement and sensation – is almost always done with the child in an incubator. It may be done by the paediatrician or it may be the responsibility of the physiotherapist. The baby may have had to travel a long distance to the hospital and has been subjected to a lot of examination and handling so it is vital for the operator to work quickly and efficiently. She needs to be very experienced and to have some knowledge of the developmental progress of a normal newborn child for comparison in order to detect the abnormal (Fig. 19/9) (Sheridan, 1969).

To carry out the assessment the examiner first records her general impressions – abnormal position of limbs, deformities present, movement (if any), etc. Reflexes are tested as far as possible and then groups of muscles as individual muscle testing is impossible in one so small in the time available (Holgate, 1970). A sensory chart is then completed and to do this the protopathic or deeper feeling is tested with a safety-pin as testing the epicritic feeling, or light touch as with cotton wool, is unsatisfactory at this stage. The most reliable test of feeling is whether the baby cries when pricked with the pin. This obviously shows that he has felt it. If the limb moves when pricked although the movement may be an uncontrolled reflex action and if that movement is repeated when the spot is pricked again, there must be some sensation to cause it.

While the baby is still in hospital, providing he is well enough, the physiotherapist turns her attention to any deformities that may be present. Most common of these is talipes equino-varus and all will be treated according to the wishes of the consultant concerned.

Talipes equino-varus may be strapped with zinc oxide or elastic

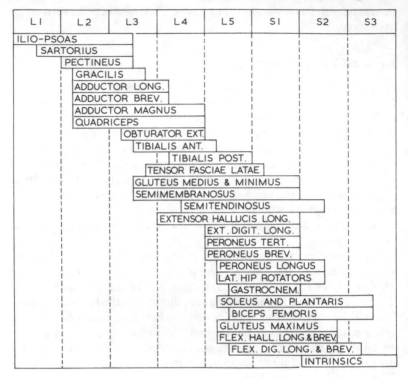

Fig. 19/9 Muscle innervation chart

strapping, or treated by splinting. Whichever is used the physiotherapist must remember that the baby has impaired sensation, poor circulation and probably limbs that are in a poor condition generally so that she must be even more careful than usual in applying corrective measures. The limb should be coated with Tinct. Benzoin Co. (to get better adhesion and prevent sores) and a length of 2.5cm strapping attached down the inside of the leg below the knee, around the heel to hold it in the correct position and up the lateral side of the leg to the knee but not over it. The second piece of strapping is to correct the forefront of the foot. It is attached to the dorsum of the foot at the level of the fifth metatarsophalangeal joint, carried across the top of the foot along the line of the joints, under the sole and again up the lateral side of the leg. This is under tension so that the deformity is corrected as far as possible. Some prefer this length of strapping to be started on the plantar side of the fifth metatarsophalangeal joint before being carried across the dorsum, but by using this method there is more danger of constricting the circulation. Short lengths of strapping are then passed around the leg (not under tension) to keep the first two in position. One length around the calf may be enough but a second piece near the ankle may also be necessary. A continuous piece of strapping used as a bandage is not advised in cases of spina bifida because of the poor skin condition and danger to the circulation. Once in position the feet must be watched for any interference in the circulation.

Different consultants like different methods of strapping for talipes equino-varus but the principle is the same – to strap the foot into eversion and dorsiflexion to correct the varus and equinus (i.e. inversion and plantar flexion) of the feet. Occasionally the feet may lie in a

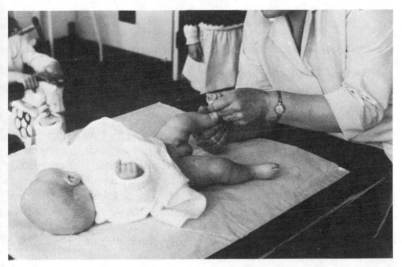

Fig. 19/10 Stretching talipes equino-varus: manipulation of the foot into dorsiflexion and eversion

calcaneo-valgus position (in eversion and dorsiflexion) when strapping or splinting, if used, is into plantar flexion and inversion. In either case the physiotherapist will be called upon to stretch the feet (Fig. 19/10).

The hips may be dislocated or 'at risk' from birth and the physiotherapist will be instructed accordingly. She will know the preferences of the consultant in charge and will only treat according to his wishes. The baby may be nursed in a splint to keep his legs in abduction and lateral rotation and again the same precautions must be taken to prevent pressure and sores especially as there is the danger of wetting and soiling from the nappy.

Some splints used to maintain the abduction and lateral rotation are

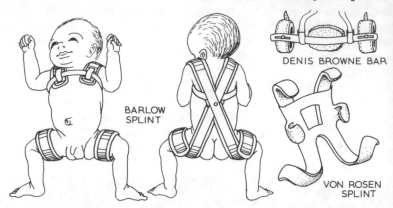

Fig. 19/11 Appliances for congenital dislocation of hip

the Barlow, Von Rosen and Denis Browne (Fig. 19/11). The Barlow and Von Rosen are made of light malleable metal suitably padded to prevent undue pressure. The Barlow is in the form of the letter X, the upper arms of which are bent over the shoulders while the lower ones are put round the legs in the correct position. The Von Rosen is very similar but is H-shaped. The Denis Browne is just a straight bar with two cuffs into which the abducted and laterally rotated legs are placed; there is an oval pad in the central back to avoid pressure on the lesion and sometimes a harness to keep the splint in position. The choice of splint is the consultant's but in every case the damaged area of the back must be avoided and this may be the deciding factor. All the precautions against any pressure must be rigorously observed. Other deformities are individual to each baby and are treated accordingly.

Subsequent Treatment

When the baby is sent home a new but equally important team of workers look after the child and his family. This will include the family doctor and probably an infant welfare doctor, the health visitor, district nurse, social services department and a physiotherapist. Later this team will be extended to include a teacher at the child's school.

The physiotherapist is an essential part of this team – she may be the one to act as liaison between the team and the hospital concerned and her work will include far more than pure physiotherapy. It will be 'healing by physical means' in the truest sense by becoming an adviser in the physical management of the child.

Most spina bifida children are treated in paediatric hospitals with a large catchment area and frequent visits to the out-patient department may be impossible; the physiotherapist becomes a vital link here as she sees the child and parents regularly for treatment. With tact and understanding she can help the family to accept the baby as he is – a normal child born with a disability.

Acceptance by the family from the beginning and their future attitude to the child are very often dependent on the attitudes of the professional people who advise them. If the physiotherapist, while not showing undue optimism, can accentuate what the child *can* do and do her best to improve what is difficult and minimise what is impossible, then not only the family but also the child himself is likely to have a practical outlook for the future.

Physiotherapy

Physiotherapy already started while the child was in hospital is continued at home for many reasons – to treat any deformities present and to prevent others developing; to encourage what movement there may be in the limbs and to strengthen the muscles producing it; to exercise limbs that the child cannot exercise himself and by so doing improve the circulation; to encourage the child to keep up with his peers in his milestones, i.e. rolling over, crawling, sitting up, and in later stages to teach him to walk in whatever calipers are necessary.

The experienced physiotherapist will be aware of any particular treatment advocated by the hospital concerned and a frequent exchange of ideas and information is helpful but the principles are the same in all cases.

Treatment of any deformities started in hospital will be continued and all joints will be exercised in their full range to prevent contractures. In general the flexor muscles are stronger than the extensors and this especially applies to the hips, even though the difference may be only slight. Hip flexion is often present and with the consent of the orthopaedic surgeon, hip extension stretching should be routine as well as teaching the mother to place the baby in a prone position during playtime, preferably on the floor. It is hip flexion that causes the marked lordosis that is characteristic of older children with spina bifida.

Any movement present must be noted and encouraged and if there is any sensation in the legs this can be used to stimulate movement by tickling or touching. There may be little or no sensation present and until the baby can respond to toys most of the movement will be passive. These passive movements must be given in as full a range as possible to all joints starting with the toes, then the tarsal joints, ankles, knees and hips. This not only helps to keep them supple but it gives the circulation the pumping action that normal babies provide by their kicking. Mothers must be taught how to carry out these movements and advised to do them each time they change the baby's nappy.

Arm movements can be started as soon as the baby responds and exercises to strengthen the shoulder girdle gradually introduced. This is necessary because most patients with spina bifida will need to rely on sticks or crutches to help them to walk and a strong shoulder girdle is very necessary.

A knowledge of the developmental progress and milestones of a normal child is necessary to be able to assess when a disabled child is ready to be encouraged to attempt another skill such as rolling over, sitting up and even his own brand of crawling (see Chapter 3). The physiotherapist must be alert to his development and start instructing him in the next step just before he is ready for it. The mother is encouraged to prop him up as soon as he shows an interest in his surroundings. In the past children have become more disabled simply because having been told that their child is disabled, the parents have not realised and have not been told that their child needs all the challenges and stimuli he can get to develop his potential to the full in the same way as any other baby.

Play therapy forms a very important part of the general physiotherapy. As soon as the baby begins to respond, brightly-coloured toys and those that make a noise are excellent to encourage any movement – squeaky toys to press on; coloured balls to push away; 'bridging' to allow a toy motor car to go under is useful for encouraging gluteal contractions (Fig. 19/12); all these activities have a useful place in treatment.

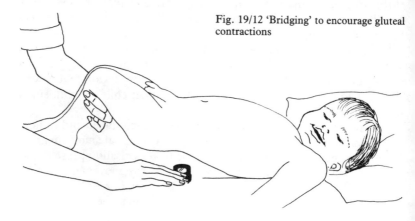

Fig. 19/12 'Bridging' to encourage gluteal contractions

As the child gets older, bigger toys can be introduced – nursery slides to pull *up* rather than slide down, to strengthen the shoulders, and small trampolines to teach the child to sit on an unsteady surface and later to stand on it.

The ingenuity of the physiotherapist will be taxed to the full to make the treatment interesting and so get the child's full cooperation because routine exercises are boring to small children and they rarely respond.

Proprioceptive neuromuscular facilitation (PNF) has very little use in the early treatment of spina bifida partly because of the lack of sensation and partly because physiotherapy is of most use when the child is too young to respond to the kind of instructions necessary. Resisted exercises can however be devised to encourage action in muscles which are innervated, i.e. putting baby's feet with knees and hips flexed on one's chest and saying 'push me away' is useful in some sacral lesions where hip and knee action is present, but weak.

If spasticity is present, treatment is given on the usual lines for cerebral palsy (Chapter 20).

Ambulation

Early ambulation is now regarded as advisable for the normal development of a spina bifida child. All babies – except some retarded ones – walk sometime between their first and second birthdays, a few a little before and some slightly later. This is the psychological time for walking and most spina bifida children, despite their slow start, are no exception. If they can be fitted with suitable appliances to help them to walk, then the physiotherapist has nature and the innate desire of the children to help her and her task is lighter. The age when each child is ready physically and psychologically for walking varies and there is no arbitrary rule. It is up to the physiotherapist to learn to use her judgement. Once this stage has passed and the children realise they are different the barrier of 'conditioned inability' creeps in. The longer walking is delayed the deeper this conviction becomes and the greater will be the work of the physiotherapist to overcome it.

It was hoped that early ambulation would reduce the tendency of adolescents with spina bifida to retire to a wheelchair. This has not been wholly realised and in spite of all the training many victims do find a wheelchair existence preferable. Many others are determined to remain ambulant against all odds while still more find an acceptable balance between the two. Whichever way the young adult finds most convenient to his way of life the choice is his. Without adequate physiotherapy and training that choice would not exist.

In order to enable children with spina bifida to walk some sort of calipers will be necessary in all but a few cases. In general the higher in the back the lesion occurs the greater will be the splintage needed. Those with a dorsal lesion often need calipers with both pelvic and chest bands, while dorso-lumbar lesions usually need calipers with a pelvic band and sacral lesions manage with only below-knee irons.

In general the physiotherapist should aim at having the child walking independently (albeit with suitable aids) by the time he is due to go to school but this may not be possible in all cases. The physiotherapist will still be necessary as adviser in management in the school as well as to prevent any deterioration in walking and for postoperative physiotherapy but the greater part of the education in walking and independence should be finished by then.

Surgery

The attitude of the general public towards disabled children has improved markedly in recent years and this, coupled with enlightened medical treatment, means that children born with a disability can look forward to finding their rightful place in the community. This especially applies to those with normal intelligence and the physical ability to obtain a good degree of independence. Many cases of spina bifida are in this category, but to do this, education and training are essential to enable the children to develop to their full potential. Doctors therefore try to arrange that all major surgery is, if possible, carried out during the pre-school years so that the child's education is interrupted as little as is practicable.

The main exception to this is when surgical intervention for scoliosis is necessary. This becomes apparent as the child develops and surgery is delayed until the extent of the deformity can be finally assessed.

This means that before he is five the child may have been in and out of hospital many times. Occasionally the shunt may block and replacement prove necessary. As the child grows the distal catheter may need to be replaced with a longer one. Orthopaedic surgery may be necessary to correct deformities, so enabling the child to wear calipers and become mobile. Lastly, the ileal loop or urinary diversion operation as described earlier may be carried out any time in the first five years.

Education

The problem of schooling has probably worried the parents from the beginning and a good physiotherapist needs to know what facilities are available in her district. She will be asked by the team to give her judgement on what type of school the child is physically best suited for. Educational suitability will be assessed by the educational psychologist but the authorities often depend on the opinion of the physiotherapist as to whether the child can cope with a normal school or whether a school for the physically handicapped would suit his disability best. Once the child starts in a normal primary school the teachers welcome the advice of the physiotherapist in his management; whereas if he goes to a school for the physically disabled there are usually physiotherapists on the staff.

Training

More and more avenues are opening for disabled adolescents and given the ability and desire (and a certain amount of adjustment by all concerned including the adolescent and his family) many trades and professions welcome disabled members.

During adolescence the full impact of his disability may hit the victim and this is the time when the early training in acceptance will help, but there is often a period of depression and withdrawal when he realises that he will never be normal. Such a teenager should be encouraged to join as much as he can in the social life of the community. There are many activities at which the spina bifida youngster can excel – horseriding, archery, table-tennis are but a few where he can compete with normal people.

There are a few training colleges specially designed to cater for the training of disabled people in many skills, but most universities, teachers' training colleges and colleges of further education are only too willing to accept disabled young adults if it is at all possible.

Marriage

The question of marriage and reproduction is another one that has occupied the thoughts of parents and is often discussed by them during physiotherapy sessions. The early treated spina bifida sufferers have now reached maturity; many have married and a few of the girls have had children. This is such an individual and personal topic that it requires specialist advice in each case. There is much more information available and advisers are able to discuss all aspects of sexuality with the person concerned.

In general it may be said that spina bifida girls can marry and have children, some of whom may be quite normal, but in men the sex act depends largely on sensation and where that is absent the man will probably be impotent, but this is a very complicated matter and other factors are involved.

Spina bifida cystica is the biggest single cause of congenital physical handicap. The invention of the shunt has had very far reaching results, the impact of which presented the medical profession in general and physiotherapists in particular with a challenging problem. Physiotherapists have accepted this challenge by widening their horizons and becoming an integral part of the various teams who work together to give such children as normal a life as their disability will allow.

REFERENCES

Holgate, L. (1970). *Physiotherapy for Spina Bifida.* Obtainable from Queen Mary's Hospital, Carshalton, Surrey.
Sheridan, M. (1975). *The Developmental Progress of Infants and Young Children*, 3rd edition. Her Majesty's Stationery Office, London.

BIBLIOGRAPHY

Anderson, E. M. and Spain, B. (1977). *Child with Spina Bifida.* Methuen and Company Limited, London.
Menelaus, M. B. (1980). *The Orthopaedic Management of Spina Bifida Cystica*, 2nd edition. Churchill Livingstone, Edinburgh.
Nettles, O. R. (1969). *The Spina Bifida Baby.* The Scottish Spina Bifida Association.
Nettles, O. R. (1972). *Growing Up with Spina Bifida.* The Scottish Spina Bifida Association.
Nettles, O. R. (1979). *Counselling Parents of Children with Handicaps.* Tappenden Print Company Limited, Crawley, Sussex.
Stark, G. (1977). *Spina Bifida: Problems and Management.* Blackwell Scientific Publications Limited, Oxford.

The following booklets are available from ASBAH, Tavistock House North, Tavistock Square, London WC1H 9HJ. Prices will be supplied on request.
Your child with spina bifida by J. Lorber
Your child with hydrocephalus by J. Lorber
The care of an ileal conduit and urinary appliances in children by E. Durham Smith
Aids and equipment
Sex and spina bifida by Bill Stewart
The handwriting of spina bifida children by J. Cambridge and E. M. Anderson
The nursery years by S. Haskell and M. Paull

ACKNOWLEDGEMENTS

The author thanks everyone who has helped her in the compilation of this chapter. In particular she acknowledges the advice of Mr D. M. Forrest, F.R.C.S. in the original writing of the chapter. She also thanks the physiotherapists at Chailey Heritage and Coney Hill for their help and suggestions.

Chapter 20

Cerebral Palsy

by S. LEVITT, B.SC. (Physiotherapy) Rand

CEREBRAL PALSY, MENTAL HANDICAP AND DEVELOPMENTAL DELAY

The physiotherapy in cerebral palsy is intimately involved with child development. Most of the techniques, therefore, are used in the field of mental subnormality and any other developmental delay in children besides that associated with cerebral palsy.

Definition

Cerebral palsy, or more accurately, the cerebral palsies are a group of motor disorders caused by damage or maldevelopment of the brain that occurs prenatally, peri-natally or postnatally. Although the lesion is non-progressive, since the brain and nervous system develop in the presence of the lesion, the clinical picture of disordered movement and posture will change as the child gets older. Despite its name the cerebral palsies present not only 'palsies', or motor problems, but many other problems in these children. They often have multiple handicaps.

Incidence

In various countries this varies between 0.6 and 5.9 per 1,000 births. In Britain the incidence is given as 1.7 per 1,000 (Asher and Schonell, 1950), 1.9 per 1,000 (Woods, 1975) and 1.99 per 1,000 (Ingram, 1964).

Multiple Handicaps

Damage or malfunction of the brain of the infant and young child may disrupt not only motor function but also other functions of the brain. The lesion is often diffuse. There may be speech and communication problems, hearing or visual disorders, epilepsy, perceptual disturbance, apraxias, mental defect and general behaviour problems. Fortunately not all of these may be present in the same child. The non-motor handicaps may be due to the original organic lesion or they may be secondary to the motor handicap. Secondary handicap occurs because the child is unable to acquire normal learning experience because he cannot move normally and explore his environment. He cannot creep, crawl or walk, nor use his hands to discover the meaning of space and direction, of textures, of shape or temperature. He may not be able to look at, reach or touch different parts of his face and body in order to learn his body image and its spatial relationships. This paucity of normal everyday experiences disrupts normal perceptual and conceptual development. This and his poor motor development affect speech and language development. If, say, he cannot even control his head, he cannot observe what makes a specific sound and he cannot easily communicate with eye to eye contact with another person. Without head control he also misses perceptual information; he cannot observe perceptual aspects such as the relationship of objects to himself and to each other which give meaning to words. He has not experienced the meaning of such words as 'far, near, up, down, in, out, beside'.

Socially and emotionally the child is handicapped as he cannot run up to join his friends at play, cannot fling his arms around his mother's neck or even push an annoying child away.

In addition, the stress on the family having a handicapped child creates emotional problems, some of which may handicap the cerebral palsied child as well. The family's attitudes and their socio-economic problems are important influences on the cerebral palsied child's function.

With all these problems to face, it is, therefore, not surprising that an intelligent cerebral palsied child may appear mentally subnormal or, if he is mentally low, may appear even more subnormal than he is. The contribution of the physiotherapist to the cerebral palsied child's motor development, therefore, has far-reaching effects on the child's total development.

Aetiology

There are many causes in pregnancy, labour and delivery which may result in cerebral palsy. The most common are those associated with abnormal labour and delivery, including forceps delivery, asphyxia of the newborn, neonatal jaundice and especially prematurity. Postnatal causes may be trauma, meningitis, encephalitis, high fever, a vascular accident or tumours. The cause may not be clear and a number of possible causes may be present or there may even be a history of normal pregnancy, labour and birth. Genetic factors may exist. Brain damage may also be associated with hydrocephalus and spina bifida and similar problems encountered as in cerebral palsy.

Clinical Features

The causes of mental subnormality or the 'clumsy child' or minimal brain dysfunction are often the same as the causes of cerebral palsy. The severity varies from severe mentally and physically handicapped children to the clumsy child who is intelligent but who has specific learning problems.

Classification

Any classification or diagnosis is only a beginning and the physiotherapist must make a detailed assessment, especially of the motor skills or functions in each child at his levels of development.

Cerebral palsied children are classified differently in different clinics. The most commonly accepted classifications are the diagnostic types given as follows.

Diagnostic Types

1. Spastics
2. Athetoids or dyskinesias
3. Ataxics
4. Rigid and dystonics (sometimes classified under the dyskinesias)
5. Mixed types.

Atonic type usually changes to become one of the above. It is more common to have some mixture in these types of cerebral palsy.

There is also:

CLASSIFICATION OF DISTRIBUTION

1. Hemiplegia. One side of the body affected.
2. Bilateral hemiplegia or quadriplegia. All limbs are affected (mainly the upper limbs).
3. Diplegia. All limbs are affected (mainly the lower limbs).
4. Triplegia. Lower limbs and one arm affected.
5. Paraplegia. Lower limbs affected.

6. Monoplegia. One limb affected (very rare).

Topographical classification should *not* be so dogmatic as to prevent the physiotherapist from checking the function of the other parts of the body.

CLASSIFICATION OF SEVERITY

This varies greatly from clinic to clinic. In general:

1. Mild. Where the child is independent and even so mild that he only appears to be clumsy. The non-motor handicaps may be the greater problem in these children.

2. Moderate. Where the child can achieve partial independence and requires aids for most activities.

3. Severe. When the child is totally or almost totally helpless and a wheelchair is inevitable. The accuracy of this classification is poor as it is too general for the physiotherapist.

SIGNS AND SYMPTOMS

Slow Acquisition of Motor Skills

Cerebral palsied babies and children have not acquired the motor skills seen in normal children of their own age.

Abnormal Performance of any Motor Skills

The few motor skills that are acquired by the child are frequently carried out in an abnormal way. The abnormal performance may simulate the pattern of posture and movements seen in infants or children younger than the cerebral palsied child. In addition there are postures and movements which are not seen at earlier levels in any normal children but are pathological. These pathological postures and movements result from spasticity, rigidity, involuntary movements of various kinds and from ataxia.

Abnormal Reflexes or Reactions

These are of four kinds.

1. The abnormal reflexes of the upper motor neurone lesion such as the brisk tendon jerks. These reflexes do not affect the physiotherapist directly and are diagnostic.

2. The reflexes or neurological reactions present in the newborn which do not disappear as in normal development. Techniques to counter these in older children may be needed.

3. The neurological reactions which appear in the maturing nervous system. Techniques to stimulate these reactions are frequently needed.

4. Pathological reflexes seen in upper motor neurone lesions, e.g. associated reactions and withdrawal reflexes, extensor thrusts, symmetrical tonic neck reflex, asymmetrical tonic neck reflex and tonic labyrinthine reflex (see Chapter 2).

The physiotherapist must know what all these reflexes look like and whether they are present in her patients. For example, in the author's experience the tonic neck and labyrinthine reflexes are rarely present as such in cerebral palsied children. However, what is even more important is to recognise only those reflexes or reactions which disrupt function or cause deformity. There are many reactions which are diagnostic and of no direct interest for physiotherapy.

The most important reactions which should appear with maturation or motor development and which require physiotherapy are the following. (The presentation is taken from Purdon-Martin (1967) who studied these postural reactions in adults.)

POSTURAL FIXATION

Maintenance of posture of the head, trunk, pelvic and shoulder girdles.

COUNTERPOISING

Maintenance of posture while counterpoising the movement of part of the body such as an arm or leg.

TILTING REACTIONS

If the child is tilted off the horizontal he adjusts his balance using his neck and trunk muscles.

SAVING OR PROTECTIVE REACTIONS

If the tilt of the child is so great that his tilt reactions cannot save him from falling, he will fling his arms and legs out to save himself.

RISING OR RIGHTING REACTIONS

These are used to rise from the floor to sitting, hands and knees, or to standing and other positions. Change of posture is dependent on these reactions.

LOCOMOTION REACTIONS

To initiate a step, continue walking and to stop walking.

SPECIFIC SIGNS AND SYMPTOMS

The Spastic Type

The clinical description of spasticity differs in different systems of treatment. In general the observations are:

RESISTANCE TO SUDDEN PASSIVE STRETCH IN SPASTIC MUSCLE GROUPS

Sudden passive stretch results in a resistance given by an increase of muscle tension. This occurs at a threshold in the passive range of movement. Such spasticity is of the 'clasp-knife' variety, also called hyperactive stretch reflex. Spasticity occurs mainly in the shoulder flexors, retractors, adductors, internal rotators, elbow flexors and pronators, wrist flexors, flexors of fingers and thumb, hip flexors, internal rotators, adductors, knee flexors, plantar flexors, evertors, and invertors of the feet.

ABNORMAL POSTURES OF A GREAT VARIETY

The spastic muscle groups above usually shorten and have a tight pull on the joints contributing to their abnormal positions (Figs 20/1 and 20/2). There is apparent weakness of their antagonists which do not counteract these abnormal joint positions. The abnormal postures must be studied in the whole child, that is, his limbs, trunk and head, as they are almost never localised to one joint. The abnormal postures are deformities, which at first are unfixed but become fixed deformities or contractures if not treated adequately.

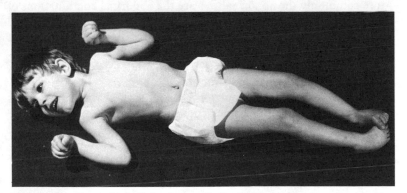

Fig. 20/1 Spastic quadriplegia (supine position) with head asymmetry, shoulders in semi-flexion/abduction, elbows in flexion-pronation, hands clenched in palmar flexion and thumbs adducted. Legs adducted and semiflexed with feet in equino-varus and toes flexed

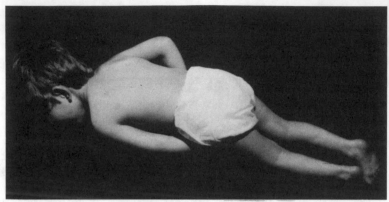

Fig. 20/2 Spastic quadriplegia (prone position) with asymmetry of head and arms; hips and knees in semiflexion and adduction; feet in equino-varus

ABNORMAL VOLUNTARY MOVEMENT

Spasticity is not paralysis; the movements are present but often laboured, weak and look abnormal.

1. **The synergies or patterns** of movements are similar to the postures and vary in each child and at different developmental levels. The following synergies are common examples. *Arm*: Shoulder protraction, adduction, internal rotation. Elbow flexion, pronation or extension-pronation. Wrist and hand flexion and ulnar deviation. *Leg*: Hip semi-flexion, adduction, internal rotation. Knee flexion. Foot plantar flexion or eversion or inversion.

Total extensor or total flexor synergies may be seen occasionally. More commonly the abnormalities are the abnormal combinations of flexion at some joints with extension at others together with abnormal abduction, adduction, internal or external rotation.

2. **Weakness** is present in the antagonists to the spastic synergies. The spastic muscle groups themselves are often weak and do not act throughout their full range of motion.

3. **Isolated movements** of one joint are difficult or impossible, thus the discrete movements of finer coordination of say, the hands, are difficult.

4. **Associated reactions.** Movement of one part of the child's body may have an associated increase in spasticity in other parts of the child's body.

The spastics may have squints, a variety of intelligence levels and perceptual problems. Poor posture-balance mechanism is present (see above). Involuntary movements occasionally occur in distal joints.

The Athetoid Type

INVOLUNTARY MOVEMENTS OR ATHETOSIS

These are purposeless slow or fast movements which may be un-patterned or patterned. They may be writhing, jerky, tremor, swiping or rotary patterns which may be present at rest, or only aroused on effort to move or speak, on excitement or even deep thinking. Some athetoids have involuntary movement at rest and on activity. Involuntary movements may be uncontrollable or the child can learn to control them. Fatigue, drowsiness, fever, prone lying or holding the child's full attention decrease the involuntary movements. Athetosis may be present in all parts of the body including the facial grimacing and tongue musculature.

VOLUNTARY MOVEMENTS

These are usually possible but may be disrupted by the involuntary movements or hypertonia, if present. Poor fine movements and weakness are common.

HYPERTONIA OR HYPOTONIA

Hypertonia or hypotonia or fluctuations of tone are possible. The hypertonia may be rigidity or dystonia which resists passive stretch throughout the range of movement, i.e. the 'lead pipe' variety (see Chapter 4). There may also be spasticity in athetoids and sudden spasms of flexion or extension.

Athetoids often have high intelligence which may be masked by the severe grimacing and involuntary movement, instability and muscle tension. Eye movements, especially upwards, may be absent. There is often a high frequency hearing loss in the athetoids due to severe neonatal jaundice (kernicterus). Poor posture-balance mechanism (see above).

SUB-CLASSIFICATION

There are many different kinds of athetoids so that one should never discuss the 'treatment of athetoids', but describe the problems. Sub-classification of these patterns varies from clinic to clinic. The tremor type of cerebral palsy is usually treated similarly to the athetoids.

The Ataxic

DISTURBANCE OF POSTURE-BALANCE MECHANISM

The absence or abnormality in the postural reactions presented above (according to Purdon-Martin) is the most significant symptom. However, this also occurs in spastics and athetoids so that a pure ataxia is rare.

VOLUNTARY MOVEMENTS

Voluntary movements are present, clumsy and uncoordinated. The child overshoots or undershoots the mark he aims for. This is also known as 'dysmetria'. An intention tremor may accompany movements.

HYPOTONIA

Hypotonia is usual.

NYSTAGMUS, LOW INTELLIGENCE, SLURRED SPEECH

These are often present.

The spastic, athetoid and ataxic are the main types and other types will be treated as subclassifications of these three.

Evolution of Signs and Symptoms

The specific signs and symptoms of the spastic, athetoid, ataxic, rigid and any other types of cerebral palsy are rarely seen in infants and babies. They may be rigid and become floppy or more often floppy and become spastic, athetoid or ataxic after a few years. Athetosis may appear as late as three years of age.

The babies are delayed in development with abnormal neurological reactions. They often have feeding problems and may be irritable. However, some normal babies start life this way and so it is difficult to know when to treat and when to 'wait and see'. On the whole physiotherapists prefer early treatment as it prevents deformity and stimulates the best possible motor performance in cerebral palsy children. In addition parents are shown how to handle their baby so that they can play, feed, dress, wash and later toilet train him. In carrying these activities out correctly there is stimulation of the best patterns of posture and movement in each child's damaged nervous system. Until medical prognosis is possible it is better to give 'developmental stimulation' to babies and correct any abnormal positioning until the diagnosis can be made.

TREATMENT

There are many systems of treatment in cerebral palsy and some of the most well-known approaches will be reviewed.

Muscle Education and Bracing

Dr W. M. Phelps, an orthopaedic surgeon in Baltimore, USA, encouraged physiotherapists, occupational therapists and speech therapists to form themselves into teams to treat cerebral palsy children. The main points of this treatment programme were as follows:

1. A specific diagnostic classification of the cerebral palsied child was the basis for specific treatment techniques. This included five types of cerebral palsy and many sub-classifications.

2. A list of fifteen 'modalities' or methods were taught to the therapists. These consisted of massage, passive motion, active assisted motion, active motion, resisted motion, rest, conditioned motion, confused motion, combined motion, balance, reach and grasp, skills, relaxation, movement from relaxation and reciprocation.

3. Braces or calipers were specially designed and developed by Phelps. He prescribed braces to correct deformity and braces to control athetosis.

4. Equipment for daily living. Many aids for dressing, washing and feeding, and for sitting and locomotion were developed.

5. Muscle education for spastics and training in joint control for athetoids was the emphasis of the largely orthopaedic view of cerebral palsy. Motor development was seldom discussed as a foundation for therapy.

Muscle education for spastics was also developed in specific ways by a number of other cerebral palsy authorities such as Pohl in America, Plum in Denmark and many orthopaedic therapists and doctors in Britain.

Although many people today dismiss Phelps' approach, there is much of interest which can still be used for these patients. Braces (calipers) are needed by some children although they need not be as extensive or used for as many years as Phelps recommended. Muscle education is necessary before and after orthopaedic surgery. Many of the aids devised at Phelps' clinic form the basis of occupational therapy today.

In Tardieu's work in Paris, there is not only neurological assessment but also detailed 'factorial analysis' of muscles in spastics to explain the abnormal movements and deformities. He recommends bracing, some muscle education, alcohol injections into the motor point of a particular spastic muscle, orthopaedic surgery and developmental training.

Progressive Pattern Movements

The main points of this approach devised by Temple Fay (1954) are:

1. The recommendation that the cerebral palsied be taught motion according to its development in evolution. Fay regards motor development as evolving from reptilian squirming to amphibian movements, through mammalian reciprocal motion 'on all fours' to the advanced skill of walking. He argues that as early movements of progression are carried out by lower animals with a simple nervous system, they can similarly be carried out in the human in the absence of a normal cerebral cortex. The primitive patterns of movement and reflexes can be stimulated in the handicapped parts of the body, through the spine, medulla, pons and mid-brain. Fay's 'pattern movements' are based on these ideas.

The author has found the pattern movements useful for coordination, reciprocal motion, concentration and rhythm.

2. The movement patterns begin with prone lying, head and trunk rotation or primitive squirming followed by a primitive creeping with a homolateral pattern of the arm and leg on the same side, then a contralateral pattern of arm and leg on the opposite sides. After creeping the child is trained to crawl on hands and knees and then 'elephant walk' on hands and feet and finally the walking pattern of man.

3. A strict sequence of this phylogenetic development is stressed.

4. The creeping movements are taught with passive motion or 'patterning' by adults. The child is much later encouraged to carry this out alone.

5. No braces and no aids are used.

6. Reflex movements or 'unlocking' reflexes are used to relax spasticity, e.g. reflex withdrawal of hip and knee into flexion abduction to 'unlock' adductor extensor spasticity.

Proprioceptive Neuromuscular Facilitation

Kabat disagrees with the training of isolated muscles or isolated joint motion which he says are almost never used as such in voluntary activities.

The main points in this approach, which have been developed by Margaret Knott, Dorothy Voss and others are:

1. Movement patterns rather than muscle education of individual

muscle groups are recommended. However, the movement patterns taught should be those used by man in such functions as rolling over, getting up, locomotion and various daily skills using the upper limb.

2. The diagonal and rotary aspects of movement patterns were observed by Kabat. Every movement pattern used in the therapeutic techniques has a diagonal direction. Internal-external rotation and flexion-extension and abduction-adduction are the elements of the patterns.

3. Sensory (afferent) stimuli were shown to stimulate motion. Proprioception is emphasised although the techniques include touch, auditory and visual stimuli as well as the stimuli from stretch, pressure and muscle contraction.

4. Resistance is used to facilitate stronger muscle action within the synergic patterns of movement. Various methods are used to adjust the degree of resistance. It is also important to know where to apply resistance to get a local effect or an effect in another part of the body associated with the movement pattern.

5. Ice treatments are used to relax or inhibit hypertonus. Relaxation techniques of a special kind are also included for selected cases.

These methods are useful in many cerebral palsied children; they are particularly good for weakness in any condition and can be used to train motor skills. Although not mentioned by most authorities writing about proprioceptive neuromuscular facilitation, the author has found that modifications should be made when treating the various types of cerebral palsy.

Neuromotor Development

Eirene Colles was a British pioneer of cerebral palsy treatment. She stressed neuromotor development as a basis for treatment. Her developmental milestones were dogmatically presented. She also considered it important to plan the whole day of the child and not rely solely on short physiotherapy sessions. Colles suggested that there should be 'cerebral palsy therapists' rather than separate professions of physiotherapists, occupational therapists and speech therapists. She thought this would help the child to have a more successful total therapeutic day, and also counteract the isolation of the different professional disciplines.

Neurodevelopmental Treatment with Reflex Inhibition and Facilitation

Dr Karel Bobath, a neuropsychiatrist, and Mrs Berta Bobath, a physiotherapist, base assessment and treatment on the premise that the fundamental difficulty of cerebral palsy is lack of inhibition of reflex patterns of posture and movement. The Bobaths associate these abnormal patterns with abnormal tone due to overaction of tonic reflex activity. These tonic reflexes and asymmetrical tonic neck reflexes have to be inhibited. Once the abnormal tone and reflex patterns have been inhibited, there should be facilitation of more mature postural reflexes. All this is carried out in a developmental context. The main features of their work are:

1. 'Reflex inhibitory patterns' specifically selected to inhibit abnormal tone associated with abnormal movement patterns and abnormal posture.

2. Sensory motor experience: the reversal or 'breakdown' of these abnormalities gives the child the sensation of more normal tone and movements. This sensory experience is believed to 'feed back' and guide more normal motion. Sensory stimuli are also used for inhibition and facilitation and voluntary movement.

3. Facilitation techniques for mature postural reflexes.

4. 'Key points of control': the inhibition of abnormal postures and movements in reflex inhibiting patterns, and the facilitation of more desirable patterns are carried out by correct manual handling of the child by skilful use of 'key points of control' and by various sensory stimuli.

5. Developmental sequence is followed and adapted to each child.

6. All day management should supplement treatment sessions. Parents and others are advised on daily management and trained to treat the children Finnie (1974).

A rather simplified example of the features of this approach may be applied to a spastic child who is excessively extended in supine. This extensor spasticity is considered to be due to the tonic labyrinthine reflex (see p. 30). In order to inhibit the spasticity one of the *reflex inhibitory patterns* might be to flex the child's head and shoulders and hips and knees manually, or in a hammock, for everyday management. The flexion may be carried out actively. The *keypoints of control* might be that if the head is held flexed, the legs may be able to flex actively or if the hips are held in flexion, as a keypoint of control, then the child may be able actively to flex his head to look at his knees. Flexion of his head, off the couch, is also part of the more *mature postural reaction* of head righting in supine. This head righting is *facilitated* while there is a reflex inhibitory pattern to inhibit the extensor spasticity. The *developmental sequence* is involved in that a reflex inhibitory pattern may be sitting with hip and knee flexion rather than the earlier level of supine lying with hip and knee flexion. In facilitating the head righting in supine, this would be possible if the child is approximately at about the six months normal developmental level when this postural reaction is expected. Once again in the all day management, the child may be carried correctly in a flexed position, placed in chairs which are designed to flex his hips and knees and have his shoulders flexed forward instead of retracted into extension. Play activities are given to motivate flexion at the child's developmental level.

Every child is individual and the above example does not apply to every child with extensor spasticity, but is only an example to clarify some of the features of this approach.

Sensory Stimulation for Activation and Inhibition

Margaret Rood, a physiotherapist and occupational therapist, bases her approach on many neurophysiological theories and the literature. The main features of her approach are:

1. Afferent stimuli: the various nerves and sensory receptors are described and classified into types, location, effect, response, distribution and indication. Techniques of stimulation, e.g. stroking, pressure, brushing (tactile); icing, heating (temperature); bone pounding; slow and quick muscle stretch; joint retraction and approximation, muscle contractions, muscle pressure (proprioception), are used to activate, facilitate or inhibit motor response.

2. Muscles are classified according to various physiological data, including whether they are for 'light work muscle action' or 'heavy work muscle action'. The appropriate stimuli for their actions are suggested.

3. Reflexes other than the above are used in therapy, e.g. tonic labyrinthine reflexes, tonic neck, vestibular reflexes. withdrawal patterns.

4. Ontogenetic development sequence is outlined and strictly followed in the application of stimuli.

   (i) Total flexion or withdrawal pattern (in supine).

   (ii) Roll over (flexion of arm and leg on the same side and roll over).

   (iii) Pivot prone (prone with extension of head, trunk and legs).

   (iv) Co-contraction neck (prone, head over edge for co-contraction of vertebral muscles).

   (v) On elbows (prone and push backwards).

(vi) All fours (static, weight shift and crawl).
(vii) Standing upright (static, weight shifts).
(viii) Walking (stance, push off, pick up, heel strike).
5. Vital functions: a developmental sequence of respiration, sucking, swallowing, phonation, chewing and speech is followed. Techniques of brushing, icing and pressure are used.

Reflex Creeping and Other Reflex Reactions

Dr Vaslav Vojta, a neurologist working in Czechoslovakia, developed an approach based on the work of Temple Fay, Kabat and his own ideas (Vojta, 1974). The main features are:
1. Reflex creeping: the creeping patterns involving head, trunk and limbs are facilitated at various 'trigger' points or 'reflex zones'. The creeping is an active response to the appropriate 'triggering' from the zones with sensory stimuli. The muscle work used in the normal creeping patterns or 'creeping complex' have been carefully analysed. The therapist must be skilful in the facilitation of these normal patterns and not provoke 'pathological patterns'.
2. Sensory stimulation: touch, pressure, stretch and muscle action against resistance are used in many of the triggering mechanisms, or in the facilitation of creeping.
3. Resistance is recommended for action of muscles. Various specific techniques are used to apply the resistance so that either a tonic or phasic muscle action is provoked. The phasic action may be provoked on a movement of a limb creeping up or downwards. The tonic action, or stabilising action is obtained if a phasic movement is fully resisted. Therefore the static muscle action of stability occurs if resistance is applied so that it prevents any movement through the range.

Conductive Education

Professor Andras Peto in Budapest, Hungary, originated Conductive Education. Since Professor Peto's death, his work has been continued by Dr M. Hari. The main features are the integration of therapy and education by:
1. A conductor acting as mother, nurse, teacher and therapist. She is specially trained in the habilitation of motor disabled children in a four-year course. She may have one or two assistants.
2. The group of children, about fifteen to twenty, work together. Groups are fundamental in this training system.

3. An all day programme: a timetable is planned to include getting out of bed in the morning, dressing, feeding, toilcting, movement training, speech, reading, writing and other school work.

4. The movements: there are sessions of movements, mainly taking place on and beside slatted plinths (table/beds) and with ladder-backed chairs. The movements are devised in such a way that they form the elements of a task or motor skill. The tasks are carefully analysed for each group of children. The tasks are the activities of daily living, hand skills including hand function, balance and loco-motion. The purpose of each movement is explained to the children. The movements are repeated, not only in the movement session of, say, the 'hand class' or 'plinth work', but also in various contexts throughout the day. The children are shown in practice how their 'exercises' contribute to daily activities.

5. Rhythmic intention: the technique used for training the ele-ments or movements is 'rhythmic intention'. The conductor and the children state the intended motion, 'I touch my mouth with my hands'. This motion is then attempted together with their slow, rhythmic counts of one to five. Motion is also carried out to an operative word such as 'up, up, up' repeated in a rhythm slow enough for their active movement. Speech and active motion reinforce each other.

6. Individual sessions may be used for some children to help them to participate more adequately in the work of the group.

7. Learning principles are basic to the programme. Conditioning techniques and group dynamics are among the mechanisms of train-ing discussed. 'Cortical' or conscious participation is stressed, as opposed to involuntary and automatic, unconscious reflex therapy.

The Eclectic Viewpoint

It is difficult to prove which treatment approach is superior to the other. All claim good results and to date no approach can be scientifically proved superior by a controlled study. There are many variables such as intelligence, home background, personality of the child and of the therapist as well as different associated handicaps, which could affect the result of physiotherapy. Untreated controls are difficult to obtain, and it is also difficult to match the treated children in a study.

Theoretical considerations are controversial and none of the approaches have the complete answer to the understanding of the cerebral palsies. The lack of a complete 'answer' is not surprising as neither what is happening in the brain of the cerebral palsied nor the effect of therapy on the neurological and psychological mechanisms is fully understood as yet. From practical experience many physiotherapists find that each child is so individual in his clinical picture and needs, that it is difficult to confine all the children to any one set of techniques or approach. The facilities for treatment will also affect what techniques can be used.

In order to draw on various schools of thought and treatment systems it may be helpful to use the following general principles. These are the common factors the author has found after a study of many different systems of treatment.

MOTOR DEVELOPMENT

Follow the normal motor developmental sequences (gross and fine motor) and *modify them* according to each child. A detailed developmental assessment of each child is essential for treatment. The motor skills at each developmental level, such as head control, rolling, creeping, crawling, sitting, standing, walking and hand function should be facilitated with techniques from any treatment system (Figs 20/3 and 20/4). A physiotherapist may invent her own methods to obtain these motor activities and she must work particularly closely with the occupational therapists.

Fig. 20/3 (*left*) Spastic quadriplegia with visual handicap unable to control head and trunk at developmental levels of an infant

Fig. 20/4 (*right*) Father carrying out home programme to develop head and trunk control for sitting. Note improvement of arm and leg postures though head asymmetry persists

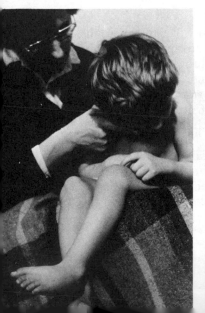
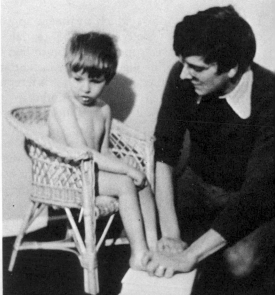

AFFERENT STIMULI

Various techniques are used with afferent stimuli to obtain desirable
activity and decrease hypertonus.

PREVENTION OF DEFORMITY

Any methods to stimulate a variety of corrective movements should be used. Splintage, bracing, correct furniture, footwear and frequent changes of posture are important in the prevention of deformity. Orthopaedic procedures, using plaster of Paris or surgery, may be indicated in selected cases.

INHIBITION AND FACILITATION

Inhibition of hypertonus can be obtained as a result of facilitation of active corrective movements and postures. These activities are best carried out within the function or context of the motor skills of child development. Correct training of, say, hand function, head control, rolling over, creeping, crawling, sitting, standing and walking will, at the same time, inhibit hypertonus and involuntary movement.

However, special techniques of inhibition of hypertonus may also be needed in some children. Both facilitation and inhibition techniques are available from many different approaches.

MOTIVATION TECHNIQUES

Motivation techniques with songs, toys, adventure playgrounds, play equipment, group games, group exercises, playgroups, music and horse riding can be subtly arranged to obtain active corrective movements, posture and equilibrium.

MOVEMENT PATTERNS AND MUSCLE WORK

Most modern systems train movement patterns rather than muscle education. However, specific muscle groups may be particularly weak or spastic or both and need concentrated therapy. They may be treated in isolation or 'in pattern', depending on the child.

TEAMWORK AND ALL DAY CARE

It is not enough to see the treatment of the child as only a half-hour session in a day. The physiotherapist should check that her aims of treatment are not hampered by incorrect management throughout the day. She must check the furniture used by the child, his toys, the way he is carried, his feeding, washing, toileting and any other activities involving posture and movement. She will have to advise parents, teachers, other therapists, housemothers, and anyone handling the child as to what postures and movements to avoid and what to encourage.

In order to understand the child as a whole, and to treat him in a total habilitation programme, it is obvious that the therapist must function as part of a team of cerebral palsy workers. It is easier if the personnel handling the child are all working in the same building so that contact can be maintained. Staff conferences are useful, but informal discussions in the staff room are as important for team work.

It is essential to explore the different ways in which various professions overlap for the sake of total habilitation of the child. It is unrealistic for each professional person of a cerebral palsy team to isolate herself in her own department. The overlapping of therapies and education does not mean that there is still not a need for the benefits of the specialised knowledge and training. Clearly the parents must be part of this team work. Where cerebral palsy teams do not exist, parent participation is the only way a child can be treated.

INCREASE GENERAL SENSORY-MOTOR EXPERIENCE

The physiotherapist should make sure that in giving the child postures and movements and added independence, he uses these achievements to explore space, textures, shapes, temperatures and other everyday experiences. If he is learning to crawl or walk he should try not only on the floor of the physiotherapy room, but on grass, rough ground, in sand, on inclines and so on. He should get into boxes, cupboards, under tables, go into different rooms in his house and so on. Any visits to shops, the country and the zoo must be encouraged.

EARLY TREATMENT

The advantages of early treatment are that not only is motion stimulated but it is stimulated in the best possible patterns. An intelligent baby can be motivated to move by an enterprising mother. However, he will move in the way which comes easiest to him. In other words, the abnormal patterns of movement will be used. If there is a potential for more normal patterns in the baby's nervous system, correct early physiotherapy can facilitate this, and prevent the abnormal patterns from being established as habitual. If abnormal patterns are used, this can lead to deformities and later contractures.

LEARNING PROCESSES

Physiotherapy systems are preoccupied with orthopaedic and neurophysiological techniques. However, this is not the only way a child learns to move. While working within multidisciplinary teams, physiotherapists should obtain information and be guided by educationalists and psychologists. The physiotherapist should also study principles of learning movement from the field of education, human movement studies, child development and psychology (see Chapter 23).

Techniques of Treatment

It is not possible to describe these in a chapter. The physiotherapist must attend courses, gain clinical experience, study the literature and carry out study visits in order to learn how to treat cerebral palsy. She must collect a repertoire of methods and understand the purpose of each method she decides to use. The methods must be relevant to each child's problems.

In selecting techniques for each child, the physiotherapist naturally selects the technique which she can carry out skilfully. Some techniques require more supervision and training than others.

In selecting techniques it is important to focus on the stimulation of motor function in daily life and the correction of the way in which they are performed. Techniques are, therefore, on three related aspects:

1. Techniques only used by specially trained paediatric physiotherapists.

2. Techniques which can be shown to parents, nurses, playgroup workers, teachers and others stimulating movement or caring for cerebral palsied children.

3. Selection of equipment to reinforce techniques, or to be used with techniques of movement training.

REFERENCES

Asher, C. H. D. and Schonell, F. E. (1950). 'A survey of 400 cases of cerebral palsy in childhood.' *Archives of Disease in Childhood*, 25, 360.

Fay, T. (1954). 'The use of pathological and unlocking reflexes in the rehabilitation of spastics.' *American Journal of Physical Medicine*, 33, 347–52.

Finnie, N. (1974). *Handling the Young Cerebral Palsied Child at Home*, 2nd edition. William Heinemann Medical Books Limited, London.

Ingram, T. T. S. (1966). *Paediatric Aspects of Cerebral Palsy*. Churchill Livingstone, Edinburgh.

Purdon-Martin, J. (1967). *The Basal Ganglia and Posture*. Pitman Medical, London.

Vojta, V. (1974). *Die Cerebralen Bewegangstorungen im Sauglingsalter*. Ferdinand Enke Verlag, Stuttgart, West Germany.

Woods, G. E. (1975). *The Handicapped Child: Assessment and Management*. Blackwell Scientific Publications Limited, Oxford.

BIBLIOGRAPHY

Bobath, B. and Bobath, K. (1975). *Motor Development in the Different Types of Cerebral Palsy*. William Heinemann Medical Books Limited, London.

Bobath, K. (1980). *A Neurophysiological Basis for the Treatment of Cerebral Palsy*. William Heinemann Medical Books Limited, London.

Cotton, E. (1974). *The Basic Motor Pattern*. The Spastics Society, London.

Cotton, E. (1975). *Conductive Education and Cerebral Palsy*. The Spastics Society, London.

Cratty, B. S. (1979). *Perceptual and Motor Development in Infants and Young Children*, 2nd edition. Lea and Febiger, Philadelphia, USA.

Decker, R. (1962). *Motor Integration*. Charles C. Thomas, Springfield, Illinois, USA.

Gillette, H. E. (1974). *Systems of Therapy in Cerebral Palsy*. Charles C. Thomas, Springfield, Illinois, USA.

Illingworth, R. S. (1974). *The Development of the Infant and Young Child: Normal and Abnormal*, 5th edition. Churchill Livingstone, Edinburgh.

Levitt, S. (1966). 'Proprioceptive neuromuscular techniques in cerebral palsy.' *Physiotherapy*, 52, 46.

Levitt, S. (1970). '*The Adaptation of PNF for Cerebral Palsy*.' Included in the Proceedings of the Sixth International Congress of the World Confederation for Physical Therapy. World Confederation for Physical Therapy, London.

Levitt, S. and Miller, C. (1973). 'The inter-relationships of speech therapy and physiotherapy in children with neuro-developmental disorders.' *Developmental Medicine and Child Neurology*, 15, 2.

Levitt, S. (1976). *Stimulation of Movement*. Chapter included in *Early Management of Handicapping Disorders*. (Oppe, T. E. and Woodford, F. P. (eds).) (A.S.P. Ltd) Elsevier Scientific Publishers Company Limited, Amsterdam.

Levitt, S. (1977). *The Treatment of Cerebral Palsy and Motor Delay*. Blackwell Scientific Publications Limited, Oxford.

Pearson, H. P. and Williams, C. E. (eds) (1978). *Physical Therapy Services in the Developmental Disabilities*. Charles C. Thomas, Springfield, Illinois, USA.

Stockmeyer, S. A. (1969). 'The Rood approach.' *American Journal of Physical Medicine*, 46, 1900.

Blencowe, S. M. (1969). *Cerebral Palsy and the Young Child*. E and S Livingstone, Edinburgh. (This book can be obtained from the Cheyne Spastic Centre, 61 Cheyne Walk, London SW3 5LX)

See also Bibliography on pp.147 and 250.

ACKNOWLEDGEMENTS

The author expresses her thanks to the photographic department of the Institute of Child Health, London for their help with the illustrations. She is also grateful to the parents of the children shown in the pictures for their permission to include them in the chapter.

Chapter 21

Muscular Dystrophy

by G. P. HOSKING, M.B., M.R.C.P., D.C.H.
and H. HAYWOOD, M.C.S.P.

A muscular dystrophy is a disorder in which there is active destruction of muscle and progressive muscle weakness. There are many forms of muscular dystrophy with onset in childhood and early adulthood. The commonest and most severe form is that described in the last century by Dr G. A. B. Duchenne and subsequently named after him. This chapter will confine itself to this Duchenne type muscular dystrophy as many of the diagnostic and management aspects of this form of muscular dystrophy apply also to the others.

Duchenne type dystrophy is an X-linked recessive condition and, therefore, only occurs in boys. Estimates of its frequency range between 13 to 33 per 100,000 live born males, which means that approximately 100 boys with the disease will be born each year in the United Kingdom.

In two-thirds of cases the mother will be a 'carrier' of the condition, although in most there will be no clinical evidence of any neuro-muscular dysfunction. Approximately half of these carriers will have a family history of muscular dystrophy – either a brother or another child affected. In a high proportion of the remainder an elevation of the muscle enzyme creatine phosphokinase (CPK) will be noted (see below).

The diagnosis of Duchenne muscular dystrophy is commonly made between the age of three and five years, although parents may well have been aware of significant abnormalities in neuromuscular function long before that time – from two to two and a half years. Often they have been 'reassured' that the child is either 'lazy', 'flat-footed' or 'clumsy'.

The presenting complaints are connected with walking, running, going up slopes or stairs; a waddling gait due to pelvic girdle weak-ness; frequent falling, and difficulty both getting up from the floor or from low chairs. In some boys the age of beginning to walk will be delayed. In the early stages significant difficulties with the arms are uncommon, but later there are complaints about the inability to raise the arms above the head while attempting specific tasks such as combing the hair.

Observations of boys getting up from the floor will reveal the characteristic manoeuvre known as the Gowers' sign. Sir William Gowers noted that the boy with Duchenne type muscular dystrophy, because of his pelvic girdle weakness, had to roll on to his front and then push against his thighs to straighten up. This is described as 'climbing up oneself' (Fig. 21/1). There is wasting in a number of muscle groups but, on the other hand, some muscles appear to be particularly bulky. The bulky muscles include those of the calf, sometimes the deltoid, the shoulder muscles and the temporalis.

It is now well known that anything up to a third of boys with Duchenne muscular dystrophy have some degree of learning difficulty or mental retardation. At times the mental retardation is of such significance that the co-existent neuromuscular dysfunction is overlooked – at least in early childhood.

Fig. 21/1 Gowers' sign in a boy with muscular dystrophy

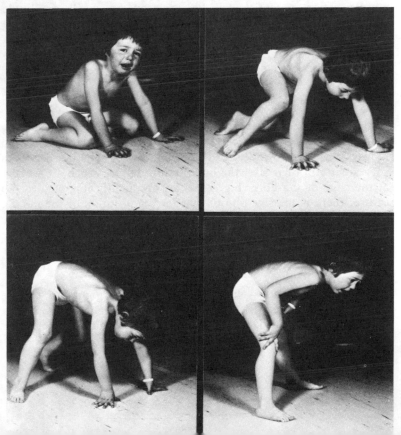

INVESTIGATIONS

The investigation of a boy with suspected muscular dystrophy is usually based upon three tests – a blood test, an electrophysiological test, and a biopsy.

Creatine Phosphokinase (CPK) Test

In all boys with Duchenne muscular dystrophy the level of CPK will be about ten times above the upper limit of the normal range. CPK is an enzyme that usually exists in high quantity within muscle and some other tissues. In the presence of a muscle disorder this enzyme will leak out into the circulation. Therefore, a high level of circulating CPK will suggest the possibility of a primary disorder of muscle. Quite why the level of CPK is so very high in Duchenne muscular dystrophy is not known. Nevertheless, this test result is diagnostically very useful.

Electrophysiological Test

An electromyographic (EMG) examination of active muscle will, with muscular dystrophy, produce abnormal results. The usual triphasic muscle action potential will be replaced by small amplitude polyphasic potentials of short duration. Some argue that the clinical picture, elevated CPK and a myopathic EMG are enough to make a positive diagnosis of Duchenne muscular dystrophy. However, diagnostic mistakes have occurred.

Muscle Biopsy

With such a 'sinister' diagnosis as Duchenne muscular dystrophy biopsy of muscle would seem to be mandatory. At whatever age the biopsy is performed profound changes are seen. The muscle fibres vary greatly in their size, the muscle fibre nuclei which are usually at the edge of the fibre (Fig. 21/2) are frequently migrated to the centre, there is massive fibrous and fatty infiltration of the muscle fibres and some evidence of attempts at regeneration (Fig. 21/3). The amount of fat and fibrous infiltration is such that muscle bulk will be increased, leading to the suggestion that, although weak, the muscle is hypertrophic. Such 'hypertrophy' is spurious and the term 'pseudo-hypertrophy' is used.

Cardiac as well as skeletal muscle is affected and this can be reflected in abnormalities seen in the electrocardiogram (ECG) in a number of boys with Duchenne muscular dystrophy.

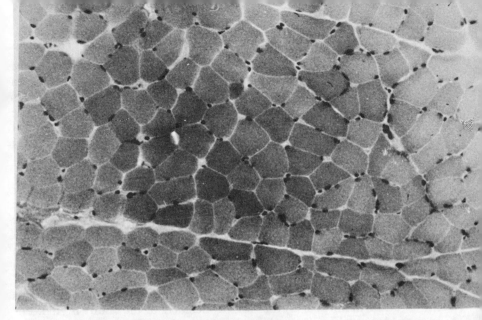

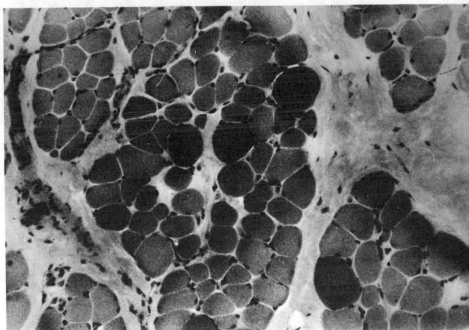

Fig. 21/2 Muscle biopsy showing normal muscle

Fig. 21/3 Muscle biopsy showing the typical findings in Duchenne muscular dystrophy

Overall the course of this disorder is one of steady deterioration in motor and, most particularly, locomotor function. However, in a small proportion of boys there may be a period of up to two years between five and seven when no functional deterioration takes place and indeed an improvement in locomotor function occurs. In these it is probable that, although there is a continuing dystrophic process, some normal muscle development is still continuing.

All boys are 'off their feet' by the age of 12 and many by 8 years. Very soon after 'going off their feet' boys with Duchenne muscular dystrophy demonstrate that by this time they have very significant upper limb weakness and, therefore, there is a need for a wheelchair which has to be electrically powered. Total dependency for virtually all day-to-day activities is usual by the early teens and death, from a respiratory infection, occurs anytime from the mid-teenage years to the early twenties.

Genetic counselling with attempts made to establish 'carrier' status of the mothers and other female members of the family is vital. For this as early a diagnosis as possible in the index case is essential.

THERAPY AND MANAGEMENT

Innumerable therapeutic trials of a variety of drugs have been undertaken, but in none has there been any convincing evidence of lasting benefit. Therefore, in the present state of our knowledge, management of Duchenne muscular dystrophy must start with the realisation that there is no specific treatment of this disorder.

Mobility is the major problem in the early years after diagnosis is made. From the early phases of the disease there is a tendency towards walking 'on the toes'. It is arguable why this should or should not be. An inequality in weakness between the below knee anterior muscles and posterior muscles may be the explanation. On the other hand, the pelvic girdle weakness will allow some rotation forward of the pelvis, and in order to maintain the centre of gravity within the axis of the body, lordosis, slight flexion at the knees, and extension of the ankles is necessary (Fig. 21/4). Contractures at the hip and ankle are common findings in the ambulant boy but this does not resolve what could be considered as a 'chicken and egg' argument.

The role of physiotherapy in the management of Duchenne muscular dystrophy has to be reviewed realistically. There is no evidence that 'exercise' programmes have any benefit, although regular moderate exercise is as desirable as it is to any individual. Immobility, for whatever reason, poses real threats to the child with a neuromuscular disorder. A period of inactivity may be followed by a

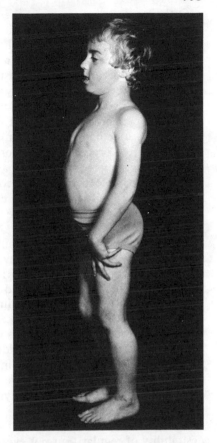

Fig. 21/4 Typical posture of a boy with Duchenne muscular dystrophy

profound decrease in mobility which may, or may not, be reversible. Thus, a boy with Duchenne muscular dystrophy should be mobilised at the very earliest opportunity after any illness or operation.

Joint contractures – hip and ankle – may be delayed, although not entirely prevented by regular passive stretching. Parents may be instructed in how stretching of the tendo Achilles can be accomplished by a regular routine of dorsiflexion of the foot with the knee flexed and in extension. This can be incorporated into a bedtime routine but must never be allowed to become a major 'issue' so that rebellion on the part of the child may make the whole procedure somewhat fraught. The management of incipient hip contractures should be with the encouragement of the boy to spend some time each day lying prone with the chest and body extended – preferably over a wedge.

Orthopaedic intervention in the ambulatory phase of Duchenne muscular dystrophy presents a difficult decision. While it still remains debatable as to why boys with Duchenne muscular dystrophy walk on their toes, a logical approach and a question as to the desirability of elongating the tendo Achilles must inevitably exist. In many boys their toe walking appears necessary for ambulation, but in others it is without reasonable doubt part of their locomotor handicap. In the authors' experience, elongation of the tendo Achilles, whether performed as a subcutaneous tenotomy under local anaesthetic, or as a more definitive procedure, has done little to improve ambulation. Nevertheless, some have argued that elongation of the tendo Achilles combined with release of possible contractures at the knee and of the ilio-tibial tract, and the fitting of calipers has improved and maintained locomotor function in those who were in danger of 'going off their feet'.

Considerable controversy surrounds the fitting of calipers to boys with Duchenne muscular dystrophy. It can be argued that well-fitting lightweight calipers in a boy with no joint contractures can aid locomotion, but it can be argued also that the benefits are very short-lived. Many boys by the time they are experiencing major locomotor difficulties are only too anxious to acquire true mobility, and the only way this is possible is with a wheelchair. Nevertheless, the fitting of calipers must be considered in any boy whose locomotor function has deteriorated to the point that continued ambulation is in question. In considering this there must be the involvement of the orthopaedic surgeon, paediatric physician, physiotherapist, orthotist, parents and the patient.

From the time of diagnosis not only is it vital to emphasise the desirability of regular, but not excessive, exercise, the avoidance of immobility for whatever reason, but also the prevention of obesity and the development of interests that do not depend upon physical well-being.

When it is clear that ambulation is no longer practical or reasonable the management of the boy with muscular dystrophy in a wheelchair has to be considered.

Using a Wheelchair

For both the boy and his parents the acquisition of a wheelchair and the dependence upon it represents a major milestone in the course of the illness. In effect, 'going off the feet' is not usually a sudden process as very often it has been found necessary to use a wheelchair for certain activities such as shopping or generally getting about outside the home and school. On the other hand, many boys, while experiencing progressive difficulty with walking, do suddenly lose their ability to walk, perhaps following an illness – or an operation.

Life in a wheelchair brings with it certain problems.

CONTRACTURES

Contractures rapidly develop at the hip and knee and they are virtually impossible to prevent. Ankle contractures are often present by the time a boy goes into a wheelchair (Fig. 21/5). Elongation of the tendo

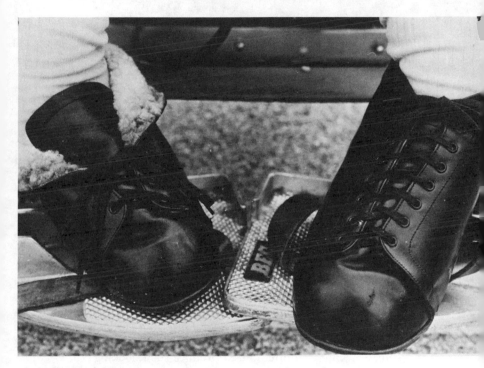

Fig. 21/5 Talipes equinovarus in a boy with Duchenne muscular dystrophy who is now confined to a wheelchair

Achilles is indicated in all boys as the progressive development of talipes equinovirus will make shoe fitting difficult, if not, in some, impossible (Fig. 21/6). This is a procedure that can be undertaken under local anaesthetic and should be followed by splinting with either plaster of Paris, below knee iron calipers, or a moulded splint for at least the first few months after surgery. Many support the wearing of night splints following surgery. Severe talipes equinovirus

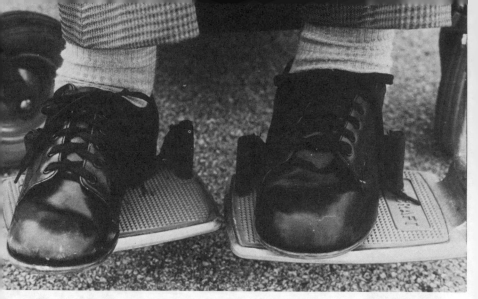

Fig. 21/6 The position of the feet after elongation of the tendo Achilles for talipes equinovarus

not only produces problems with shoe fitting, but also positioning in bed and transferring from chair to toilet, chair or bed.

SCOLIOSIS

One of the major problems for the boy with severe muscular dystrophy using a wheelchair is the development of a scoliosis. There is no doubt that this is a problem that develops only after going into a wheelchair, although scoliosis is described in some boys with muscular dystrophy who are still ambulant. Quite why some boys develop a scoliosis after becoming immobile and others do not, is not really understood. Observations have been made that if there is a significant lordosis the intervertebral facets are 'locked' and thus the spine is fixed. This observation has led to developing one form of spinal bracing that attempts to produce such 'locking'.

Severe scoliosis will lead, not only to major postural difficulties, but also to real respiratory difficulties – in themselves life-threatening. A careful watch must be kept on the possible development of scoliosis and, when seen, early bracing is essential. Often it is difficult to persuade the boys – and their parents – that bracing is necessary and, together with this, it may be that the spinal braces are too restrictive for adequate respiratory function. Gibson in Toronto has described what appears to be an effective brace that is neither significantly restrictive to the chest nor uncomfortable to wear.

The problem of scoliosis raises a major question – that of wheelchair design and fitting. If scoliosis is first considered – it has been suggested that if a wheelchair has a 10 to 15° back slope the scoliosis may well be prevented or delayed in developing. On the other hand, it is hardly functional to be in a chair in which one is sitting well back, and most boys prefer to lean forward and lean on one or other arm of the chair. Soft wedges placed inside the chair on either side of the trunk help in giving support.

The prevention of foot deformities depends to a great degree on the resting position of the feet while in the wheelchair. It is, therefore, vital that the footplates on the wheelchair are correctly adjusted. Wedges placed between the side of the chair and the thighs help to keep the knees from flopping outwards (Fig. 21/7).

As referred to above, an electric wheelchair is needed very soon after ambulation is lost as upper limb weakness by then becomes very significant.

The control system of the chair will be situated on one or other arm of the chair. Studies have been undertaken as to whether posture may be improved in the chair if the control is in the centre. So far there is little to suggest that a centrally situated control confers any definite advantage.

The cause of death in Duchenne muscular dystrophy is virtually always from a respiratory infection. At times this may be combined with cardiac failure because of cardiomyopathy. Breathing exercises

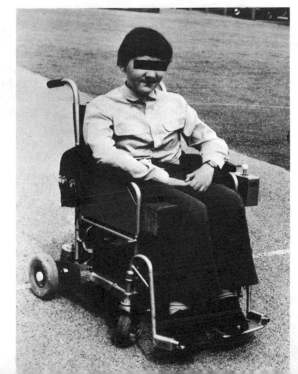

Fig. 21/7 Positioning of a boy with Duchenne muscular dystrophy in a wheelchair

are desirable for all boys and should be instituted at the very latest at the stage of going into a wheelchair. Together with this, active treatment with antibiotics and physiotherapy for any chest infection is essential.

Social Problems

There can be few conditions that pose such strains on parents, therapists, teachers, doctors and patients, as Duchenne muscular dystrophy. From the time of diagnosis to the time of death both patient and parents need a great deal of support. Diagnosis brings with it a major trauma to any family. While the temptation may exist to 'spare' the parents the full details of the disease, it is the opinion of the authors that they should be told everything from the initial diagnosis. Following the initial telling full support and the willingness to talk through all the implications of the diagnosis must be offered. The involvement and support of an informed social worker can be invaluable.

As time passes the true realisation of the extent of the handicap will dawn on the family. Thus, support is a continuous need. The time of diagnosis is the first crisis in the life of the family; invariably the next crisis comes when the boy finally and completely takes to a wheelchair. The degree of dependency then becomes very great; assistance is needed for dressing, toileting, turning in bed, and later for feeding. As the natural history of this disease is well known and reasonably consistent, the problems associated with dependence should be anticipated. Where necessary, applications for adaptation to the home should be made well in advance of the stage of major dependence and an occupational therapist should undertake a careful and comprehensive review of the aids that will be needed within the home.

School placement depends partly upon the wishes of the parents, the attitude of the staff at the ordinary school and the architecture of the school. There are certainly advantages in a physically handicapped school in that it is likely that it will be on a single level and relevant therapy staff are available. On the other hand, the educational standard at many physically handicapped schools may be lower than that of an ordinary school.

The strain on families who have a boy with severe muscular dystrophy is immense and, as stated above, support is essential. Parent groups can be very helpful. Marital break up is frequent; the mother so often being left to cope with the physical and emotional demands of a totally dependent adolescent. If the physical demands are not enough there is need also to recognise that, in spite of a progressive physical disease, the emotions of a young teenager remain throughout. Some years ago one of us was moved when told by a 16-year-old boy with muscular dystrophy that what he most wanted to do was to 'drink beer and chase women'. He could do neither.

BIBLIOGRAPHY

Dubowitz, V. (1978). *Muscle Disorders in Childhood.* Holt-Saunders Ltd, Eastbourne.
The Muscular Dystrophies (1980). *British Medical Bulletin,* 36.
Walton, J. N. (ed) (1974). *Disorders of Voluntary Muscle,* 3rd edition. Churchill Livingstone, Edinburgh.

Chapter 22

Physiotherapy in some Psychiatric Conditions

by J. M. DODGSON, M.C.S.P., O.N.C.

In the ever-changing field of psychiatry, the physiotherapist is taking an increasingly active part. The purpose of this chapter, however, is not only to be of assistance to the serious student of psychiatric physiotherapy, but, it is hoped, to be of some value to the physiotherapist in a general department.

We have all met the patient who, in spite of many courses of different types of physical treatment, fails to improve. There may, or may not, be obvious signs of tension or anxiety in the patient. After a while, when all investigations have failed to produce a physical origin for the complaint, the patient is labelled 'neurotic', or the condition labelled 'psychosomatic' and he is referred to the psychiatrist.

In the Physical Medicine Department, the therapist who can recognise and understand the underlying psychiatric problems at an early stage will be of much greater value to the patient than the one who is concerned solely with the physical problems. Persistence of symptoms of, for example, osteo-arthrosis may be due to over-anxiety caused by association of the term osteo-arthrosis with progressive and unavoidable crippling. Prolonged physical treatment, without the recognition and understanding of the underlying anxieties associated with any physical illness, can only be harmful. In fact, it has been said that 'the essential link between psychiatry, general medicine, surgery and obstetrics lies in the ultimate impossibility of treating states of mind apart from states of body, or states of body apart from states of mind'.

PSYCHOSOMATIC INTERACTIONS

The word 'psychosomatic' is used in various ways, commonly in reference to specific diseases, such as asthma, peptic ulcers, menstrual disorders etc, in which emotional factors are considered to be of definite aetiological significance; but sometimes as a synonym for psychoneurotic.

Pearson in *Fundamentals of Psychiatry* defines it as representing a point of view on the study of disease as a whole. He says: 'The investigation of disease from the psychosomatic point of view is the study of illness in terms of the emotional factors (feelings, moods, conflicts, attitudes, interpersonal relationships and personality developments), as well as of the physical factors (constitution, immunity, bacterial or viral invasion, trauma, degeneration and neoplasm formation)'.

Man owes his survival and his power over his environment to the flexibility of his adaptive capacity. When the individual's mental resources are not enough to meet the demands on him, and adaptation is incomplete, a state of internal disharmony occurs. This manifests itself in symptoms of physical or mental dysfunction, or, more commonly, in both.

Thus, a psychosomatic illness is one in which psychological factors appear to play an important part in producing a disorder of the function or structure of the body. There are several types of psychosomatic disorders:

1. Where various physical symptoms exist, but no physical cause can be found.

2. Where physical disease exists, but the structural changes are a result of emotional factors.

3. Where actual organic disease exists, but some of the presenting symptoms arise not from this disease, but from mental factors. Here the disability is often out of proportion to the physical disease.

PHYSICAL CHANGES IN EMOTIONAL STATES

All emotions are expressed through physiological processes and all are accompanied by physiological changes. Thus we show sorrow by weeping, amusement by laughter and shame by blushing. Emotional situations arising from interaction with other people give rise to nervous impulses which influence the complex muscular interactions that take place in the body. Thus fear produces palpitation of the heart; anger produces increased heart activity, elevation of blood pressure, and changes in carbohydrate metabolism; and despair causes sighing (i.e. deep inspiration followed by deep expiration).

These changes in the body as reactions to acute emotion are of a passing nature and return to normal when the emotion disappears. If the emotion is repressed, however, or unduly prolonged, the functional disturbance produced in any organ may lead finally to definite anatomical changes, and to the clinical picture of severe organic illness. For example, hyperactivity of the heart may lead to hypertrophy of the heart muscle, or hysterical paralysis of a limb may lead to certain degenerative changes in the muscles and joints because of inactivity.

Two emotional states which commonly give rise to psychosomatic illness are anxiety and tension.

Anxiety

Anxiety in its simplest form may be considered as a normal reaction to danger, or the threat of danger. Biological changes occur in the individual which improve his responsiveness to external stresses. A small amount of anxiety increases alertness and efficiency of performance, but an increase in the amount of anxiety will eventually lead to a deterioration of the level of response. When anxiety develops as an abnormal state, not necessarily related to stress, it is regarded as a symptom or part of a broader-based psychiatric syndrome. It reaches a pathological degree only when it surpasses the inherent ability of the subject to bear it.

The physical manifestations of an anxiety state resemble those of fear, with excessive activity of the autonomic nervous system. There may be symptoms associated with any of the bodily systems:

Cardiac – tachycardia and palpitation

Respiratory – breathlessness and tightness of the chest

Gastro-intestinal – nausea, vomiting, diarrhoea and abdominal cramps

Genito-urinary – frequency, urgency, enuresis

Vasomotor – sweating, shivering and dizziness

Neuromuscular – weakness, tension.

The anxious patient shows signs of apprehension and assumes a tense posture with furrowing of the brow and wringing of hands. The voice may be uneven or strained, and the pupils widely dilated. There may be sweating of the hands and face and weakness, nausea and tremor may be present.

In a moderate degree of emotional stress only a few of these signs and symptoms may be present. However, long-continued emotions of fear, shame, anger, resentment etc, may produce more symptoms and if they become exaggerated and established they may continue even after the original situation has disappeared and may eventually lead to structural changes in the organ or viscus through which the anxiety is expressed ('The sorrow which has no vent in tears may make other organs weep': Henry Maudsley). Disorders of bodily functions are the clinically dominant features and a patient will rarely complain or even recognise his anxiety, tension or depression.

Tension

Tension is a component of anxiety and may be confused with the effect of anxiety. It arises when an individual is torn between contradictory desires and strivings.

In tension the patient has a continuing feeling of tautness, both emotionally and in his muscles. He senses a restlessness, dissatisfaction and dread. He presents a strained, tense facial expression, has tremor of the hands and his movements are abrupt. He probably will complain of tightness or other unpleasant sensations in the head and other bodily pains – usually in the neck and shoulders, back and chest. The pain in the head may be described as 'dull', 'nagging', 'an ache', or 'tight' and occasionally 'stabbing'. There is usually difficulty in concentration, broken sleep and fatigue. Among other symptoms of tension are: abdominal pain (particularly in children), amenorrhoea, dysmenorrhoea, menorrhagia, constipation, diarrhoea, frequency of micturition, migraine, and various skin changes such as itching and flushing.

Hyperventilation

Much has been written about hyperventilation, or habitual over-breathing. In the psychiatric department, many patients will be found to be suffering from this breathing disorder. Although it is usually considered to be one of the numerous manifestations of an anxiety state, it is probable that in many cases the continuous distress caused by the respiratory alkalosis arising from chronic hyperventilation has, in itself, given rise to the state of anxiety.

Many bodily functions are affected by respiratory alkalosis apart from the psychic. Cardiac, neuromuscular, gastro-intestinal and respiratory functions may all be affected in varying degrees. The symptoms may become very marked, and may give rise to mis-diagnosis such as intestinal disorders, heart disease or epilepsy.

Observation of the patient at rest will usually show an irregular breathing pattern, mainly upper thoracic, with frequent sighing, and often noisy or heavy breathing. There may be a marked variability in the size of individual breaths, and in the rate and rhythm of breathing. Other signs include:

dizziness and headache

chest pain, mimicking angina (due to overuse of the upper
   thoracic muscles)
tachycardia and palpitations
indigestion
air swallowing or frequent saliva swallowing
general feeling of weakness and fatigue.

AIMS OF TREATMENT

1. To teach general relaxation
2. To make the patient aware of faulty breathing habits
3. To convert the habitual thoracic breathing to diaphragmatic.

TREATMENT

1. Make an accurate assessment of the patient's symptoms.
2. Explain to the patient exactly what he is doing wrong.
3. Teach general relaxation in lying and sitting.
4. Teach diaphragmatic breathing in standing, walking, and on the
stairs.
5. Show the patient how to slow down his breathing rate, by
putting in a pause at the end of each expiration. The taking of
occasional extra breaths must be discouraged.
6. Teach home instruction: the patient is told to practise breathing
and relaxation for a few minutes each hour, and also to have two or
three longer practise sessions of about 20–30 minutes each day.
7. The effectiveness of the treatment should be reinforced by
getting the patient to over-breathe for one to two minutes, to repro-
duce his symptoms. He will then become confident of his ability to
eliminate his symptoms by relaxing and correcting his breathing.

Treatment should continue over a period of several weeks, at first
daily, then reducing to weekly or fortnightly, as his confidence
increases.

INFLUENCE OF EMOTIONAL FACTORS ON SOME SPECIFIC ILLNESSES

Rheumatoid Arthritis

There are many theories concerning the cause of rheumatoid arthritis,
none of which establishes sufficient proof to be fully acceptable.
Probably several factors, including infections, local trauma, debilitating states and emotional disturbances may precipitate or aggravate the
disease. Often direct temporal relationships between the onset of the
arthritic symptoms and emotional crises are observed, and exacerba-

tions and remissions can often be linked with changes in the environmental stress under which the patient lives.

While some authorities hold the view that rheumatoid arthritis is an organic psychosomatic disease others suggest that the emotional factors apparently affecting the disease are only part of the picture, and should be looked upon as only one of several possibly provocative agents.

Sufferers from rheumatoid arthritis tend to fit into a particular personality pattern which is frequently associated with psychosomatic disorders. They show emotional inhibition, probably stemming from early childhood when they were shy and retiring, possibly due to restrictive overprotective parental influence in infancy. Many aspects of their emotional lives are repressed and they grow up into meticulously orderly, overconscientious people, well adjusted to emotional life, but showing restrictions of feelings and emotions.

Whatever the cause of the disease, or its exacerbations, it must be remembered that any chronically disabling disease is likely to produce serious emotional problems. Many patients develop a sense of hostility due to the threat of dependency, and the frustrations associated with the condition (disruption of social life, interference with earning power etc) tend to produce neurotic symptoms. Others tend to cling to their position of dependency. Either of these reactions to the limiting factors of the disease is damaging to the confidence of relationships with others, even (or perhaps especially) those who are trying to help. The type of person whose mobility and muscular ability is essential to his adaptation will suffer deeply and have less inner strength to deal with the enforced regression which the limitations of the disease impose.

Asthma

Because of the close relationship between emotional tensions and respiratory function, as instanced by crying, laughing, screaming or speaking, it is probable that in most diseases of the respiratory system, psychological factors play an important role.

It has long been known that emotional factors play a large part in the asthmatic attack, although the spasm of the bronchioles, which is the immediate cause of the attack, is often precipitated by exposure to a specific allergen, such as pollen, animal fur, or paint. Usually both these factors co-exist to produce an attack but either may be the precipitating factor.

The emotional disturbances leading to an asthmatic attack are many and varied, and include almost any sudden intensive emotional stimulus, such as anger, jealousy, rage, or sexual excitement. It has been found that anything which threatens to separate the patient from the protective mother or her substitute is apt to precipitate an attack. For example, the birth of a sibling is often found to be the initiating factor of the asthmatic condition. This repressed dependence upon the mother is a constant feature around which different types of character defences may develop. Among asthma sufferers may be found many types of personalities – aggressive, ambitious, argumentative, or hypersensitive aesthetic types, all of which develop from the conflict surrounding the excessive unresolved dependence on the mother.

The theory has been advanced that the asthmatic attack represents symbolically both a protest against separation from the mother, and also the wish to re-establish this relationship through crying; this is considered equivalent to a repressed cry and in fact the sounds made in asthma resemble those of a whining cry or repressed sobbing. This view is substantiated by the fact that most asthma patients spontaneously report difficulty in crying and observe that asthmatic attacks have terminated when the patient could give vent to his feelings of crying.

In other patients, an asthmatic attack may occur as a conditioned reflex to a conditioned stimulus. For example, a patient who had previous attacks precipitated by pollen from a certain plant may develop further attacks when shown a picture of that plant.

Thus it can be seen that emotional factors play an important part in the production of the illness though the relative importance of the physiological and psychological elements is variable. Treatment is directed towards both these elements, though it has been found that the elimination of only one of them will usually effect a remission of symptoms.

SPECIAL ASPECTS OF PSYCHIATRIC PHYSIOTHERAPY

The physiotherapist working with psychiatric patients, whether in a small unit attached to a general hospital or in a large psychiatric hospital is not 'another being' in 'another world'. It is true that there are some small differences in the tasks before the physiotherapist but the basic situation is the same, i.e. a patient is a person with an illness and the physiotherapist is a member of a team committed to restoring that person to full health.

With modern techniques and drugs in psychiatry the tendency is for more patients to be returned to the community and in a much shorter time; therefore the number of chronically sick is diminishing, although there will always be some patients who need constant and long-term care. With this in mind, the present policy is for patients with acute psychiatric illnesses to be treated in small units which form an integral part of the general hospital, many of them attending as day patients, and returning home each evening. This, it is hoped, will help to banish the stigma which is still attached, to a greater or lesser degree, to being a psychiatric patient.

While the main function of the physiotherapist in psychiatry is still the management of the physical condition of the patient, she is also a member of the team whose function is to restore the patient to full mental and physical health. So she is concerned not only with the physical effects of treatment but also with the psychological, social and economic adjustment of the patient to illness and disability.

Nurses, physiotherapists, occupational therapists and other staff who are in constant personal contact with the patients are in an excellent position to observe any changes in their mood or behaviour, which may be caused by the pattern of the illness. Physical changes may be due to medication. Parkinsonism is a common side-effect of drugs. As an overall picture of the patient's behaviour is an essential part in the planning or changing of treatment schedules by the psychiatrists, any such change must be reported to them. Liaison among the staff is augmented by frequent inter-disciplinary meetings, in addition to the consultant's ward round.

All staff at these meetings know the personal as well as the medical background of each patient and so are able to note even small physical or mental changes. With this full knowledge of the patients' personal backgrounds, avoidance of over-involvement of any member of staff with any one patient is essential.

TREATMENTS

Exercises

Many psychiatric patients, either because of the nature of their illness or because of the drugs prescribed, need much firm persuasion to become involved in anything physically active. Apart from their natural reluctance to join in anything as 'childish' as organised games or class exercises, they often have a genuine feeling of lethargy or tiredness. Once persuaded, however (often by other patients who have previously had to overcome their own inertia), they usually enjoy the classes and the sense of well-being produced.

Classes of general exercises should be organised to suit the varying needs of the individual patients – grouped according to either age or general physical fitness. The aims of all such classes must be:

1. To prevent or overcome physical deterioration
2. To improve precision and coordination
3. To promote relaxation of tense muscles
4. To relieve feelings of aggression and hostility

Classes for older or less physically fit patients should consist of simple rhythmical exercises, perhaps performed to music. If music is used it should be carefully chosen, with a simple but positive rhythm and it should be borne in mind that a patient may occasionally be upset by a particular record, because of previous associations, but this cannot be foreseen, and the situation must be dealt with as it arises.

The scheme of exercises should include a selection for all parts of the body, special attention being paid to the muscles controlling head, neck and shoulders as it is in these muscles that tension associated with the majority of mental disorders is found. Free swinging exercises should be given at intervals throughout the session in an attempt to break the physical tension.

Sometimes patients on certain drugs find that head movements produce vertigo and even nausea, but this usually decreases as the medication is stabilised, and can be controlled by deep breathing exercises, which should form part of the programme.

Postural training in sitting and standing should also be included. Younger, fitter patients should have more vigorous exercises, more suited to their superior physical fitness, and ball games may be included; although it may be more beneficial both physically and psychologically for the more formal exercises to be performed at the beginning of the day, and ball games and apparatus work taken as an additional activity later in the day.

Apparatus work should be as varied and stimulating as possible, and include such things as weight-lifting, static rowing, punch ball as well as team games with small apparatus such as ropes, small balls or bean bags. Outdoor games are to be recommended wherever possible, as these give active youngsters the opportunity to 'let off steam' without disturbing other patients.

It is interesting to note how, at all levels, the performance of individual patients alters as the mental condition improves. Often the improvement noticed in the performance of exercises is one of the first indications that the patient is beginning to recover mentally.

Relaxation

Relaxation therapy is an invaluable part of the treatment prescribed for many psychiatric patients, most of whom exhibit some signs of physical tension. Their diagnoses may vary considerably, from depressive illnesses to personality disorders or phobias, but tension is common to all.

The timing of the class is important as some patients, e.g. those with anxiety states, are most tense in the morning and improve as the day goes on, whereas others will derive more benefit from an afternoon session, as their tension increases as the day progresses.

Relaxation therapy may be requested by the psychologist for patients undergoing a course of aversion therapy, i.e. a treatment aimed at inducing a conditional aversion to, say, alcohol or drugs by associating the taking of them with repeated nausea and vomiting. In this case relaxation is given immediately prior to the treatment.

In general, patients who are very aware of their tensions, and have a strong desire to relax, are the ones who start to improve most quickly. They require a more concentrated effort to relax and usually learn the technique more readily. On the other hand some patients may increase their tension by trying too hard! If some time is devoted to explaining to the patient the particular relaxation technique to be used, before treatment commences, the stage is well set for the therapy to begin. The patient will accept the treatment more readily, and knowing what is expected of him, will be in a less apprehensive, and therefore more receptive, frame of mind. Even so, it is unlikely that he will achieve relaxation at the first session. Often several sessions are required before the patient, having learnt the technique, is able to use it as a conscious weapon against the tensions arising in his muscles.

The physiotherapist will have her own relaxation technique, but the one most commonly used is the rhythmical contraction-relaxation movement of each group of muscles from toes to head. The patient must concentrate on each movement so that he learns to distinguish between the feelings of tension and relaxation in each muscle group.

Whatever the technique used, the prerequisites are the same:

1. The patient must be lying comfortably! It is useless to try to teach a patient to relax if he is uncomfortable. The patient should choose his own lying position, though if the side lying position is adopted, the top leg must be flexed and supported by a pillow, *not* by the other leg. Similarly, the lower arm should be behind the trunk, not having to support it, or be crushed by it. If the patient prefers to lie on his back, a pillow should be placed under the knees to avoid strain on the lumbar spine.

2. The mattress should be on a firm base, or even on the floor as long as there are no draughts.

3. The room should be darkened, as much as is consistent with the therapist's ability to observe the patient, and as quiet as possible.

4. The patient should be covered with a blanket, both for warmth and added security.

5. Commands should be given in a low, monotonous voice.

6. At the end of the instruction time, the patient should be encouraged to concentrate his thoughts on breathing in and out slowly. This in itself helps to promote relaxation, and channels the patient's thoughts away from any external factors which may produce tension.

7. The session should last for at least an hour, during which time the patient is observed for signs of increasing tension such as tightening of the face muscles. If this occurs the procedure should be repeated from the beginning. It may be necessary for a patient to leave before the full time has elapsed, as sometimes lying in a quiet, darkened room may increase the tension.

8. Treatment should be reviewed frequently, as some patients may derive more benefit from other forms of treatment, or relaxation sessions could become just an 'escape to sleep'.

9. Progression of relaxation from lying to sitting should be practised, so that if at any time the patient becomes aware of increasing muscular tension, he is able to relax at will, without the need for retiring to bed!

Facial massage may be a useful adjunct for extremely tense patients, sometimes with dramatic results. Some patients, however, are unable to tolerate any tactile stimulation, and derive no benefit from it.

RELAXATION USING ELECTROMYOGRAPHIC BIOFEEDBACK

For some patients, particularly those with tension headaches, anxiety neuroses and chronic pain, a quantitative measure of relaxation such as obtained by the use of electromyographic (EMG) biofeedback, is useful.

Electrodes are placed on the frontalis muscle, the EMG of which is recorded, amplified and rectified, and used to drive an oscillator that emits a tone or a series of clicks. The frequency of the tone or clicks varies with the amount of tension in the muscle, and the patient can consciously lower this by further relaxation of the muscle.

Once the patient has been taught to relax at will, further feedback information may also be obtained by placing electrodes on the palms of the hands or fingertips, and recording the degree of sweating. Any increase in the level of anxiety of the patient will produce an excess of sweating, and, by being made aware of this, the patient can be taught to reduce his own anxiety level.

Electro-Sleep Therapy

There are many different types of electro-sleep apparatus at present in use in hospitals in this country. They have been designed for use in re-establishing a normal sleep pattern in a patient whose pattern has been disturbed by either physical or psychiatric illness. Most developments in this field have taken place in the USSR and Germany over the past few years. It is not yet known how electrically-induced sleep works, but experiments have shown that the electrical impulses are carried into the central nervous system and have an inhibitory effect.

Electro-sleep therapy is used in the treatment of anxiety, tension and insomnia, and claims have been made for its beneficial use in many medical and surgical conditions, as well as in psychiatric conditions, and psychosomatic illnesses.

Sleep is induced by applying small modulated impulses to the skull, by means of three or four electrodes, usually incorporated in rubber goggles. The positive electrodes are placed on the closed eyelids, and the counter-electrodes placed on the mastoid processes. Some designs have only one counter-electrode, which is then placed at the nape of the neck.

The prerequisites of treatment are the same as those for relaxation therapy, but it is even more important here, for the procedure to be explained to the patient, and the expected effect. This is to minimise feelings of apprehension when the electrodes are applied. He will merely feel a slight tingling sensation under the electrodes, and (with some machines) hear a musical note throughout the treatment, designed to exclude any extraneous sounds. He will feel very relaxed during treatment, will become drowsy, and finally enjoy a relaxing sleep, though because of the initial apprehension this might not be so in the first treatment or two. It should be pointed out to the patient that the machine is independent of the mains current. When he is lying on the bed in the normal sleeping position, the rubber goggles are placed on the patient's head, and the connecting leads are plugged into the machine which is then switched on. The output control is turned up slowly until the patient reports that he can feel a tingling sensation under the electrodes, and then left. The first session should be of 20 minutes duration, this time being increased at each daily session until each session lasts one to two hours.

The number of sessions required varies with the individual, but optimum effect is usually reached in 10–15 sessions, though some patients need a longer course, and will continue to derive benefit even after 30–40 treatments.

As there are no side-effects to the treatment, it can be used to replace drugs for night sedation if the treatment is given at the normal bedtime, and a normal sleep pattern is re-established.

Continuous Narcosis

Continuous narcosis is now rarely used, but may still be the treatment of choice for some patients in states of acute anxiety following recent severe stress. Modified narcosis may still be used for drug dependents who are being withdrawn from their drugs, though this has largely been replaced by neuro-electric therapy.

The treatment aims to produce light sleep for most of each 24 hour period, the sleep only being interrupted at five-hourly intervals for feeding, toilet requirements, exercise and general nursing care. The duration of the treatment varies from a few days to a few weeks. Before the narcosis commences, breathing exercises are taught to the patient and practised at each waking interval thereafter. Care of the chest is of prime importance, as with the enforced inactivity secretions may collect in the lungs. Postural drainage with clapping and shaking is carried out daily. Simple abdominal and postural exercises are also given, and the treatment is concluded with a brisk walk. This improves circulation and reduces the risk of venous thrombosis. Nursing staff supervise the exercises and walking at each wakeful period when the physiotherapist is not on duty. A sudden drop in blood pressure sometimes occurs, which can cause severe vertigo, and this must be taken into account at all exercise sessions. Chest and circulatory disturbances are not uncommon in patients undergoing narcosis therapy.

Neuro-Electric Therapy

During the last decade a new method of treatment for drug dependence has been more widely used. Neuro-electric therapy owes its origin to the practise of electro-acupuncture analgesic techniques, where drug addicts reported that, while undergoing the treatment for neurosurgical conditions, their craving for heroin disappeared and any withdrawal symptoms they were experiencing at the time diminished rapidly.

Now, transcutaneous stimulation applied over the left and right mastoid areas is found to be effective not only in reducing these symptoms, but also in the early restoration of a normal, drug-free sleep pattern. The stimulation is given continuously for the first five days and nights, then intermittently for another five days. During this period, the patient is usually very unwilling to participate in anything active, and the physiotherapist's persuasive powers are taxed to their utmost, in getting the patient to participate in even the simplest forms of exercise or games.

Individual schemes of exercises and activities must be carefully planned to not only take account of the initial physical state of the patient (usually very poor due to the continued self-neglect associated with drug dependence), but also to overcome the inertia arising from the inadequacy, and the sense of emptiness and meaninglessness which produced the addiction.

The physiotherapist, along with the other members of the therapeutic team, must always be aware of the manipulative skills of this type of patient and be prepared to deal with the considerable acting skills that are often exhibited when an easy, short-term answer to his needs is preferable to the disciplining necessary to achieve long-term physical and mental rehabilitation.

A good working relationship between the therapist and the patient must be established, and is only possible when the therapist has sufficient confidence in her own clinical acumen to recognise and cope with such deceits as the feigning of withdrawal symptoms in order to escape the chores of an active programme.

A compassionate but firm approach is necessary to help the patient overcome the physical problems produced by the addiction, and hopefully the increased self-esteem engendered will eventually lead to the patient becoming re-integrated into constructive family and social relationships.

Other Treatments

Statistics show that there is a higher percentage of physical ailments among psychiatric patients than among the general population. All of these are treated in the prescribed manner, but it must be borne in mind that in these patients there may be more psychological overlay.

Hysterical paralysis must be mentioned, although physical treatment is usually contra-indicated for these patients, as is any treatment which draws further attention to the 'paralysed' limb or limbs. In some cases, however, treatment is prescribed in order to prevent muscular atrophy or contractures arising from disuse.

Any treatments planned by the psychiatric physiotherapist must take into account the possible side-effects of any drugs prescribed for the patient. Many of these drugs can produce side-effects such as heat or light sensitivity which are incompatible with normally acceptable physiotherapy procedures. For instance, treatment by ultraviolet light is contra-indicated for patients who are taking chlorpromazine and particular caution must be used in the application of any form of heat therapy to patients on antidepressants such as imipramine hydrochloride which also produces heat/light sensitivity.

CONCLUSION

The physiotherapist, being in such close and constant contact with the patient, is in an excellent position to recognise and elicit any signs of anxiety or tension and in many cases to allay the fears and apprehensions of the patient.

For example, in a general department, while it is no part of the physiotherapist's role to reveal the prognosis of a chronic or incurable disease, it is her duty to promote physical and mental rehabilitation, by demonstrating at an early stage of the illness that the patient can lead a life which is as full and independent as possible. It is also important that she is able to recognise that a 'simple' condition such as a Colles' fracture can produce, in some patients, as much anxiety and distress as an apparently more serious illness.

In a psychiatric hospital, the emphasis is shifted somewhat in that a diagnosis of an anxiety state or other psychiatric disorder has usually been made, and the physiotherapist's role is as a member of the psychiatric team whose aim is to restore the patient to a life of physical, mental and emotional stability. This means that, although a far smaller proportion of the day is concerned with physical treatments there is much closer involvement with the patients, their social background, and their overall treatment. This close involvement makes the work of the psychiatric physiotherapist a very stimulating and rewarding experience.

SOME TERMS USED IN PSYCHIATRY

Psychosis and Neurosis

These terms are used to differentiate between two groups of mental illnesses which correspond approximately to the commoner expressions 'madness' or insanity (psychosis) and the milder 'nervousness' (neurosis). The distinction between the two terms is by no means clear-cut, and it is often difficult to decide in which group a particular patient belongs.

However, the chief points of difference are as follows:
1. Psychosis is a severe disorder of the mind which seriously inter-

feres with the patient's relationships with other people. Neurosis is a less severe disorder.

2. A psychosis may be brought about by organic factors, or by psychological factors, or by a combination of the two. A neurosis is brought on by psychological factors, e.g. a reaction to stressful circumstances in a personality predisposed as a result of adverse experiences in childhood.

3. A psychosis is usually characterised by the presence of one or more such specific symptoms as delusions, illusions or hallucinations. A neurosis is not usually characterised by these, but the clinical picture often includes one or more specific symptoms such as conversions, phobias and obsessions.

4. A psychosis involves severe disorganisation of the various personality functions such as memory, perception, judgement etc. A neurosis involves decreased efficiency of one or more of these functions but less disorganisation of them.

5. Psychotics are usually not aware of the fact that they are psychiatrically ill – they lack 'insight'. Neurotics are usually aware of their illness – they have 'insight'.

6. In psychosis there is a loss of contact with reality, whereas in neurosis there is normal contact.

Schizophrenia

This is a generic name for a group of mental disorders which have certain characteristics in common. It is probably the most common of all psychoses.

The condition is characterised by an emotional coldness and a loss of connection between thoughts, feelings and actions. It occurs in people with a particular type of temperament characterised by reticence, aloofness, and partial divorcement from reality. The schizoid personality expriences many adaptive difficulties from childhood onwards, and often becomes more and more aloof, and less interested in other people, or in events which interest other people. His shyness leads to exclusiveness and an inability to make human contacts. Not everyone with this type of personality breaks down into illness. Indeed, many manage to find a niche for themselves in which they can work and indulge in fantasy. The poorer the contact with reality the greater the liability to schizophrenic breakdown.

The onset of symptoms usually coincides with a period of emotional stress, such as that of puberty, though increasingly strange behaviour over a period of time has usually been noted by relatives. The patient appears preoccupied and withdraws interest from life. This inward attitude is often associated with the emergence of delusions of being watched or influenced in uncanny ways. His behaviour may become peculiar and unpredictable, and apathy and lack of interest in normal activities develop. This may be progressive throughout the course of the illness, and then contributes to the severe degree of deterioration found in so many chronic patients.

Diagnostic features include severe thought disorder, delusions supported by hallucinations, stupor alternating with frenzy, and in the later stages a marked emotional indifference.

Schizophrenic disorders are often classified into four varieties, the simple, hebephrenic, catatonic and paranoid types. There is often overlapping of symptoms from one type to another, and during the course of his life a patient may have a number of schizophrenic illnesses, the forms of which may vary and at different times may fit better into one category than another.

SIMPLE SCHIZOPHRENIA

In this disorder, which usually develops insidiously throughout adolescence and early adulthood, there are no highlights of gross behaviour disorder, hallucinations, or delusions. For some time the only manifestations may be lack of drive, an odd manner and an emotional impoverishment. The patient becomes increasingly solitary and detached and eventually may withdraw from society, refusing to go to work, and neglecting his appearance. His physical health may deteriorate as a result of lack of exercise and adequate nourishment and he may need admission to hospital. Many of these people, however, continue to exist in the community but often are alone, friendless and on a very low economic level.

HEBEPHRENIC SCHIZOPHRENIA

This disorder also tends to develop in young people, but is characterised by more obvious symptoms, and comes closer to the popular idea of 'madness'. Often after a period of insidious withdrawal, the patient enters a phase of wild excitement during which he shows many florid symptoms of mental disorder. Hallucinations are common and the patient may be preoccupied with voices which he hears, often accusing him of misdeeds, or ordering him to perform actions which he may consider to be quite alien to his nature. If he realises that there is no one about, he tends to blame 'wireless' or 'electricity' for the voices. The voices may command him to perform anti-social actions, such as attacking others, and he may become so preoccupied with them that he is incapable of any normal activity.

Some patients find it difficult to express their ideas in words, and often thoughts do not follow each other in the normal manner and connections appear illogical and bizarre. The episode of acute disturbance is usually short, and the patient is often left feeling bewildered and perplexed. With or without treatment the patient may recover sufficiently to resume normal life although relapses are likely to occur, each attack leaving him less well than the previous time, until finally he withdraws from reality and lives in a world of fantasy.

CATATONIC SCHIZOPHRENIA

This disorder comes on later than the previous two, but the first attack usually occurs in young adulthood. The prognosis is somewhat better, especially if the patient's previous personality was mature and well integrated. The extremes of catatonic behaviour are stupor, where the patient remains motionless in bed, apparently unaware of what is going on around him, and an attack of excitement and wild senseless activity. The transitions from one state to the other may be very sudden and occur almost without forewarning. These extremes of behaviour can, nowadays, usually be modified by treatment with appropriate drugs.

PARANOID SCHIZOPHRENIA

This disorder begins later in life, usually between 30 and 40 years. It is characterised by delusions of a fairly coherent nature, which may change rapidly. There is often a discrepancy between the disturbing delusions and hallucinations on the one hand, and the poor emotional response which they evoke on the other. The onset is usually gradual, and the personality is better preserved than in the other types of schizophrenia.

The prognosis in schizophrenic disorders is less favourable than in many other mental disorders, though with the aid of modern drugs, many patients recover from their acute schizophrenic attacks and remain apparently well for long periods, often leading a useful and happy existence in the community.

Dementia

Irreversible impairment of intellectual ability, memory and personality, due to permanent damage or disease of the brain, occurs in this disorder. It also accompanies degenerative changes which occur in some apparently hereditary conditions, like Huntington's chorea. The patient's performance in intelligence tests deteriorates, though his vocabulary usually remains good. He may retain the ability to solve concrete problems but is unable to think in the abstract. For example, he may be unable to add up figures, but able to count beads.

His understanding of other people's actions and feelings declines, and he may become irritable and stubborn, with rapid changes of mood. Often there is a decline in moral standards, and the patient eventually becomes helpless and totally dependent.

BIBLIOGRAPHY

Ackner, B. C. G. (1964). *Handbook for Psychiatric Nurses*, 9th edition. Baillière Tindall, London.

Curran, D., Partridge, M. and Storey, S. (1976). *Psychological Medicine: Introduction to Psychiatry*, 8th edition. Churchill Livingstone, Edinburgh.

Hamilton, M. (ed) (1978). *Fish's Outline of Psychiatry for Students and Practitioners*, 3rd edition. John Wright, Bristol.

Kolb, L. C. (1977). *Modern Clinical Psychiatry*, 9th edition. Holt-Saunders Ltd, Eastbourne.

Mereness, D. A. and Taylor, C. M. (1978). *Essentials of Psychiatric Nursing*, 10th edition. C. V. Mosby Co, St Louis, Missouri.

Snell, H. (1977). *Mental Disorder: An Introductory Textbook for Nurses*. George Allen and Unwin, London.

Trethowan, W. H. (1979). *Psychiatry*, 4th edition. Baillière Tindall, London.

ACKNOWLEDGEMENTS

The author thanks Dr D. Gander, Dr D. C. Beatty and Dr A. Edwards for their helpful criticism. She also thanks Mr A. G. Boddington, M.C.S.P., Superintendent Physiotherapist, Queen Elizabeth II Hospital, Welwyn Garden City, and all the physiotherapy staff for their support and encouragement. Finally she thanks Mrs C. Davidson for the typing of the chapter.

Chapter 23

Applied Psychology for Physiotherapists

by D. A. HILL, B.SC., M.C.S.P., DIP.T.P.

The behavioural science course objectives for students of physiotherapy have been revised by a panel which has frequently sought advice from behavioural scientists. Final minor modifications were made in the light of comments from principals and teachers of physiotherapy schools and the result is a syllabus inspired by the expressed needs of physiotherapy teachers, and formally structured with the assistance of behavioural scientists. This chapter gives an interpretation of the agreed course objectives as best applied to students of physiotherapy. 'A good student will probably soon become a good physiotherapist, with or without a knowledge of psychology. But psychology may help her to become an even better physiotherapist even sooner' (Hill, 1974).

DEFINITION

Psychology may be defined as the study of behaviour and experience. Consideration of this definition reveals that there are few, if any, areas of human activity without a psychological component. The scope of the subject necessitates division into areas, and some of these areas are now listed.

Physiological psychology deals with the relationship between physiological processes and behaviour. Activity within the nervous system is closely related to behaviour, and neuropsychology is an important area of physiological psychology.

Comparative psychology compares behaviour between different animal species, and frequently correlates structural differences with differences in behaviour.

Social psychology studies the way in which members of a species, especially man, interact with each other.

Developmental psychology considers the changing processes in organisms as they mature, and whether such changes are due to inherited genetic factors or acquired environmental factors.

Educational psychology deals with those areas of study which have significant parts to play in the learning process, with some emphasis on children of school age.

Clinical psychology is concerned with the study and treatment of those members of society whose behaviour is abnormally undesirable, whether due to inherited or environmental factors.

Occupational psychology is the study of man in relation to his working environment, and deals with organisations in industry, hospitals, offices and the armed forces.

Human behaviour has attracted the attention of experts from many academic disciplines. Biologists, medical practitioners, philosophers, engineers, sociologists, physical scientists and mathematicians have all contributed to the fund of knowledge. It is not surprising, therefore, that various schools of thought have arisen in attempts to explain and ultimately predict human behaviour (Woodworth, 1970). The hard scientific approach of the behaviourist school attempts to explain behaviour in strictly definable and measurable terms and is not much concerned by notions of mind and consciousness which are difficult to define and measure. At the other extreme are the analytical schools which are mainly centred on Freudian psychology. Although at first the conflicting schools appear irreconcilable, deeper study frequently shows that they are looking at similar problems from different viewpoints, and it is unwise to accept blindly the teachings of any one school to the exclusion of all others.

DEVELOPMENTAL PSYCHOLOGY

Literature dealing with anatomical and physiological development reveals that the differences between child and adult are more than differences in body dimensions. Differences in body proportions and composition also exist. Likewise, differences in the quantity and quality of behaviour and mental experience are extensive. The physiotherapist working with children should be aware of these differences, and the approximate ages of transition of development from one stage to another, so that she can tell whether the child's failure to understand the world in adult terms is due to lack of maturity appropriate to the child's age, or due to genuine mental retardation.

The most valuable recent contribution to developmental psychology has come from Jean Piaget of Geneva. His work deals with the development of a child's understanding of the events which occur in the world around him. A brief description of the observed stages follows.

THE SENSORY MOTOR STAGE

This lasts from birth to two years. Early behaviour is mainly reflexive, and this implies that certain nerve pathways are innate, and the child arrives in the world with certain abilities (see Chapter 3). These innate reflexes combine to give more complex, purposive movements during the first few months of life. The term 'sensory motor' is self-explanatory. The child responds to sensory stimuli with fairly specific motor responses. Towards the end of this stage the use of language and the development of play and imitation reveals that the child is developing real understanding, and not just responding reflexly.

THE PRE-OPERATIONAL STAGE

This lasts from two to seven years. During this stage the child becomes increasingly skilled at handling objects in the material world, but his perception of these objects is still at a very different level from that of the mature adult. For example, if fluid from a container is poured into a container of a different shape, the child will state that the amount of fluid is either more than previously, or less than previously, but not the same. The conservation of volume with change of shape is not appreciated. Similarly it can be demonstrated that there is lack of appreciation of conservation of mass and number. The rules of simple arithmetic as we know them are just not accepted. Evidence to date suggests that practice and training have little if any effect in speeding up a child's progress through this stage. Presumably one has to wait for appropriate neurological maturation.

THE CONCRETE OPERATIONAL STAGE

This follows and extends to the age of eleven. The child now realises that properties such as weight, volume, number, mass, and area are conserved, even though dimensions of objects may be changed. In this stage the child also learns to classify groups of objects according to colour, size, shape and other properties.

THE FORMAL OPERATIONAL STAGE

This starts at eleven years. The child learns to transfer his knowledge and skill from concrete objects to ideas and concepts of a more abstract nature. For example, practical experience with weights and volumes gives rise to the concept of density or specific gravity. Generalisation of the properties of objects enables the child to appreciate scientific laws concerning such phenomena as buoyancy, the laws of reflection of light, and other laws of physics and chemistry.

The above stages demonstrate a progressive understanding of the properties of the physical world.

The development of moral and ethical values has also been studied by Piaget. He simply read stories to children in order to determine a child's sense of right and wrong (Brown, 1966). Children under seven judge naughtiness by the consequences of an act while older children and adults tend to make moral judgements based on the intentions leading to the act. Thus a child who accidentally broke fifteen cups was judged by young children to be naughtier than a child who broke one cup while stealing some jam. It is unlikely that a child possesses a conscience, or knowledge of right and wrong as understood by adults. He knows that certain acts will result in punishment if discovered. Distinguishing between different types of naughtiness is difficult for young children. They classify both swearing and the telling of untruths as lying. Both are undesirable forms of verbal behaviour, and therefore go together. As the child matures, the idea of reciprocity develops, in which the level of punishment is equated with the severity of the crime. By the time adolescence is reached ethical values are frequently well developed. Whole complexes of abstract ideas and concepts may be fervently advocated, and may be of a religious, political or social nature. Not only can the adolescent appreciate abstract concepts and laws concerning the material world, but he also feels strongly about how this material world should be manipulated for moral reasons in order to provide, for example, a socialist or a capitalist society.

Learning

Learning is the adaptive change in an organism as a result of experience. It is a change which is inferred because of changes in behaviour. The physiotherapist should be familiar with certain aspects of learning theory, since the majority of patients are required to learn at some stage in their treatment, whether it be breathing exercises, muscle strengthening, or re-education of walking. Some types of learning are more relevant to physiotherapy, and appropriate consideration of these types follows.

CLASSICAL CONDITIONING

This was studied in great detail by Pavlov. His best known experiment involved a bell repeatedly rung in the presence of a dog. Food was presented to the dog shortly after each bell ring. After several such episodes the dog salivated to the sound of the bell in anticipation of the food. Humans show evidence of classical conditioning. We may salivate at the sound of a dinner gong, or experience an increased pulse rate when we hear a police siren. We, in common with Pavlov's dogs, have learned to associate or pair stimuli and events, and the autonomic nervous system responds in a manner appropriate to the anticipated event. Many psychologists believe that classical conditioning plays an important part in attitude formation, and in this respect has some relevance to physiotherapy. Many patients are apprehensive, and a few are possibly terrified on their first visit to the department. The signs of stress will be demonstrated by the activity of the sympathetic nervous system. It is up to the physiotherapist to ensure that favourable attitudes are developed towards therapy. A friendly approach and a comfortable, effective treatment are essential in the early stages. Attitudes are rapidly formed and slow to decay. Imagine the attitude of Pavlov's dog if the bell had been followed by painful stimuli. Further sounds from the bell would have resulted in stress and anxiety.

OPERANT CONDITIONING

This has been investigated by B. Skinner. In this type of learning the organism works for a reward. A rat may learn to press a lever and be rewarded by a pellet of food. A child may run an errand and receive a tip. An adult will work for a month to receive a pay cheque. Operant conditioning involves the use of the voluntary skeletal muscles to create the conditions in which a reward is earned. The therapist can train the patient by operant conditioning to improve his skill level when voluntary movements are involved (O'Gorman, 1975). The most effective rewards will probably be praise and encouragement from the therapist and a realisation of improvement in the patient's condition.

AVOIDANCE CONDITIONING

This is a sophisticated term for punishment, and has little part to play in physiotherapy. The function of punishment is to suppress undesired behaviour, and although the therapist does not usually physically attack an uncooperative patient, it must be remembered that words and facial expressions of disapproval may act as avoidance conditioners, especially to sensitive patients. Punishment is unreliable as an avoidance conditioner, whereas operant conditioning by rewarding a correct response is usually highly successful (Wright and Taylor, 1972).

The three types of conditioning described are all examples of associative learning, in which specific stimuli are paired with specific responses. The timing of reward or punishment is critical. If presented long after the paired behaviour, the links may not be forged and learning will not occur. Consideration of conditioning processes in isolation gives the impression of man as a machine, responding when the appropriate button is pushed, but much evidence exists to suggest that man also learns with conscious understanding. Latent learning takes place when no apparent reward or punishment is involved. You probably know the make of your neighbour's car, the name of the pub at the bottom of your road, and the colour of the walls of the department in which you work. Such learning has gone in as an impression received and retained, simply by existing as part of your environment.

INSIGHT LEARNING

This occurs when the learner receives a flash of inspiration, which results in the solution of a problem. We all know the feeling when 'the pieces all fall into place'. Evidence exists to suggest that many higher mammals enjoy insight learning (Hilgard et al, 1975). Creativity is probably the most advanced form of mental activity, in which a series of mental processes result in a completely new solution to a particular problem in science, or a new form of expression in art, literature or music (Vernon, 1970). Because man is capable of the cognitive processes, the physiotherapist should explain in suitable terms the relevant details of the patient's pathology and the aims and objectives in treatment, in order to harness greater cooperation and higher motivation from the patient.

HABITUATION

This is a form of learning in which a repeated stimulus eventually produces a reduced response. For example, a doctor may take a patient's blood pressure two or three times, and the successive reductions in recorded pressures indicates habituation to the process of taking blood pressure. Patients will habituate to successive physiotherapy treatments and will cooperate more fully and perform at a higher level as their anxiety is reduced.

To return briefly to the theme of child development, we can now consider some of the learning processes involved during the process of socialisation, when the child acquires the accepted values, traditions, and behaviour norms of the culture in which he is reared, and acquires what we loosely refer to as a conscience.

The American sociologist, Talcott Parsons, has called the birth of new generations a recurrent barbarian invasion (Brown, 1966). Behaviourists claim that these barbarians become civilised by conditioning processes applied during maturation of the nervous system. Behaviour is shaped by various mixtures of rewards and punishment until culturally desirable behaviour is elicited. Love-oriented techniques, using the social rewards of praise and affection, and the withdrawing of these rewards for undesired behaviour, produce superior results to object-oriented techniques of tangible rewards and physical punishment. Superior, in that the children have fewer feeding and toilet training problems, and possess a stronger conscience, whereas physical punishment produces individuals low in self-esteem, aggressive and unfriendly (Hilgard et al, 1975). Innate tendencies to certain forms of behaviour do exist, but they can be profoundly modified by conditioning processes.

Biofeedback

During recent years psychologists have developed an interesting area of study known as biofeedback. Originally the term referred to studies in which it was demonstrated that it was possible to exercise voluntary control over certain bodily functions that had previously been described as involuntary. N. E. Miller and others demonstrated that animals could learn to control at will such functions as heart rate, blood pressure, diameter of arterioles, and contractions of the musculature of the digestive tract. Even EEG rhythms could be altered voluntarily.

Much research has now been conducted on human subjects, demonstrating that man can also learn to control these same physiological variables. All this is possible provided that, in the learning stage, rapid feedback of information concerning the physiological parameter under investigation is provided to the subject. These findings have obvious application in the control of some circulatory and neurological disorders such as hypertension, migraine and epilepsy (Harvey, 1978).

The realm of biofeedback has now been extended to include techniques which increase the level of control over voluntary muscles. Here the applications for physiotherapists include training in local and general relaxation, and in rehabilitation of patients suffering from conditions such as hemiplegia, spasmodic torticollis and peripheral nerve injuries (Hurrell, 1980).

It must be emphasised that feedback is information. Treatments involving biofeedback therefore increase the amount of information available to the patient, usually by means of sophisticated electronic

apparatus. This additional information facilitates voluntary contro'
by the patient.

Intelligence

It is a matter of common observation that some people are more clever
than others. But when we attempt to define intelligence a hard-and-
fast definition seems impossible. This is because intelligence is an
abstract idea which is assumed to exist, and yet remains intangible.
Such intangibles are known as constructs. We assess intelligence by
observing intelligent behaviour. Hence the rather cynical definition
that 'intelligence is what intelligence tests measure'. An intelligence
test samples behaviour of individuals. Heim defines intelligence as
'grasping the essentials in a given situation and responding appro-
priately to them' (Child, 1977). The grasping cannot be assumed until
the responding has been observed. Detailed consideration of intelligence testing and measuring is not appropriate in this chapter, and the
interested reader should consult standard references (Vernon, 1964).
One name which stands out in the history of intelligence testing is
Binet, a Frenchman who devised test items which, with slight modifications, are still included in some current tests. Briefly, he identified
abilities of average children of all age groups. He then measured the
abilities of individual children, and described their mental ages
according to the level of test items they could pass. Thus a child of
chronological age twelve years who performed at the level of an
average nine year old would be said to have a mental age of nine. From
this data the intelligence quotient could be calculated as

$$\frac{\text{Mental Age}}{\text{Chronological Age}} \times \frac{100}{1} = \frac{9}{12} \times \frac{100}{1} = 75$$

After the age of sixteen years intelligence does not increase in the
same manner as during maturation, but the idea of a spread of ability
among the population persists. The precise ranges of scores in a
population varies with the type of test, but as a broad generalisation
two-thirds of the population have IQs between 85 and 115, the population mean being, by definition, 100. There is strong evidence indicating that intelligence is due to genetic, inherited factors to a much
greater extent than environmental factors. For example, genetically
identical twins reared apart have closer IQ scores than genetically
different twins reared together (Mittler, 1971).

Spearmen identified a general (g) factor (Wiseman, 1967). This g
factor contributes to all areas of intellectual activity. The result is that

he more intelligent the individual is, the more likely he is to be above
average in all areas of ability. In addition to the g factor, possession of
specific abilities raises one's performance to higher levels in some
areas than in others, so that some excel in maths, others in history or
art.

The trained physiotherapist should remember that her proven
ability in passing the pre-entry requirements for physiotherapy train-
ng, plus her ability to pass the qualifying examinations indicate that,
together with other professional people, she is of above average
intelligence. Her colleagues at school, work, and in social contexts are
also probably of above average intelligence. But if the patients she
treats form a typical cross-section of the community, half of them
must by definition be of below-average intelligence. They will less
easily understand the pathology of their condition and the principles
of treatment. It is easy to interpret this inability as stubbornness or
lack of cooperation.

Personality

Personality is that area of psychology most concerned with individual
differences. When an acquaintance is described as generous, aggressive, kind, greedy or sulky, he is being compared with some mythical
averages of these qualities, or behaviour tendencies, which exist in
varying degrees in all individuals. Not only do individuals differ from
each other in the strength of these tendencies, but the strength varies
from time to time within the same individual. The behaviour tendencies are referred to as traits, and one of the aims of students of
personality is to identify and measure such traits. Each trait adjective
has an opposite, so that a person's score for kindness would exist on a
dimension between kindness and cruelty.

Eysenck (1970a) has developed tests which identify two important
traits on the dimensions of extroversion-introversion and stability-
neuroticism. He describes extroverts and introverts as follows:

'The typical extrovert is sociable, likes parties, has many friends,
needs to have people to talk to, and does not like reading or
studying by himself. He craves excitement, takes chances, often
sticks his neck out, acts on the spur of the moment, and is generally
an impulsive individual. He is fond of practical jokes, always has a
ready answer, and generally likes change; he is carefree, optimistic,
and likes to "laugh and be merry". He prefers to keep moving and
doing things, tends to be aggressive, and loses his temper quickly.
Altogether, his feelings are not kept under tight control, and he is
not always a reliable person.

'The typical introvert, on the other hand, is a quiet, retiring sort of person, introspective, fond of books rather than people; he is reserved and distant except with intimate friends. He tends to plan ahead, "looks before he leaps" and distrusts the impulse of the moment. He does not like excitement, takes matters of everyday life with proper seriousness and likes a well-ordered mode of life. He keeps his feelings under close control, seldom behaves in an aggressive manner, and does not lose his temper easily. He is reliable, somewhat pessimistic, and places great value on ethical standards.'

The behaviour patterns of these two groups may be broadly summarised by saying that the extrovert seeks continuous stimulation, variety, and change, while the introvert avoids these. Eysenck proposes a neurological explanation of these behaviour patterns which should appeal to physiotherapists with their background of neurophysiology. Briefly, the extrovert has an underactive ascending reticular activating system, and he is, therefore, continually seeking stimuli to arouse and alert the cerebral cortex to optimum efficiency. The introvert has an overactive reticular system, and surplus stimuli result in over-arousal of the cortex, with consequent discomfort and loss of efficiency.

A strong case can also be presented for an organic basis of the stability-neuroticism dimension, with manifestations demonstrated via the autonomic nervous system.

These two independent dimensions can interact to give four extreme types. Thus there are neurotic introverts, stable introverts, neurotic extroverts and stable extroverts. Before the reader tries to force himself into one of these categories, it is important to stress that these groups are extreme, and the majority of the population are near to the centre of the dimensions. When large specific groups are studied certain tendencies can be observed. Physiotherapists tend to be slightly extroverted and slightly neurotic when compared with the population mean (Child, 1977). Such a person prefers contact with people and is anxious to do a good job. Physical educationalists, on the other hand, tend to be stable extroverts, which equips them for the stressful conditions of competitive performance (Kane, 1968). Other professional groups also display typical personality profiles.

The neurotic extrovert displays hysterical symptoms of a physical nature when under stress. Examples are functional aphasia, hysterical paralysis, and asthma of psychosomatic origin. Such symptoms provide the individual with an escape route away from the stress-producing situation. Thus a man who is required to talk in his job can escape by precipitating aphasia, while a clerk would develop hysterical paralysis of his writing arm.

The neurotic introvert under stress is more likely to develop obsessional neuroses, which consists of unnecessarily repetitive behaviour which is time-absorbing and takes his thoughts away from the stress-or anxiety-producing circumstances. It will be appreciated that a neurosis is not so much an illness as an individual's personal solution to a problem. Furthermore, cure of the symptoms without removal of the stressful cause may result in substitution by an even more severely handicapping set of symptoms. Much tact must, therefore, be employed when treating neurotic patients. When the stress is removed spontaneous recovery frequently follows, but the symptoms may persist as habits, in which case they may be cured without risk of substitution.

Sometimes whole clusters of personality traits appear together to form a personality type. Combinations or clusters of traits can be detected by special tests designed to measure personality types. For example the authoritarian type demonstrates a clustering of patriotism, conservatism, prejudice, tough-mindedness and rigid thinking (Brown, 1966; Eysenck, 1970b).

The importance of early influences on the way in which adults behave is emphasised in an area of development in psychology known as Transactional Analysis. Advocates of this approach point out that our responses to verbal comments from others demonstrate three possible states within us, and that changes from one state to another are apparent in manner, appearance, words and gestures. The three states are known as Child, Parent and Adult and it is assumed that all three states exist in us, waiting to be elicited by appropriate stimuli.

The child is demonstrated by the type of reactions expected from a small child, such reactions being emotional in nature (Berne, 1970; Harris, 1973).

The parent is represented by beliefs and values which were received from parental figures, and internalised without being subjected to logical analysis.

The adult grows in us as a result of our ability to find out for ourselves, taking in data from the real world and submitting it to our own analytical processes.

When interacting with others, an individual's response may be that of the child, the parent, or the adult in him.

Psychotherapy based on transactional analysis usually aims at bringing out the adult in the patient. This does not mean that child and parent responses are always undesirable. Indeed, they provide much of the variety and richness in the quality of life. Treatment is only needed when they exhibit themselves so frequently and emphatically that they impair an individual's relationships and coping abilities.

If a therapist talks to a patient in the manner of parent to child, the patient may accept this relationship as appropriate, or he may resent it, thus erecting a barrier to further fruitful communication.

Motivation

Without a motivating or driving force the human organism is totally inactive. Something has motivated the reader to cast his eyes across this page! Motivations or drives may be regarded as inner forces compelling us to action. The hunger and thirst drives compel us to eat and drink. Without such drives we would soon die from malnutrition or dehydration. Such physiological drives ensure our continued survival. The sex drive ensures the perpetuation of the species. Once the biological drives are satisfied we have time for drives ensuring safety and comfort, such as seeking a warm, safe place to live and suitable clothes to wear. Social drives compel us to seek companionship, to obtain a sense of belonging, and to exchange love and affection with other people, and be respected by them. If the physiological and social drives are satisfied man can rise to higher drives in creative spheres and find satisfaction in art, music or other aesthetic or philosophical activities.

This brief description of drives suggests a hierarchical structure, and has been proposed by Maslow (1969). The higher drives are unlikely to receive attention unless the lower ones are satisfied. A man dying from starvation is unlikely to be appreciative of fine art or music. Similarly a patient deprived of the social satisfaction obtained from family and friends, and restricted to a ward bed, may show a regression in behaviour because his motivations have changed. If he is in pain his motivations may appear selfish, but will be concerned with escape from pain. When he is well on the way to recovery he may be more concerned with escape from hospital and the medical team can capitalise on the driving force. Most patients want to be breadwinners and homemakers, but the occasional patient finds life rather pleasant when the physiological drives of hunger and thirst are satisfied by the tender loving care of attentive young nurses. It is the task of the hospital team to shift his motivations higher up the hierarchical list. He should be encouraged to help in routine ward activities or sent to a convalescent or rehabilitation centre where a more independent lifestyle is possible and the circle of interests may be enlarged. It is imperative that during this stage the patient should experience feelings of success and achievement whenever progress is made towards greater independence. Praise should be meted out generously for each step forward, whether the patient is a young motorcyclist with a fractured femur, a middle-aged amputee or an aged hemiplegic. In many ways motivation is the core of psychology. Without it man is virtually lifeless. When present its nature determines our choice of behaviour.

THE ACQUISITION OF MOTOR SKILL

Definitions of skill are many and varied, some experts regarding almost every activity of any living creature as an act of skill. For the purposes of this chapter Guthrie's definition is the most suitable. Skill is defined as 'the learned ability to bring about predetermined results with maximum certainty, often with the minimum outlay of time or energy or both'.

If car driving is taken as an example of a skill, the highly skilled driver is more likely to complete the journey (predetermined result) in a relaxed manner (minimum energy) and shorter time than the learner driver.

Not all skills are 'learned' abilities in some senses of the word. A baby crawls and walks as a result of neurological maturation rather than learning but continued effort increases the ability level. We may, therefore, use the term maturational skill to describe crawling, walking or running as distinct from learned skills such as driving, cycling, swimming or using mechanical apparatus such as a camera or a piano.

The majority of students and practitioners of physiotherapy are more concerned with skill acquisition than with any other area of psychology. The student is required to learn to handle apparatus and equipment which is very unlike anything she has ever used before. In addition she must develop the skill of manipulating the body tissues of the patients in her care. The practitioner of physiotherapy is, in the vast majority of cases, concerned with encouraging the development of new skills, or reviving lost skills in her patient. The majority of treatment sessions include some form of exercise, and for this the cooperation and motivation of the patient are essential. But even with optimum motivation, much of the energy put into skill acquisition may be wasted if the therapist does not follow certain principles.

The first of the principles is guidance during the practice of the skill. Practice may be undertaken for one of three reasons – to acquire a new skill, to improve an existing skill, or to maintain an existing high level of skill. The student is concerned with the first two, the qualified therapist will be fulfilling the second throughout her daily routine, and may become involved with the first when new treatment techniques are introduced. The third reason concerns individuals at peak levels of performance of a skill, such as professional sportsmen or musicians. The patient may be concerned with the first two. Some patients may never have used the diaphragm correctly, and will, therefore, be concerned with a new skill, whereas other patients will be concerned with relearning (re-education) of existing skills such as walking.

Guidance of the learner is most important. Proper guidance results in quicker and more effective skill acquisition. Lack of guidance may mean that the skill learner will never realise his otherwise potential skill level (Knapp, 1967). Usually the initial guidance is verbal, that is an explanation of the nature and requirements of the skill. This should usually be followed by visual guidance, or demonstration, which will assist the learner by providing the opportunity of imitation. Finally, manual or mechanical guidance may be used, as when the teacher places her hands on the student's hands when teaching massage manipulations. Spring or weight-assisted exercises, and plaster slabs to enable patients to use their limbs, are all examples of mechanical guidance. Learning without guidance is learning by trial and error, and this is seldom satisfactory. The learning is slower and less effective, and the maximum possible skill level is seldom achieved. There is little to recommend 'being thrown in at the deep end'. Motivation will certainly be high, but the end result may be fatal!

Having got the learner practising with appropriate guidance, the teacher should provide a continuous feedback of information to the learner concerning progress. To modify a truism, 'practice with feedback makes perfect'. The patient learning to walk with crutches will require continual corrections in the early stages. Length of pace, timing of pace, position of head, general posture, weight on wrists, and many other points will need frequent attention. If the patient is sent to the far end of the gymnasium to practise on his own, the faults will become ingrained and may prove difficult to eliminate. The best feedback is praise for good performance whenever possible. Blame and criticism, if too frequent, are demotivating, and can cause the sensitive learner to give up completely.

The next considerations are spacing, duration, and timing of practice sessions. The optimum duration and frequency for maximum skill level may conflict with administrative desirability. If a new skill is practised for ten minutes without a break the total gain in learning will probably be less than if the skill is practised for two sessions of five minutes. Learning by massed practice results in what is known as reactive inhibition, which reduces total learning (Eysenck, 1970a). Briefer periods of spaced practice suffer less in this way. Two five-minute sessions of diaphragmatic breathing, or quadriceps exercises, although inconvenient because of time spent travelling by the therapist to and from the ward, will result in more total learning than one ten-minute session. Perhaps a compromise could be reached by going round the patients in a ward twice during one visit, spending less time during each treatment.

Transfer of skill must be considered in most learning situations. Transfer is concerned with what happens when a skill is practised in a different context. Strictly speaking it is impossible to repeat a movement. Even a simple repetitive task, such as throwing darts at a board results in different scores with successive throws. The goal may be the same on each occasion, but success at approximating to the goal varies due to minor modifications in the interpretation of perceptual cues, and variations in muscle action. In skill learning the aim is to achieve maximum positive transfer. This will mean that skill will be performed at a high level even though the environment or stimulus situation is different. Many skill-training situations necessitate transfer. Air pilots are required to make their initial mistakes in a dummy cockpit before being trusted with a planeload of passengers. The extent to which the skills learned in the simulator can be utilised when placed in the real situation is a measure of the degree of positive transfer. Students practise massage and other therapeutic techniques on each other before they are allowed to treat patients. The greater the similarity between the practice environment and the treatment environment, the larger will be the amount of positive transfer. A student who has only practised a certain treatment technique on the left arm of a healthy, thin, young fellow student sitting on a chair will not enjoy much positive transfer when faced with treating the right arm of a sick, obese, elderly bedridden patient.

Transfer is also important from the patient's point of view. He may have learnt to walk up and down the gymnasium steps, which have a rise of five inches and a tread of ten inches, and a handrail on the right. Confident that he can manage stairs, he is discharged. He then realises that his own stairs have a seven-inch rise, a nine-inch tread, a hand rail on the left, and a spiral at the top. The importance of students and patients practising skills in different contexts is obvious, but this aspect of skill acquisition is frequently neglected.

Perception

Perception is sometimes considered to be synonymous with vision, but this is a rather limited view of what is really a wide-ranging and complex area of study.

The author chooses to define perception as the organism's interpretation of the environmental stimuli impinging on its sensory receptors. Much laboratory work in perceptual research has been performed on animals and the word organism embraces them. The environment includes internal and external environments. One fascinating area of perception deals with determination of innate perceptual abilities and acquired perceptual abilities. The nature-nurture controversy ranges throughout most areas of psychology. The philosophers Locke and James assumed that the neonate's perceptual awareness was analogous with a blank slate, waiting for impressions to be made by experience. 'A big, booming, buzzing confusion' was how James described the infant's consciousness (Vernon, 1970). Confusion was assumed to decrease as perceptual learning occurred. More recent work by skilled psychologists has demonstrated that the newborn infant possesses many perceptual abilities which earlier workers had been unable to detect. Recognition of human faces, distances, and other perceptual abilities either exist at birth or develop very rapidly (Gregory, 1977). Such abilities are rapidly lost if visual stimuli are absent or distorted, so an interaction between the organism and a normally stimulating environment is essential. There is also much evidence that cultural factors affect perception profoundly. Tribesmen reared in visually restricted jungle environments interpret small retinal images as being necessarily produced by small objects, instead of large distant objects. They are less susceptible to illusions involving straight lines typical of the Westerner's 'carpentered' environment.

The internal environment can also play perceptual tricks. Hungry subjects perceive pictures of food as brighter than other equally illuminated pictures. This is known as perceptual set, and similar forms of set affect us all far more than we normally realise. Southerners have a stereotyped picture of northerners and vice versa. Each will tend to perceive in the other that which they expect to perceive. A special form of set is perceptual defence. This occurs when we raise the threshold of perception to stimuli that we do not wish to be aware of, because we find them embarrassing or annoying. We turn a convenient subconscious blind eye if it suits us.

Pain

Pain is a topic which merits consideration in this chapter, for it is frequently the symptom which first motivates a patient to seek treatment. Relief of pain is often one of the primary aims in physiotherapy treatments. A proper understanding of the psycho-physiology of pain is therefore important.

It has been known for many years that pain impulses travel to the higher centres of the central nervous system via the lateral spinothalmic tracts. Recent research (Melzack, 1973) suggests the existence of a 'pain gate' in the substantia gelatinosa region of the dorsal horn of the spinal cord. Activity in this area is responsible for suppression, amplification, or variation in the quantity and quality of pain experienced. Such activity is profoundly influenced by the psychological state of the patient.

The therapist should bear in mind that fear, stress, apprehension and ignorance concerning his condition can all increase the amount of pain actually experienced by the patient.

Emotion

Human emotions have interested man throughout history. The supposed anatomical sites of the origin of emotions have varied through the ages from the womb, heart, guts and spleen until present-day theories developed by electrical stimulation techniques point to the brain as the seat of emotion. The mid-brain and hypothalamus are the pleasure centres, while stimulation of discrete regions of the temporal lobe gives rise to feelings of anger and rage.

Brain damaged patients frequently appear in the physiotherapy department and emotional disorders are sometimes present in a subtle form, and may even be wrongly attributed to distress concerning the accompanying physical symptoms such as those of hemiplegia or Parkinson's disease. But depending on the specific areas of brain involvement, signs of depression, anger, distress and weeping, euphoria and rapid swings of mood can be directly due to brain damage. To complicate the issue even further, the displayed behaviour may not even match the mood experienced. Some hemiplegics display uncontrolled weeping even though they report feeling quite cheerful. Close relatives will sometimes report changed moral values in the patient. He may have started telling lies or stealing. The therapist will tend to assume that the patient has always been so inclined unless informed to the contrary.

The physiotherapist is not concerned with treatment of the psychologically abnormal unless she is employed in a hospital unit which specially caters for such patients, in which case she would be well advised to attend courses and refer to books dealing with the psychologically abnormal. For those readers who are interested some suitable textbooks are recommended. Much controversy exists even between experts in the complex area of abnormal psychology. Analytic techniques aim at probing the mental life of the patient and restructuring the personality brick by brick, while behaviourists consider many behaviour disorders as consequences of faulty learning, and the treatment consists of eradication of such learning by avoidance conditioning and substituting correct learning by operant conditioning. The efficacy of treatment frequently seems to be more related to a satisfactory relationship between the patient and clinician than to any particular treatment technique!

Stress

Few people are unaware of the increasing attention paid to stress by psychologists and the medical world generally. We all experience periods of stress from time to time, and stress is blamed for much of the unhappiness in today's technological society. Yet to define stress poses certain problems. Definitions vary depending on the angle from which stress is being considered.

Some definitions are stimulus based. For example, stress can result from extremes of temperature, pain, hunger, or noise. Varying the level of stimulus is therefore equated with varying the level of stress. Other definitions are response based, and variations in responses such as heart rate and blood pressure are taken as indications of changes in stress levels. A more complex but more useful model is one in which stress is regarded as an imbalance between the perceived demands being made on an individual, and the perceived coping ability of the individual (Cox, 1978). According to this model, if a man does not realise that he cannot cope, he will not be stressed. On the other hand, if he is capable of coping, but thinks he cannot cope, he will be stressed. The conscious state and perceptions of the individual are therefore most important.

Cox continues by describing some of the many pathologies which can arise from continued uncontrolled stress, such as cardiac disease disorders of the digestive tract, and other psychosomatic disorders. Management of stress may include the following: reduction in the demands being made on the individual, increasing the individuals coping ability, counselling, and the use of certain drugs.

With progress in neurology and biochemistry more and more mental disorders are being recognised as physiological in origin, and the controversy over cause and appropriate treatment recedes.

The day may come when it will be possible to explain all psychology in terms of physiology, but it may not prove to be the most useful and productive way of explaining behaviour. A multi-disciplinary approach to the study of man results in a balanced rounded view of homo sapiens, the organism at the top of the evolutionary tree.

REFERENCES

Beard, R. M. (1969). *An Outline of Piaget's Developmental Psychology.* Routledge and Kegan Paul Limited, London.
Berne, E. (1970). *Games People Play: Psychology of Human Relationships.* Penguin, Harmondsworth.
Brown, R. (1966). *Social Psychology.* (Free Press, US). Collier Macmillan, West Drayton.
Child, D. (1977). *Psychology and the Teacher,* 2nd edition. Holt-Saunders, Eastbourne.
Cox, T. (1978). *Stress.* Macmillan Press, London.
Eysenck, H. J. (1970a). *Fact and Fiction in Psychology.* Penguin, Harmondsworth.
Eysenck, H. J. (1970b). *Uses and Abuses of Psychology.* Penguin, Harmondsworth.
Gregory, R. L. (1970). *Eye and Brain: The Psychology of Seeing,* 3rd edition. Weidenfeld and Nicolson, London.
Harris, T. A. (1973). *I'm O.K. – You're O.K.* Pan Books, London.
Harvey, P. G. (1978). 'Biofeedback – trick or treatment?' *Physiotherapy,* **64**, 333.
Hilgard, E. R., Atkinson, R. C. and Atkinson, R. L. (1975). *Introduction to Psychology,* 6th edition. Harcourt Brace Jovanovich Limited, London.
Hill, D. A. (1974). 'The psychology syllabus for students of physiotherapy.' *Psychology Teaching,* 2, 2, 186.
Hurrell, M. (1980). 'Electromyographic feedback in rehabilitation.' *Physiotherapy,* **66**, 293.
Kane, J. (1968). PhD Thesis, University of London (unpublished). Personal Communication.
Knapp, B. (1967). *Skill in Sport.* Routledge and Kegan Paul Limited, London.
Maslow, A. H. (1969). *Toward a Psychology of Being.* Van Nostrand Reinhold Co Limited, Wokingham.
Melzack, R. (1973). *The Puzzle of Pain.* Penguin, Harmondsworth.
Mittler, P. J. (1971). *The Study of Twins.* Penguin, Harmondsworth.
O'Gorman, G. (1975). 'Anti-motivation.' *Physiotherapy,* **61**, 176.
Vernon, M. D. (1970). *Psychology of Perception.* Penguin, Harmondsworth.
Vernon, P. E. (1964). *Intelligence and Attainment Tests.* University of London Press.
Vernon, P. E. (1970). *Creativity.* Penguin, Harmondsworth.
Wiseman, S. (1967). *Intelligence and Ability.* Penguin, Harmondsworth.
Woodworth, R. S. (1970). *Contemporary Schools of Psychology.* Methuen and Co Limited, London.
Wright, D. S. and Taylor, A. (1972). *Introducing Psychology: An Experimental Approach.* Penguin, Harmondsworth.

BIBLIOGRAPHY

Gillis, L. (1980). *Human Behaviour in Illness: Psychology and Interpersonal Relationships*, 3rd edition. Faber and Faber, London and Boston.

Holding, D. H. (1965). *Principles of Training*. Pergamon Press Limited, Oxford.

Rachman, S. J. and Phillips, C. (1978). *Psychology of Medicine*. Penguin, Harmondsworth.

Shakespeare, R. (1975). *The Psychology of Handicap*. Methuen and Co Limited, London.

Spielberger, C. (1979). *Understanding Stress and Anxiety*. Harper and Row, London.

Stafford-Clark, D. (1970). *Psychiatry Today*. Penguin, Harmondsworth.

Williams, M. (1979). *Brain Damage, Behaviour and the Mind*. Wiley and Sons Limited, Chichester.

ACKNOWLEDGEMENTS

The author would like to thank Mr A. T. Scowcroft, M.C.S.P., DIP.T.P., for information and advice concerning the formulation of a suitable syllabus in psychology for students of physiotherapy.

He also thanks Mrs Pamela McDowell of the Ulster Polytechnic for her secretarial assistance.

Glossary of Neurological Terms

A selection of neurological terms – symptoms, signs, and names of diseases – which may be encountered and which are not defined elsewhere in this book are listed here.

agnosia inability to recognise a perceived object

akinesia difficulty in initiating movement (common in Parkinson's disease)

Alzheimer's Disease a frequently occurring degenerative brain disease of later life, producing dementia

amyotrophic lateral sclerosis motor neurone disease, q.v.

amyotrophy muscle wasting

aneurysm an expanded segment of an artery. In the brain, its rupture causes subarachnoid haemorrhage

aqueduct stenosis congenital blockage of the pathway for cerebrospinal fluid in the brainstem: an important cause of hydrocephalus

arachnoiditis inflammation of the leptomeninges; a cause of spinal and nerve root disorders

astereognosis inability to perceive shape by touch

astrocytoma the most important primary brain tumour of adults; a glioma, q.v.

basal ganglia disorders movement disorders due to disease of basal ganglia, e.g. Parkinsonism, athetosis, chorea, dystonia

brachial neuritis pain in an arm due to irritation of a cervical nerve root

Brown-Séquard Syndrome weakness on one side, loss of pain and temperature sensation on the other, due to damage to one side of the spinal cord

bradykinesia slowed voluntary movement, as in Parkinson's disease

catatonia freezing of movement. Occurs in Parkinson's disease

Charcot joints severely damaged joints resulting from loss of pain sensation

Charcot-Marie-Tooth Disease peroneal muscular atrophy

clonus rhythmic rapid repetitive muscle contraction, associated with increased tone

Creutzfeldt-Jakob Disease a dementing disease of adults due to a transmissible agent

demyelinating disease disorders – like multiple sclerosis – in which the white matter of brain and spinal cord is damaged

dermatomyositis inflammatory disease of muscle, with skin involvement

diplegia, congenital weakness and spasticity, present from birth, affecting all limbs but legs more than arms

Down's Syndrome mongolism. A chromosomal abnormality and most important cause of mental retardation

dysphagia difficulty in swallowing

dystrophia myotonica slowly progressive muscular dystrophy in which myotonia, q.v., may be prominent

embolism, cerebral a blood clot from elsewhere in the circulation blocking an artery in the brain; one of the causes of a stroke

encephalopathy disorder of the brain substance, producing coma and fits, with many causes

ependymoma tumour of brain and spinal cord, often benign

extrapyramidal disorders synonym for basal ganglia disorders

facio-scapular-humeral dystrophy mild variety of muscular dystrophy mainly affecting face and shoulder muscles

fasciculation visible involuntary contraction of bundles of muscle fibres; may be a prominent feature of motor neurone disease

fibrillation involuntary contraction of individual muscle fibres; visible in tongue

general paresis of the insane meningoencephalitis occurring in the late stages of syphilis, and producing dementia

glioma the most important group of brain tumours, derived from the connective tissue (glia) of the brain

Guillain-Barré Syndrome an acute form of polyneuritis, from which recovery usually occurs

haematoma, intracerebral blood clot in the brain

haematoma, subdural or extradural blood clot inside the skull, compressing the brain

haemorrhage, cerebral bleeding into the brain, causing a stroke. Subarachnoid haemorrhage is bleeding into the coverings of the brain

hemianopia loss of half of the field of vision

hemiballismus violent involuntary movements of a limb

hemiparesis weakness of one side of the body

infarction, cerebral death of brain tissue following blockage of the artery supplying it with blood; one cause of stroke

Kugelberg-Welander Disease late onset, relatively benign form of spinal muscular atrophy, q.v.

Landry's Paralysis old term, often regarded as synonymous with Guillain-Barré syndrome

leuko- (as in leukoencephalitis) affecting the white matter of brain

limb girdle dystrophy moderately severe variety of muscular dystrophy, affecting shoulder and pelvic-girdle muscles

medulloblastoma important malignant cerebellar tumour of children

Menière's Disease disease of the inner ear in middle life, causing giddiness and deafness

meningioma tumour of coverings of brain and spinal cord, usually benign

meningoencephalitis inflammation of the brain and its coverings

monoparesis weakness of one limb

motor neurone disease fatal, progressively paralysing disease of adults due to degeneration of motor nerve cells

myasthenia gravis muscle disease in which weakness results from blockage of transmission of nerve impulses to muscle

myelitis inflammation of the spinal cord

myoclonus brief shock-like involuntary muscular contraction

myopathy disorder of muscle, producing weakness, and resulting from many causes

myotonia state of persistence of muscle contraction and slowed relaxation after a voluntary movement

neuralgic amyotrophy pain, weakness and wasting in shoulder muscles due to inflammation of cervical nerves

neurofibroma benign tumour of nerve

neurofibromatosis (von Recklinghausen's Disease) congenital disorder with skin pigmentation, multiple neurofibromas and other abnormalities

neuromyelitis optica demyelinating disease affecting optic nerves and spinal cord

ocular myopathy variety of muscular dystrophy in which eye movements are affected

oligodendroglioma slow-growing form of glioma, q.v.

ophthalmoplegia paralysis of eye movements

optic neuritis inflammation of optic nerves

paraparesis weakness of both legs

polio- (as in poliomyelitis) referring to grey matter of brain and spinal cord

polymyositis inflammatory disorder of muscle

progressive muscular atrophy variety of motor neurone disease, q.v.

quadriparesis   weakness of all four limbs

radiculitis   inflammation of nerve roots

Refsum's Disease   inherited form of polyneuropathy due to defective lipid metabolism; a cause of hypertrophic neuropathy

retrobulbar neuritis   inflammation of optic nerves

Schilder's Disease   white matter disease of various causes, producing brain damage in children

schwannoma   benign   nerve   sheath   tumour,   similar   to neurofibroma, q.v.

scotoma   area of defective vision

spinal muscular atrophy   group of inherited disorders of motor nerve cells producing wasting and paralysis of muscle

striatal disorders   basal ganglia disorders, q.v.

subacute combined degeneration of cord   demyelinating disorder of spinal cord, affecting mainly legs, due to vitamin B_{12} deficiency

subacute sclerosing panencephalitis   slowly progressive, usually fatal encephalitis due to persistent measles virus infection

syringomyelia   cavitation of spinal cord producing loss of function in limbs

tabes dorsalis   inflammation of nerve roots occurring in late stages of syphilis, affecting function of limbs, eyes and bladder

tetraparesis   quadriparesis, q.v.

torticollis   contraction of neck muscles, sustained or spasmodic, resulting in tilt of head

vertebrobasilar insufficiency   impairment of blood supply to brainstem, often due to cervical spondylosis

Werdnig-Hoffmann Disease   fatal form of spinal muscular atrophy, q.v., in infants

Wernicke's Encephalopathy   damage to central areas of grey matter in brain, due to vitamin B_1 deficiency, affecting eye and limb movement

Wilson's Disease   inherited disorder affecting copper metabolism, producing basal ganglia disease and dementia

Useful Organisations

These organisations which are listed are only a few of the many who offer information, advice and counselling. In addition the following two reference books will be useful source references.

Directory for the Disabled edited by A. Darnbrough and D. Kinrade, 2nd edition, 1979. Published by Woodhead-Faulkner, Cambridge CB2 3PF

The King's Fund Directory of Organisations for Patients and Disabled People compiled by K. Sayer, 1979. Produced and distributed for King Edward's Hospital Fund for London, by Pitman Medical Publishing Co Limited, Tunbridge Wells, Kent TN1 1XH

Chest, Heart and Stroke Association
Tavistock House North
Tavistock Square, London WC1H 9JE   01–387 3012

Multiple Sclerosis Society of Great Britain and Northern Ireland
286 Munster Road
London SW6 6AP   01–381 4022

Action for Research into Multiple Sclerosis (ARMS)
71 Gray's Inn Road
London WC1X 8TR   01–568 2255

Parkinson's Disease Society of the United Kingdom
81 Queen's Road, Wimbledon
London SW19 8NR   01–946 2500

Spinal Injuries Association
5 Crowndale Road
London NW1 1TU   01–388 6840

Scottish Paraplegic Association
3 Cargill Terrace
Edinburgh EH5 3ND   031–552 8459

Muscular Dystrophy Group of Great Britain
35 Macaulay Road
London SW4 0QP   01–720 8055

Association for Spina Bifida and Hydrocephalus (ASBAH)
Tavistock House North
Tavistock Square, London WC1H 9HJ   01–388 1382

Scottish Spina Bifida Association
190 Queensferry Road
Edinburgh EH4 2BN   031–332 0743

Spastics Society
12 Park Crescent
London W1N 4EQ   01–636 5020

Scottish Council for Spastics
22 Corstophine Road
Edinburgh EH12 6DD   031–337 2804

Western Cerebral Palsy Centre
Bobath Centre, 5 Netherhall Gardens
London NW3 5RN   01–794 6084

National Association for Mental Health (MIND)
22 Harley Street
London W1N 2ED   01–637 0741

National Schizophrenia Fellowship
29 Victoria Road, Surbiton
Surrey KT6 4JT   01–390 3651

Open Door Association
c/o 44 Pensby Road, Heswall
Merseyside L61 9PQ   051–648 2022

Disabled Living Foundation
346 Kensington High Street
London W14 8NS   01–602 2491

Royal Association for Disability and Rehabilitation (RADAR)
25 Mortimer Street
London W1N 8AB   01–637 5400

Scottish Information Service for the Disabled
19 Claremont Crescent
Edinburgh EH7 4QD   031–556 3882

British Sports Association for the Disabled
Stoke Mandeville Stadium
Harvey Road, Aylesbury
Buckinghamshire HP21 8PP   0296 84848

Scottish Sports Association for the Disabled
c/o Fife Institute of Physical Recreational Education
Viewfield Road, Glenrothes, Fife KY6 2RA   0592 771700

Riding for the Disabled Association
Avenue R, National Agricultural Centre
Kenilworth, Warwickshire CV8 2LY   0203 56107

Committee on Sexual Problems of the Disabled (SPOD)
c/o RADAR, 25 Mortimer Street
London W1N 8AB   01–637 5400

Index